50 Studies Every Psychiatrist Should Know

50 STUDIES EVERY DOCTOR SHOULD KNOW

50 Studies Every Doctor Should Know: The Key Studies that Form the Foundation of Evidence Based Medicine, Revised Edition
Michael E. Hochman

50 Studies Every Internist Should Know
Kristopher Swiger, Joshua R. Thomas, Michael E. Hochman, and Steven Hochman

50 Studies Every Neurologist Should Know
David Y. Hwang and David M. Greer

50 Studies Every Pediatrician Should Know
Ashaunta T. Anderson, Nina L. Shapiro, Stephen C. Aronoff, Jeremiah Davis, and Michael Levy

50 Imaging Studies Every Doctor Should Know
Christoph I. Lee

50 Studies Every Surgeon Should Know
SreyRam Kuy, Rachel J. Kwon, and Miguel A. Burch

50 Studies Every Intensivist Should Know
Edward A. Bittner

50 Studies Every Palliative Care Doctor Should Know
David Hui, Akhila Reddy, and Eduardo Bruera

50 Studies Every Psychiatrist Should Know

EDITED BY

Ish P. Bhalla, MD
Forensic Psychiatry Fellow
Law and Psychiatry Division
Yale School of Medicine
Connecticut Mental Health Center
New Haven, CT

Rajesh R. Tampi, MD, MS, DFAPA
Professor, Psychiatry
Case Western Reserve University School of Medicine
Vice Chairman for Education and Faculty Development
Residency Program Director and Chief of Geriatric Psychiatry
Metrohealth
Cleveland, OH
Associate Clinical Professor, Psychiatry
Yale School of Medicine
New Haven, CT

Vinod H. Srihari, MD
Associate Professor, Psychiatry
Associate Residency Program Director
Yale School of Medicine
New Haven, CT

SERIES EDITOR

Michael E. Hochman, MD, MPH
Associate Professor, Medicine
Director, Gehr Family Center for Health Systems Science
USC Keck School of Medicine
Los Angeles, CA

OXFORD
UNIVERSITY PRESS

OXFORD
UNIVERSITY PRESS

Oxford University Press is a department of the University of Oxford. It furthers the University's objective of excellence in research, scholarship, and education by publishing worldwide. Oxford is a registered trade mark of Oxford University Press in the UK and certain other countries.

Published in the United States of America by Oxford University Press
198 Madison Avenue, New York, NY 10016, United States of America.

Library of Congress Cataloging-in-Publication Data
Names: Bhalla, Ish P., editor. | Tampi, Rajesh R., editor. | Srihari, Vinod H., editor.
Title: 50 studies every psychiatrist should know /
Edited by Ish P. Bhalla, Rajesh R. Tampi, Vinod H. Srihari.
Other titles: 50 studies every doctor should know (Series)
Description: New York, New York : Oxford University Press, Inc., [2018] |
Series: 50 studies every doctor should know
Identifiers: LCCN 2017058659 | ISBN 9780190625085 (pbk. : alk. paper)
Subjects: | MESH: Mental Disorders—therapy | Psychiatry—methods | Clinical Studies as Topic
Classification: LCC RC454.4 | NLM WM 400 | DDC 616.89—dc23
LC record available at https://lccn.loc.gov/2017058659

9 8 7 6 5

Printed by Webcom Inc., Canada

CONTENTS

Preface xi
Acknowledgments xiii
About the Editors xv
Contributors xvii

SECTION 1 Anxiety Disorders

1. Cognitive Behavioral Therapy, Imipramine, or Their Combination for Panic Disorder 3
Amanda Sun and Tobias Wasser

2. Fluoxetine, Comprehensive Cognitive Behavioral Therapy, and Placebo in Generalized Social Phobia 9
Erin Habecker and Tobias Wasser

SECTION 2 Bipolar Disorder

3. Lithium Plus Valproate Combination versus Monotherapy for Relapse Prevention in Bipolar I Disorder (BALANCE) 19
João Paulo De Aquino and Robert Beech

4. Mood Stabilizer Monotherapy versus Adjunctive Antidepressant for Bipolar Depression: The STEP-BD Trial 24
João Paulo De Aquino and Robert Beech

5. Suicide Risk in Bipolar Disorder: Comparing Lithium, Divalproex, and Carbamazepine 30
Rachel Katz and Robert Beech

6. The Long-Term Natural History of Bipolar I Disorder 35
Zachary Engler and Robert Beech

SECTION 3 Child and Adolescent Disorders

7. The Multimodal Treatment Study of Children with Attention Deficit/Hyperactivity Disorder (MTA) 43
Michael H. Bloch

8. Adolescents with SSRI-Resistant Depression: The TORDIA Trial 50
Amalia Londono Tobon and Hanna E. Stevens

9. Treatment of Early-Onset Schizophrenia Spectrum Disorders (TEOSS) Study 55
J. Corey Williams and Hanna E. Stevens

10. Cognitive Behavioral Therapy, Sertraline, or a Combination in Childhood Anxiety: CAMS 61
David Saunders, Andres Martin, and Jerome H. Taylor

11. Predictors of Suicidal Events: The Treatment of Adolescent Suicide Attempters (TASA) Study 67
Michael Maksimowski and Zheala Qayyum

12. Cognitive Behavior Therapy, Sertraline, and Their Combination for Children and Adolescents with OCD 73
Falisha Gilman and Zheala Qayyum

13. Initial Treatment of Bipolar I Disorder in Children and Adolescents: The TEAM Trial 79
Stephanie Ng and Andres Martin

14. The Treatment for Adolescents with Depression Study (TADS) 84
Zachary Engler and Zheala Qayyum

SECTION 4 Cognitive Disorders: Delirium/Dementia

15. Effectiveness of Atypical Antipsychotic Drugs in Patients with Alzheimer's Disease: CATIE-AD 93
Adam P. Mecca and Rajesh R. Tampi

16. Risk of Death with Atypical Antipsychotic Medications for Dementia 100
Adam P. Mecca and Rajesh R. Tampi

17. Treatment of Delirium in Hospitalized AIDS Patients: A Double-Blind Trial of Haloperidol, Chlorpromazine, and Lorazepam 106
Amanda Sun and Rajesh R. Tampi

18. Memantine in Patients with Moderate to Severe Alzheimer's Disease Already Receiving Donepezil 112
Brandon M. Kitay and Rajesh R. Tampi

SECTION 5 Epidemiology

19. Global Burden of Mental and Substance Use Disorders 121
Stephanie Yarnell and Ellen Edens

20. Prevalence and Severity of Psychiatric Comorbidities: The National Comorbidity Survey Replication (NCS-R) 127
Stephanie Yarnell and Ellen Edens

SECTION 6 Insomnia

21. Behavioral and/or Pharmacotherapy for Older Patients with Insomnia 135
Robert Ross and Rajesh R. Tampi

SECTION 7 Major Depressive Disorder

22. Treatment of Depression in Patients with Alcohol or Drug Dependence: A Meta-Analysis 143
J. Corey Williams and Gustavo A. Angarita Africano

23. Suicidality in Pediatric Patients Treated with Antidepressant Drugs: FDA Meta-Analysis 149
David Saunders and Michael H. Bloch

24. National Institute of Mental Health (NIMH) Treatment of Depression Collaborative Research Program 155
Joseph J. Taylor and Robert Ostroff

25. Efficacy and Safety of Electroconvulsive Therapy in Depressive Disorders: A Systematic Review and Meta-Analysis 161
Joseph J. Taylor and Robert Ostroff

26. Initial Severity and Antidepressant Benefits: A Meta-Analysis of Data Submitted to the Food and Drug Administration 167
Michael Maksimowski and Zheala Qayyum

27. Sequenced Treatment Alternatives to Relieve Depression: STAR*D 173
Eric Lin and Pochu Ho

28. Cognitive Therapy versus Medication in the Treatment of Moderate to Severe Depression 179
Daniel Barron and Robert Ostroff

SECTION 8 Obsessive-Compulsive Disorder

29. Exposure and Ritual Prevention, Clomipramine, or Their Combination for Obsessive-Compulsive Disorder 187
Brandon M. Kitay and Michael H. Bloch

30. Meta-Analysis of the Dose–Response Relationship of SSRIs in Adult Patients with Obsessive-Compulsive Disorder 192
Eunice Yuen and Michael H. Bloch

SECTION 9 Personality Disorders

31. Psychotherapy for Borderline Personality Disorder: A Multiwave Study 201
David Grunwald, Erica Robinson, and Sarah Fineberg

32. Dialectical Behavior Therapy versus Community Treatment by Experts for Reducing Suicidal Behaviors among Patients with Borderline Personality Disorder 207
David Saunders, Erica Robinson, and Sarah Fineberg

33. Ten-Year Course of Borderline Personality Disorder: The Collaborative Longitudinal Personality Disorders Study 213
Kevin Johnson, Erica Robinson, and Sarah Fineberg

SECTION 10 Psychiatry in Primary Care

34. Depressive Symptoms and Health-Related Quality of Life: The Heart and Soul Study 221
Amalia Londono Tobon and Catherine Chiles

35. The Canadian Cardiac Randomized Evaluation of Antidepressant and Psychotherapy Efficacy (CREATE) Trial 226
Nikhil Gupta and Catherine Chiles

SECTION 11 Women's Mental Health

36. Buprenorphine versus Methadone During Pregnancy: The MOTHER Trial 233
Rachel Wurmser and Kirsten Wilkins

SECTION 12 Schizophrenia

37. QTc-Interval Abnormalities and Psychotropic Drug Therapy in Psychiatric Patients 241
Amanda Sun and Vinod H. Srihari

38. Tardive Dyskinesia with Atypical versus Conventional Antipsychotic Medications 247
Emma Lo and Cenk Tek

39. Effectiveness of Antipsychotics in the Treatment of Schizophrenia: CATIE Phase 1 253
Chadrick Lane and Mohini Ranganathan

40. Clozapine for Treatment-Resistant Schizophrenia 260
Chadrick Lane and Vinod H. Srihari

41. Effectiveness of Clozapine versus Other Atypical Antipsychotics: Clinical Antipsychotic Trials for Interventions Effectiveness (CATIE) 266
Eunice Yuen and Cenk Tek

42. Atypical Antipsychotic Drugs and the Risk of Sudden Cardiac Death 274
Hamilton Gaiani and Cenk Tek

43. Switching Antipsychotics to Reduce Metabolic Risk: The CAMP Trial 279
Eric Lin and John Cahill

44. Cost Utility of Atypical Antipsychotics: CUtLASS-1 285
Nikhil Gupta and John Cahill

45. North American Prodrome Longitudinal Study 290
Nikhil Gupta and Vinod H. Srihari

46. Clozapine for Suicidality in Schizophrenia: The International Suicide Prevention Trial (InterSePT) 295
Daniel Barron and Noah Capurso

47. A Cohort Study of Oral and Depot Antipsychotics after First Hospitalization for Schizophrenia 300
Stephanie Ng and Cenk Tek

SECTION 13 Substance Use Disorders

48. Methadone Maintenance versus Detoxification and Psychosocial Treatment for Opioid Dependence: The M180 Study 309
Hamilton Gaiani and Srinivas Muvvala

49. Combined Pharmacotherapies and Behavioral Interventions for Alcohol Dependence: The COMBINE Study 314
Kevin Johnson and Srinivas Muvvala

50. Levomethadyl Acetate versus Buprenorphine versus Methadone for Opioid Dependence 321
Robert Ross and Brian Fuehrlein

Index 327

PREFACE

If you are a psychiatry resident who feels overwhelmed by the task of catching up on all the seminal articles in the field, while simultaneously keeping up with whatever study the radio or newspapers seem to have gotten to before you, then this book was written with you in mind. When one of us (IB) was in your position, he took the intrepid step of converting this feeling into what one of his teachers (VS) thought at the time was a Quixotic proposal: assembling a summarized list of 50 articles that would catch him up. After much discussion and guidance from the series editor, Michael Hochman, we settled into a three-year-long process that resulted in the book you are now holding.

How did we assemble these papers? We consulted widely with faculty in our department and collated their lists of articles they would classify as essential reading for trainees. We edited and submitted this long list (far more than 50) to a group of independent reviewers selected by Oxford University Press (OUP), who helped with the painful process of trimming the list. Further changes followed when we discovered a more relevant update or a gap in coverage of a subject. We chose to exclude narrative reviews and instead focused on primary research or systematic reviews. We tried to maximize participation from residents across training years and assigned senior faculty authors who were willing to take on the task of using this writing exercise as an opportunity to teach critical appraisal of the literature. If this sounds like a process that might produce an arbitrary list that would not have been replicated by a different set of editors—or indeed, by the same team if we tried again—that would be a fair assessment! This is not, we hope, the *only* 50 Studies you read during your residency training, but we do hope it gives you a foothold as you begin the long and remarkably gratifying journey of lifelong learning in psychiatry. These 50 studies are certainly not the end of this journey, but they are as good a beginning as any.

The process of generating each chapter was designed to advance a longstanding priority in our residency training program: enabling trainees to develop the capacity to translate research knowledge into their clinical practice. While the format of each chapter is consistent with the concise and informative templates used across this OUP series, all trainees had some exposure to an ongoing curriculum in evidence-based medicine (EBM). At Yale we have fledgling clinicians ask three questions of every study, in the tradition of EBM: (a) Are the results valid? (b) are the results important? (How big? How precise?), and (c) will these results help me in caring for my patient? More than 30 residents in our department appraised articles and presented draft abstracts to more than 20 faculty who edited and added commentaries to contextualize the original research for clinical application. All study authors were contacted, and the majority graciously offered suggestions. As educators with a deep investment in engaging trainees in the pedagogical practice of EBM, both RT and VS were inspired by this vast exercise in collaborative learning. While attempting to name (only) 50 important papers in psychiatry remains a foolhardy quest, getting any list read and discussed in this way was a unique and valuable educational experience.

We hope this book is also useful to anyone who wants to learn about important research studies in psychiatry—be it an individual diagnosed with a psychiatric disorder, a caregiver, or even seasoned clinicians.

Psychiatric disorders are a leading source of suffering and disability worldwide. While knowledge of how best to understand and treat these illnesses continues to grow, translation of existing evidence into practice is often delayed and inconsistent. We believe that the research-literate practitioner will be an essential part of any effort to close this implementation gap. We hope this book adds one small push to that effort.

Research relevant to psychiatric practice is growing at a rapid pace. We expect that the papers assembled here will face stiff competition for inclusion in future shortlists as new, rigorous, and relevant research expands our knowledge base. The list may need to be completely remade. This is as it should be. Indeed, our patients deserve nothing less.

Ish P. Bhalla, MD
Rajesh R. Tampi, MD, MS, DFAPA
Vinod H. Srihari, MD

ACKNOWLEDGMENTS

This book is a product of the synergy between residents, fellows, and faculty at the Department of Psychiatry, Yale School of Medicine. We want to extend our sincere gratitude to each contributor of this volume for their thoughtful work. Special thanks to Dr. Robert Rohrbaugh, Professor of Psychiatry and Deputy Chair for Education and Career Development at Yale's Department of Psychiatry, for his support of this project and mentorship to each of the editors and the several generations of trainees involved in producing this book.

Additionally, we would like to thank Drs. Emily Ansell, Andres Barkil-Oteo, Michael Bloch, Hillary Blumberg, Catherine Chiles, Paul Desan, Ellen Edens, Matthew Goldenberg, Robert Ostroff, Ismene Petrakis, Zheala Qayyum, Rajiv Radhakrishnan, Judah Weathers, Scott Woods, and Howard Zonana, who provided important input when we developed a preliminary list of papers to include. We would also like to thank Dr. Michael Hochman, the series editor, for giving us the opportunity to contribute a volume to this important educational series. In addition, we are grateful for the OUP editorial team of Andrea Knobloch, Rebecca Suzan, Emily Samulski, and Tiffany Lu for their support. We thank the team of expert reviewers chosen by the OUP who helped us select the final list of studies to be included in this book.

On a personal note, Dr. Bhalla would first like to thank his wife, Nitya, for her love and support during the writing of this book. He would also like to acknowledge his parents (Vipan and Anita), sisters (Vandana, Archena, and Puja), brothers in-law (Daudi and Michel), in-laws (Subramaniam, Renuka, Ramya, and Apoor), and nieces and nephews (Matai, Arya, Amira, Kairav, and Alina). Dr. Tampi would like to thank his wife Deena and their children (Lexi, Vaish, Julia, Livi, Poki, Smoki, and Ori) for their love and support during the writing of this book. Dr. Srihari wishes to remember David Sackett whose books and articles made it possible for him to imagine becoming a research literate physician.

David had once counted Alvan Feinstein at Yale as a mentor, and we are pleased to add one small thread to the enormous educational mission they pioneered.

Finally, we would like to thank the corresponding authors of the original studies that we have showcased in this book for their expert review of our summaries, valuable time, and words of wisdom:

- David H. Barlow, PhD
- Scott W. Woods, MD
- M. Katherine Shear, MD
- Jack M. Gorman, MD
- Professor John Geddes
- Gary Sachs, MD
- David Brent, MD
- Joan L. Luby, MD
- Karen Dineen Wagner, MD, PhD
- Lon Schneider, MD
- William S. Breitbart, MD
- Pierre N. Tariot, MD
- Harvey Whiteford, PhD
- Ron Kessler, PhD
- Charles M. Morin, PhD
- Irene Elkin, PhD
- Irving Kirsch, PhD
- Robert J. DeRubeis, PhD
- Edna Foa, PhD
- Michael H. Bloch, MD, MS
- Mary Whooley, MD
- François Lespérance, MD, MBA
- Hendrée Jones, PhD
- T. Scott Stroup, MD, MPH
- John Kane, MD
- Professor Peter B. Jones
- Tyrone D. Cannon, PhD
- Herbert Meltzer, MD
- Sharon Hall, PhD
- Raymond Anton, MD

ABOUT THE EDITORS

Dr. Ish P. Bhalla earned his BS cum laude from Case Western Reserve University and his MD from the University of Toledo College of Medicine. He completed his psychiatry residency from Yale University and is currently a forensic psychiatry fellow at Yale. He plans to pursue a career in medical education, academic psychiatry, health-care policy, and services research. He will be pursuing a health policy fellowship as a National Clinician Scholar at the University of California, Los Angeles.

Dr. Rajesh R. Tampi is Professor of Psychiatry at Case Western Reserve University School of Medicine and the Vice Chairman for Education and Faculty Development, Residency Program Director, and the Chief of Geriatric Psychiatry at MetroHealth, Cleveland, Ohio. He is also the president of the International Medical Graduates Caucus of the American Psychiatric Association and the Secretary and Treasurer of the American Association for Geriatric Psychiatry.

Dr. Vinod H. Srihari developed and oversees Yale University's Evidence-Based Mental Health curriculum, which has been recognized as a national model by the American Association of Directors of Psychiatric Residency Training. He continues to enjoy the challenge of using population-based evidence in the care of individual patients, teaching and learning how to make better use of the evidence, and designing clinical research in response to public health challenges.

CONTRIBUTORS

Gustavo A. Angarita Africano, MD
Associate Research Scientist
Associate Inpatient Chief of the Clinical Neuroscience Research Unit (CNRU)
Medical Director, Forensic Drug Diversion Clinic (ForDD)
Department of Psychiatry
Yale School of Medicine
New Haven, CT

Daniel Barron, MD
Psychiatry Resident
Neuroscience Research Training Program
Department of Psychiatry
Yale School of Medicine
New Haven, CT

Robert Beech, PhD, MD
Assistant Professor of Psychiatry
Department of Psychiatry
Yale School of Medicine
New Haven, CT

Michael H. Bloch, MD, MS
Associate Professor in the Yale Child Study Center
Associate Director, Albert J. Solnit Integrated Training Program
Associate Director of the Tic and OCD Program
Department of Psychiatry
Yale School of Medicine
New Haven, CT

John Cahill, MBBS
Assistant Professor of Psychiatry
Department of Psychiatry
Yale School of Medicine
New Haven, CT

Noah Capurso, MD, MHS
Assistant Professor
Department of Psychiatry
Yale School of Medicine
New Haven, CT

Catherine Chiles, MD
Associate Clinical Professor
Department of Psychiatry
Yale School of Medicine
New Haven, CT

João Paulo De Aquino, MD
Resident
Department of Psychiatry
Yale School of Medicine
New Haven, CT

Ellen Edens, MD
Assistant Professor of Psychiatry
Associate Fellowship Director, Addiction Psychiatry
Department of Psychiatry
Yale School of Medicine
New Haven, CT

Zachary Engler, MD
Resident
Child Psychiatry Residency Training Program
The Warren Alpert Medical School
Brown University
Providence, RI

Sarah Fineberg, MD, PhD
Instructor
Connecticut Mental Health Center
Department of Psychiatry
Yale School of Medicine
New Haven, CT

Brian Fuehrlein, MD, PhD
Assistant Professor of Psychiatry
Yale School of Medicine
Director, Psychiatric Emergency Room
Veterans Affairs Connecticut Healthcare System
New Haven, CT

Falisha Gilman, MD
Resident
Department of Psychiatry
Yale School of Medicine
New Haven, CT

David Grunwald, MD
Child and Adolescent Psychiatry Trainee
Stanford School of Medicine
Stanford, CA

Nikhil Gupta, MBBS
Resident
Department of Psychiatry
Yale School of Medicine
New Haven, CT

Erin Habecker, MD
Resident
Department of Psychiatry
Yale School of Medicine
New Haven, CT

Hamilton Gaiani, MD
Resident
Department of Psychiatry
Yale School of Medicine
New Haven, CT

Pochu Ho, MD
Assistant Professor
Psychological Medicine (PM) Service
Yale School of Medicine
New Haven, CT

Kevin Johnson, MD
Resident
Department of Psychiatry
Yale School of Medicine
New Haven, CT

Rachel Katz, MD
Clinician
Department of Psychiatry
Yale Psychiatric Hospital
New Haven, CT

Brandon M. Kitay, MD, PhD
Resident
Yale Depression Research Program
Department of Psychiatry
Yale School of Medicine
New Haven, CT

Chadrick Lane, MD
Resident
Department of Psychiatry
Yale School of Medicine
New Haven, CT

Eric Lin, MD
Resident
Department of Psychiatry
Yale School of Medicine
New Haven, CT

Emma Lo, MD
Resident
Department of Psychiatry
Yale School of Medicine
New Haven, CT

Michael Maksimowski, MD, MA
Psychosomatic Medicine Fellow
Department of Psychiatry
Yale School of Medicine
New Haven, CT

Andres Martin, MD, MPH
Riva Ariella Ritvo Professor and Professor of Psychiatry
Deputy Chair and Director of Medical Studies, Yale Child Study Center
Yale School of Medicine
Medical Director, Children's Psychiatric Inpatient Service
Yale-New Haven Children's Hospital
New Haven, CT

Adam P. Mecca, MD, PhD
Instructor
Geriatric Psychiatry and the Alzheimer's Disease Research Unit
Yale School of Medicine, Department of Psychiatry
New Haven, CT

Srinivas Muvvala, MD, MPH
Assistant Professor of Psychiatry
Yale School of Medicine
Medical Director of the Substance Abuse Treatment Unit
Connecticut Mental Health Center
New Haven, CT

Stephanie Ng, MD
Child Psychiatry Fellow
Yale School of Medicine
New Haven, CT

Robert Ostroff, MD
Medical Director, Mood Disorders Unit
Co-Medical Director, Interventional Psychiatry Service
Yale Psychiatric Hospital
New Haven, CT

Zheala Qayyum, MBBS
Assistant Clinical Professor
Department of Psychiatry
Yale School of Medicine
New Haven, CT

Mohini Ranganathan, MBBS
Associate Professor
Department of Psychiatry
Yale School of Medicine
New Haven, CT

Erica Robinson, MD
Resident
Department of Psychiatry
Yale School of Medicine
New Haven, CT

Robert Ross, MD, PhD
Resident
Department of Psychiatry
Yale School of Medicine
New Haven, CT

David Saunders, MD, PhD
Clinical Fellow in the Child Study Center
Department of Psychiatry
Yale School of Medicine
New Haven, CT

Hanna E. Stevens, MD, PhD
Assistant Professor
Department of Psychiatry
Carver College of Medicine University of Iowa Health Care
Iowa City, IA

Amanda Sun, MD
Resident
Department of Psychiatry
Yale School of Medicine
New Haven, CT

Jerome H. Taylor, MD
Child and Adolescent Psychiatrist and Research Scientist
Department of Psychiatry
University of Pennsylvania School of Medicine
Philadelphia, PA

Joseph J. Taylor, MD, PhD
Resident
Neuroscience Research Training Program
Department of Psychiatry
Yale School of Medicine
New Haven, CT

Cenk Tek, MD
Associate Professor of Psychiatry
Department of Psychiatry
Yale School of Medicine
Director, Psychosis Program
Connecticut Mental Health Center (CMHC)
New Haven, CT

Amalia Londono Tobon, MD
Clinical Fellow in the Child Study Center
Department of Psychiatry
Yale School of Medicine
New Haven, CT

Tobias Wasser, MD
Assistant Professor
Associate Director, Public Psychiatry Fellowship
Department of Psychiatry
Yale School of Medicine
New Haven, CT

Kirsten Wilkins, MD
Associate Professor and Clerkship Director
Department of Psychiatry
Yale School of Medicine
New Haven, CT

J. Corey Williams, MA, MD
Resident
Department of Psychiatry
Yale School of Medicine
New Haven, CT

Rachel Wurmser, MD
Clinical Fellow in Child and Adolescent Psychiatry
New York-Presbyterian Hospital
Columbia University College of Physicians & Surgeons and Weill Cornell Medicine
New York, NY

Stephanie Yarnell, MD, PhD
Law and Psychiatry Fellow
Neuroscience Research Training Program (NRTP)
Yale School of Medicine
New Haven, CT

Eunice Yuen, MD, PhD
Clinical Fellow in the Child Study Center Department of Psychiatry
Yale School of Medicine
New Haven, CT

50 Studies Every Psychiatrist Should Know

SECTION 1

Anxiety Disorders

1

Cognitive Behavioral Therapy, Imipramine, or Their Combination for Panic Disorder

AMANDA SUN AND TOBIAS WASSER

> Combining imipramine and CBT appeared to confer limited advantage acutely but more substantial advantage by the end of maintenance. Each treatment worked well immediately following treatment and during maintenance; CBT appeared durable in follow-up.
>
> —Barlow et al.[1]

Research Question: When treating adults with panic disorder, is imipramine in combination with cognitive behavioral therapy (CBT) more effective than monotherapy with either treatment alone?

Funding: National Institute of Mental Health

Year Study Began: 1991

Year Study Published: 2000

Study Location: Four anxiety research clinics

Who Was Studied: Adults with panic disorder with or without mild agoraphobia

Who Was Excluded: Patients with psychotic or bipolar disorders, suicidal ideation, significant substance abuse, and significant medical illnesses. In addition, patients with contraindications to CBT or imipramine, with history of poor response to similar treatments, receiving competing treatment, and those with pending disability claims.

How Many Participants: 312

Study Overview: See Figure 1.1 for a summary of the study design.

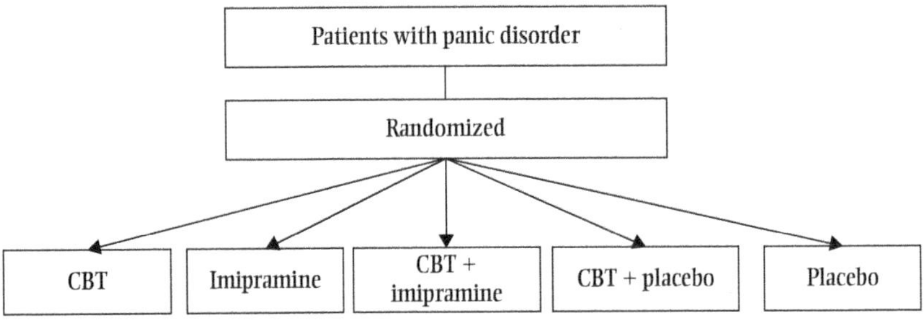

Figure 1.1 Summary of Study Design
NOTE: CBT = cognitive behavioral therapy.

Study Intervention: During the three-month acute treatment phase, those receiving CBT participated in 11 sessions lasting approximately 50 minutes each over 12 weeks. Those in combined treatment saw two therapists for a total of 75 minutes weekly. Maintenance phase treatment involved six monthly appointments involving treatment similar to the acute phase. Those who were responders were randomized to either treatment discontinuation or an extended maintenance pilot project and were reassessed after an additional six months of follow-up.

Participants randomized to imipramine or placebo received their interventions in a double-blind, fixed flexible-dose design, in which patients started imipramine (or placebo equivalent) at 10 mg/day, increased every other day by 10 mg until they were given 50 mg/day. Then, the dose was increased to 100 mg/day by week 4, and to 200 mg/day by week 5 unless the patient experienced intolerable side effects. The dose was further increased up to 300 mg/day by week 5 if the patient was still experiencing significant symptoms.

Follow-Up: Acute (three months after treatment initiation), maintenance (nine months after initiation), and follow-up (six months after treatment discontinuation).

Endpoints: Panic Disorder Severity Scale (PDSS) response rate, defined as a 40% reduction from baseline scores. Clinical Global Impressions (CGI) response rate, defined as the percent of subjects who scored a 2 (much improved) or better while also having less than 3 (mild) on the CGI severity.

RESULTS

- CBT alone and imipramine alone versus placebo:
  - Both imipramine and CBT were significantly superior to placebo in both acute and maintenance phases of treatment based on PDSS.
  - Post-acute CGI scores were not significantly different between imipramine or CBT and placebo, but after six months of maintenance, imipramine and CBT were both significantly superior to placebo for both the PDSS and CGI.

Table 1.1 SUMMARY OF STUDY FINDINGS

Outcome	CBT (%)	P value[a]	Imipramine (%)	P value[b]	CBT + Imipramine (%)	P value[c]	Placebo (%)
Acute PDSS response	48.7	0.03	45.8	0.05	60.3	0.03	21.7
PDSS response at six months	39.5	0.02	37.8	0.02	57.1	0.03	13.0
PDSS response six months after treatment ended	32.4	0.05	19.7	0.34	25.0	0.41	9.1

[a] P value of CBT compared to placebo.
[b] P value of imipramine compared to placebo.
[c] P value of CBT+impiramine compared to imipramine alone.
NOTE: PDSS = Panic Disorder Severity Scale.

- There was no significant difference in acute or maintenance analyses for CBT alone versus imipramine alone, but follow-up analyses favored CBT over imipramine.
- In the acute phase, combined therapy (CBT and imipramine) did not produce higher efficacy compared to CBT and placebo or to imipramine alone but did demonstrate superiority in maintenance analysis.
- Among treatment responders, imipramine produced a higher quality response than CBT; however, among those randomized to the no-treatment follow-up period, those who received CBT alone or CBT and placebo fared significantly better than responders to imipramine (Table 1.1).

Criticisms and Limitations: This study began when selective serotonin reuptake inhibitors (SSRIs) were not yet considered first line for panic disorder because of their favorable side-effect profile compared to tricyclic antidepressants. Thus, there was no comparator arm of patients receiving SSRIs.

Other limitations of this study include its generalizability to patients with higher levels of phobic avoidance, as the study only included patients with none or mild agoraphobia.

Other Relevant Studies and Information:

- See the Cochrane Database articles on psychological therapies in the treatment for panic disorder[1] and on combined psychotherapy plus antidepressants in panic disorder[2] to obtain more information on these topics.
- There have been other trials that studied psychotherapy,[3,4] pharmacotherapy[5,6,7] and both.[8] These studies have demonstrated conflicting evidence regarding the superiority of a combination of medication and psychotherapy.
- Based on this evidence, the American Psychiatric Association (APA) guidelines recommend psychotherapy such as CBT and antidepressants such as SSRIs in the treatment of panic disorder[9] in most circumstances.

Summary and Implications: This study found that imipramine, CBT, as well as a combination of the two treatments are superior to placebo in the treatment of panic disorder. Combination treatment was superior to each treatment alone, though it took time for this advantage to emerge. The study also showed that while imipramine produced a higher quality of response, CBT appears to exhibit more durability and is better tolerated. Notably, this study also indicates that initiating antidepressants might diminish the long-term durability of CBT after treatment withdrawal, though this finding requires replication. Based on this study and subsequent trials, the APA supports the use of antidepressants such as SSRIs and/or psychotherapy in the treatment of panic disorder.

CLINICAL CASE: TREATMENT OF PANIC DISORDER

Case History

A 21-year-old woman with a history of unspecified anxiety disorder presents to an outpatient psychiatrist after being referred by her primary care physician with complaints of increasing frequency of panic attacks. She describes frequent, almost daily, episodes of severe anxiety, palpitations, shortness of breath and gastrointestinal distress lasting about 15 minutes each. She was diagnosed with panic disorder without agoraphobia. Her primary care physician had prescribed her clonazepam for the treatment of her panic disorder, but the patient experienced only partial response and was also concerned about benzodiazepines' addictive potential. She asked about whether she could transition to an alternative treatment.

Based on this study, what therapeutic approaches should the outpatient psychiatrist take?

Suggested Answer

This study found that in the long run, CBT in combination with an antidepressant (such as imipramine) is indicated in the treatment of panic disorder.

The patient described in the vignette fits the criteria for inclusion in this study, and considering the severity of her illness, an antidepressant along with referral for CBT should be started. Of course, side effects and efficacy should be monitored closely in the acute period.

References

1. Barlow, D. H., Gorman, J. M., Shear, M. K., & Woods, S. W. (2000). Cognitive-behavioral therapy, imipramine, or their combination for panic disorder. *Journal of the American Medical Association, 283*(19), 2529–2536.
2. Pompoli, A., Furukawa, T. A., Imai, H., Tajika, A., Efthimiou, O., & Salanti, G. (2016). Psychological therapies for panic disorder with or without agoraphobia in adults: A network meta-analysis. *Cochrane Database Systematic Reviews, 4*, CD011004.
3. Furukawa, T. A., Watanabe, N., & Churchill, R. (2007). Combined psychotherapy plus antidepressants for panic disorder with or without agoraphobia. *Cochrane Database Systematic Reviews, 1*, CD004364.

4. Clark, D. M., Salkovskis, P. M., Hackmann, A., Middleton, H., Anastasiades, P., & Gelder, M. (1994). A comparison of cognitive therapy, applied relaxation and imipramine in the treatment of panic disorder. *British Journal of Psychiatry, 164*(6), 759–769.
5. Ballenger, J. C., Burrows, G. D., DuPont, R. L., Lesser, I. M., Noyes, R., Pecknold, J. C., . . . & Swinson, R. P. (1988). Alprazolam in panic disorder and agoraphobia: Results from a multicenter trial: I. Efficacy in short-term treatment. *Archives of General Psychiatry, 45*(5), 413–422.
6. Woodman, C. L., & Noyes, R. (1994). Panic disorder: Treatment with valproate. *Journal of Clinical Psychiatry, 55*(4), 134–136.
7. Pande, A. C., Pollack, M. H., Crockatt, J., Greiner, M., Chouinard, G., Lydiard, R. B., . . . & Shiovitz, T. (2000). Placebo-controlled study of gabapentin treatment of panic disorder. *Journal of Clinical Psychopharmacology, 20*(4), 467–471.
8. Gould, R. A., Ott, M. W., & Pollack, M H. (1995). A meta-analysis of treatment outcome for panic disorder. *Clinical Psychology Review, 15*(8), 819–844.
9. American Psychiatric Association. (2009). *Practice guideline for the treatment of patients with panic disorder*. Washington, DC: Author, p. 11.

2

Fluoxetine, Comprehensive Cognitive Behavioral Therapy, and Placebo in Generalized Social Phobia

ERIN HABECKER AND TOBIAS WASSER

> In adults with GSP, this study demonstrated efficacy for fluoxetine, and comprehensive cognitive behavioral therapy relative to placebo, but no evidence for greater benefit of combined treatment over monotherapies.
>
> —DAVIDSON ET AL.[1]

Research Question: For generalized social phobia (GSP), are fluoxetine and comprehensive cognitive behavioral therapy (CCBT) efficacious? How do their efficacies compare? And is there an advantage to combination therapy?

Funding: National Institute of Mental Health

Year Study Began: 1995

Year Study Published: 2004

Study Location: Outpatient Clinics at Duke University Medical Center and University of Pennsylvania

Who Was Studied: English-speaking adults between the ages of 18 and 65 meeting DSM-IV criteria for GSP

Who Was Excluded: Patients with any of the following: comorbid anxiety disorder, history of schizophrenia or bipolar disorder, major depression within the previous six months, substance abuse within the previous year, developmental disability, unstable medical condition, history of prior failure of response to fluoxetine at 60 mg/d for at least four weeks or to 12 weekly sessions of CCBT for GSP, concurrent psychiatric treatment or other psychoactive medications, positive urine drug screen, inability to maintain two weeks' psychotropic drug-free washout, pregnancy, or lactation.

How Many Participants: 295

Study Overview: See Figure 2.1 for a summary of the study design.

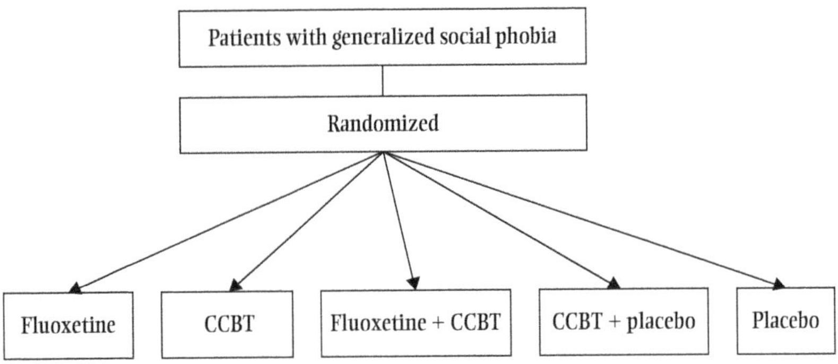

Figure 2.1 Summary of Study Design
NOTE: CCBT = comprehensive cognitive behavioral therapy.

Study Intervention: For those randomized to receive fluoxetine (FLU), treatment was started at 10 mg daily, with the goal of increasing to 40 mg. Dose could be further increased to 60 mg in patients who were tolerating the medication and had not achieved a Clinical Global Impressions (CGI) Improvement score of 1 or 2.

CCBT is a form of group CBT in which social skills training is added to exposure therapy and cognitive restructuring, developed specifically for GSP. Those randomized to the weekly CCBT groups completed a 14-week group treatment including specific social skills training and psychoeducation. A role-play test was used to evaluate patients' social skills before and after treatment.

This was a randomized controlled trial with all medications and placebo being administered in double-blinded fashion and utilizing a blinded independent rater to conduct primary outcome assessments.

Follow-Up: 14 weeks

Endpoints: Primary outcome: response rate defined as the scoring either a 1 ("much" to "very much" improvement) in the CGI Improvement scale, the CGI severity scale, and the Brief Social Phobia Scale. Secondary outcome: Social Phobia and Anxiety Inventory.

RESULTS

- 211 subjects of the 295 randomized completed the 14 weeks of treatment. The placebo (PBO) group had significantly more dropouts than the CCBT group in pairwise contrasts; otherwise, there were no significant differences in dropout rates between the groups.
- All active treatments were superior to PBO by week 14 (see Table 2.1).
- There was a stronger response from weeks 0 to 4 in the FLU group as compared to all other groups.

Table 2.1 SUMMARY OF THE GSP TREATMENT STUDY'S RESULTS

14 week outcomes	FLU	CCBT	FLU/CCBT	CCBT/PBO	PBO	P value
Response rate	50.9%	51.7%	54.2%	50.8%	31.7%	Significant for all comparisons vs. PBO
CGI Severity Scale Effect size vs PBO (95% CI)	0.42 (0.04 – 0.80)	0.27 (–0.10 – 0.64)	0.30 (–0.07 – 0.67)	0.42 (0.04 – 0.79)	N/A	
BSPS score effect size vs. PBO (95% CI)	0.40 (0.02 – 0.77)	0.30 (–0.07 – 0.66)	0.24 (–0.13 – 0.60)	0.52 (0.14 – 0.89)	N/A	

NOTES: GSP = generalized social phobia. FLU = fluoxetine. CCBT = comprehensive cognitive behavioral therapy. PBO = placebo. CGI = Clinical Global Impression. BSPS = Brief Social Phobia Scale.

- In the last 10 weeks of treatment, the group receiving combined CCBT and fluoxetine showed more improvement in rating scale scores than the fluoxetine monotherapy group.
- At the conclusion of the study, there were no significant differences in the active treatment arms as assessed by the ratings scales; combination therapy was not superior to monotherapy.
- The Subjective Units of Distress Scale scores before and after a behavioral task (exposure scenario) improved in the CCBT groups but not in the FLU or PBO groups.
- Side effects: symptoms possibly attributable to the treatment included insomnia, headaches, nausea, anorgasmia, and erectile dysfunction. Anorgasmia was more commonly seen in the groups containing FLU (Table 2.1).

Criticisms and Limitations: The trial excluded subjects with inflexible schedules, which may have led to selection bias.

Some studies have suggested that group cognitive behavioral therapy may be less effective than individual cognitive behavioral therapy in the treatment of social phobia.[2,3]

The study is restricted to looking at the effects of a single selective serotonin reuptake inhibitor (SSRI; fluoxetine), which has been shown in some studies of GSP not to be superior in efficacy to placebo.[4,5]

The study excludes comorbidities including depression, which limits generalizability of the sample.

No long-term follow-up was conducted after the conclusion of active treatment, so effects of treatment over time are unable to be assessed.

Other Relevant Studies and Information:

- A number of trials have previously suggested benefit from a combination of medication and psychosocial intervention in patients with GSP.[3,6,7]
- SSRIs are the most extensively studied medication for the treatment of GSP.[8]
- Only one prior study has compared SSRI with CCBT, similarly finding that SSRI alone and SSRI in combination with CCBT were superior to placebo.[9]
- A number of studies have investigated various SSRIs (fluoxetine, paroxetine, and sertraline) in the treatment of GSP, but no head-to-head SSRI comparison trials have been conducted.[9,10,11,12,13,14]

- A prior study of CCBT and phenelzine treatment demonstrated similar response rates to this study.[7]
- Although there have not been specific guidelines from the American Psychiatry Association about treatment of social phobia/social anxiety disorder, the National Institute for Health and Care Excellence (United Kingdom) suggests CBT as a first line treatment, followed by augmentation with SSRI, with initial SSRI therapy reserved for patients who decline CBT.[15]

Summary and Implications: This landmark trial compared head-to-head treatments of GSP including medication management with an SSRI, psychotherapy, and combined treatment. It found efficacy for both treatment with an SSRI (fluoxetine), group cognitive behavioral therapy (CCBT), and combined treatment. However, there was no evidence that combination treatment was superior to monotherapies after 14 weeks. All active treatment groups were superior to placebo. This study supports National Institute for Health and Care Excellence (NICE) guidelines for the treatment of GSP, which recommend CBT as a preferred first line treatment, followed by SSRI augmentation if necessary.

CLINICAL CASE: TREATMENT OF GENERALIZED SOCIAL PHOBIA OR SOCIAL ANXIETY DISORDER

Case History

A patient comes to clinic with symptoms of anxiety and fear of embarrassment in classroom settings and at parties. Anxiety symptoms are particularly bothersome when the patient is expected to speak or present in classroom settings and include sweaty palms, shaking hands, and flushing. The patient has started to avoid going to class to avoid these symptoms. She recognizes that this fear is excessive and likely not reality-based. She was diagnosed with GSP. The patient is interested in medication or psychotherapy. Based on the results of this study, what is indicated?

Suggested Answer

This study found that group CBT was as efficacious as fluoxetine when treating GSP after 14 weeks, though fluoxetine may have worked faster. There was no added benefit of combined medication and psychotherapy based on this study.

The patient in this vignette would have met inclusion criteria for this study. Treatment with CBT or medication, preferably an SSRI, would both be reasonable options depending on patient preference. The psychiatrist should discuss treatment options with the patient, including the risks and benefits of each intervention and help the patient arrive at an informed decision.

References

1. Davidson, J. R. T, Foa, E. B., Huppert, J. D., Keefe, F. J., Franklin, M. E., Compton, J. S., . . . Gadde, K. M. (2004). Fluoxetine, comprehensive cognitive behavioral therapy, and placebo in generalized social phobia. *Archives of General Psychiatry, 61*(10), 1005–1013.
2. Stangier, U., Heidenreich, T., Peitz, M., Lauterbach, W., & Clark, D. M. (2003). Cognitive therapy for social phobia: Individual versus group treatment. *Behaviour Research and Therapy, 41*(9), 991–1007.
3. Ingul, J. M., Aune, T., & Nordahl, H. M. (2014). A randomized controlled trial of individual cognitive therapy, group cognitive behaviour therapy and attentional placebo for adolescent social phobia. *Psychotherapy and Psychosomatics,* 83(1), 54–61.
4. Clark, D. M., Ehlers, A., McManus, F., Hackmann, A., Fennell, M., Campbell, H., . . . Louis, B. (2003). Cognitive therapy versus fluoxetine in generalized social phobia: A randomized placebo-controlled trial. *Journal of Consulting and Clinical Psychology, 71*(6), 1058–1067.
5. Kobak, K. A., Greist, J. H., Jefferson, J. W., & Katzelnick, D. J. (2002). Fluoxetine in social phobia: A double-blind, placebo-controlled pilot study. *Journal of Clinical Psychopharmacology, 22*(3), 257–262.
6. Mayo-Wilson, E., Dias, S., Mavranezouli, I., Kew, K., Clark, D. M., Ades, A. E., & Pilling, S. (2014). Psychological and pharmacological interventions for social anxiety disorder in adults: A systematic review and network meta-analysis. *The Lancet Psychiatry, 1*(5), 368–376.
7. Blanco, C., Heimberg, R. G, Schneier, F. R, Fresco, D. M., Chen, H., Turk, C. L., . . . Liebowitz, M. R. (2010). A placebo-controlled trial of phenelzine, cognitive behavioral group therapy, and their combination for social anxiety disorder. *Archives of General Psychiatry, 67*(3), 286–295.
8. Hidalgo, R. B., Barnett, S. D., & Davidson, J. R. (2001). Social anxiety disorder in review: Two decades of progress. *International Journal of Neuropsychopharmacology, 4*(3), 279–298.
9. Blomhoff, S., Haug, T. T., Hellstrom, K., Humble, M., Madsbu, H. P., & Wold, J. E. (2001). Randomised controlled general practice trial of sertraline, exposure therapy and combined treatment in generalised social phobia. *British Journal of Psychiatry, 179*(2), 23–30.
10. Van Ameringen, M. A., Lane, R. M., Walker, J. R., Bowen, R. C., Chokka, P R., Goldner, E. M., . . . Swinson, R. P. (2001). Sertraline treatment of generalized social phobia: A 20-week, double-blind, placebo-controlled study. *American Journal of Psychiatry, 158*(2), 275–281.

11. Katzelnick, D. J., Kobak, K. A., Greist, J. H., Jefferson, J. W., Mantle, J. M., & Serlin, R. C. (1995). Sertraline for social phobia: A double-blind, placebo-controlled cross-over study. *American Journal of Psychiatry, 152*(9), 1368–1371.
12. Allgulander, C. (1999). Paroxetine in social anxiety disorder: A randomized placebo-controlled study. *Acta Psychiatrica Scandinavica, 100*(3), 193–198.
13. Baldwin, D., Bobes, J., Stein, D. J., Scharwachter, I., & Faure, M. Paroxetine in social phobia/social anxiety disorder: Randomised, double-blind, placebo-controlled study. Paroxetine Study Group. *British Journal of Psychiatry, 175*, 120–126.
14. Stein, M. B., Liebowitz, M. R., Lydiard, R. B., Pitts, C. D., Bushnell, W., & Gergel, I. (1998). Paroxetine treatment of generalized social phobia (social anxiety disorder): A randomized controlled trial. *JAMA, 280*(8), 708–713.
15. National Institute for Health and Care Excellence. (2013). *Social anxiety disorder: Recognition, assessment and treatment.* NICE Clinical Guidelines No. 159. London: Author.

SECTION 2

Bipolar Disorder

3

Lithium Plus Valproate Combination versus Monotherapy for Relapse Prevention in Bipolar I Disorder (BALANCE)

JOÃO PAULO DE AQUINO AND ROBERT BEECH

Our results suggest that patients should be advised that a better outcome would be likely with combination therapy with lithium plus valproate semi-sodium or lithium alone.

—The BALANCE Investigators[1]

Research Question: Is lithium plus valproate better than monotherapy with either drug alone for relapse prevention in bipolar I disorder?

Funding: Stanley Medical Research Institute; Sanofi Aventis

Year Study Began: 2001

Year Study Published: 2010

Study Location: 41 sites in the United Kingdom, United States, Italy, and France

Who Was Studied: Patient aged 16 and older with a DSM-IV diagnosis of bipolar I disorder who required long term drug therapy to prevent relapse

Who Was Excluded: Patients who were having an acute episode or had a medical disorder that precluded use of either lithium or valproate

How Many Participants: 330

Study Overview: See Figure 3.1 for a summary of the study design.

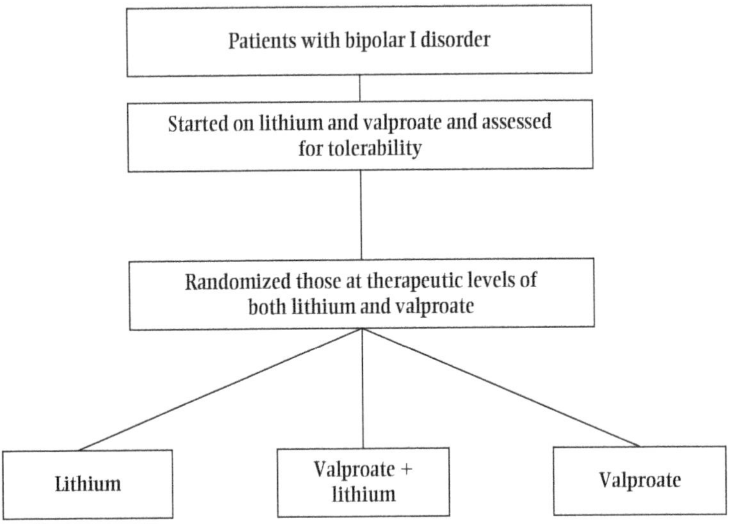

Figure 3.1 Summary of Study Design

Study Intervention: First, there was a "run-in phase" of four to eight weeks where patients were given short-term trials of both medications to assess tolerability. Lithium was titrated to serum levels of 0.4 and 1 mmol/L, and valproate was given up to a target dose of 1,250 mg daily, or the highest tolerated dose. Those patients who had therapeutic lithium levels, valproate dose of at least 750 mg daily or concentration of 50 ug/mL, and were 70% compliant on medications were allowed to participate in the study phase.

In the study phase, patients were randomized in an open-label fashion to receive either medication as monotherapy or a combination of lithium and valproate.

Follow-Up: 24 months

Endpoints: The primary outcome was whether or not patients required a new intervention for an emergent mood episode. New interventions included adding or increasing medication dose or admission to the hospital. Secondary outcomes included global assessment of functioning, deliberate self-harm, quality of life, adverse events, and adherence to the assigned treatment.

RESULTS

- The hazard ratio of the primary outcome (the need to start a new intervention to address a mood disturbance) was significantly lower in the participants allocated to combination therapy compared to those allocated to valproate monotherapy but not those allocated to lithium monotherapy.
- The hazard ratio of the primary outcome was significantly lower in the group allocated to lithium monotherapy compared to those on valproate monotherapy.
- The risk for hospital admission was lower for participants allocated to combination therapy compared to patients allocated to valproate monotherapy but was not significantly lower for those on lithium alone.
- Discontinuation of allocated treatment, self-harm, quality of life, and global functioning did not differ significantly between groups (Table 3.1).

Table 3.1 Summary of BALANCE Trial's Key Findings

Outcome	Combination therapy	Lithium monotherapy	P value	Valproate monotherapy	P value
% with an emergent mood episode	54%	59%	0.23	69%	0.0014
Hazard ratio vs. combination therapy	n/a	0.82	0.27	0.59	0.0023
Hazard ratio vs. lithium monotherapy				0.71	0.0472

Criticism and Limitations: Treatment allocation was not blinded from the investigators or participants. Therefore, performance and ascertainment biases could have arisen if clinicians or participants had behaved systematically differently dependent on the treatment allocation. Furthermore, around 21% of patients withdrew from the trial, although the reasons for withdrawal did not differ significantly between groups.

It is worthy of mention that the dose of valproate used was lower than is recommended for treatment of acute mania (1,200–1,500 mg/day), and increased doses might have improved its effectiveness. Finally, there was no placebo comparator group in this trial.

Other Relevant Studies and Information:

- A previous smaller randomized trial compared lithium monotherapy with a combination of lithium plus valproate in patients with rapid cycling disorder and comorbid substance abuse.[2] The estimate of the hazard ratio was in favor of combination therapy similar and to that recorded on BALANCE.[1]
- There have been other studies investigating differences between lithium and valproate in the treatment of bipolar disorder,[2,3] which found mixed results favoring the use of lithium over valproate in bipolar disorder.
- According to the American Psychiatric Association (APA) *Practice Guideline for the Treatment of Patients with Bipolar Disorder, Second Edition,*[4] the medications with the best empirical evidence to support their use in maintenance phase include lithium and valproate, although this study supports efficacy of lithium over valproate as monotherapy. Alternatives include lamotrigine, carbamazepine, antipsychotics, or oxcarbazepine.

Summary and Implications: The BALANCE trial was a landmark study that found that combination of lithium and valproate was not substantially superior to lithium alone in the treatment of bipolar disorder. The study did find some benefit of using lithium in combination with valproate, compared with valproate alone. Based on the results of this and other trials on this topic, the APA recommends using lithium and valproate as prophylactic treatment for episodic mood disturbances in people with bipolar disorder.

CLINICAL CASE: LITHIUM PLUS VALPROATE VERSUS MONOTHERAPY IN THE MAINTENANCE TREATMENT OF BIPOLAR I DISORDER

Case History

A 32-year-old woman with bipolar I disorder has been relatively stable for 3 months on valproate but over the last week has been irritable and agitated around the house and at work. She is uncertain about switching or optimizing the mood stabilizer would be the best course of action in her treatment.

Based on the results of BALANCE trial, how should this patient be treated?

Suggested Answer

The BALANCE trial found that combination of lithium and valproate is superior to valproate alone, but not lithium alone, in the maintenance treatment of bipolar disorder.

When planning long-term pharmacological interventions to prevent relapse, physicians should take into account drugs that have been effective during manic or depressive episodes, discussing with the person the possible benefits and risks of each drug for them. A thorough discussion with the patient should follow aiming to clarify whether the patient prefers to continue this treatment or switch to lithium, as lithium is the most effective long-term treatment for bipolar affective disorder. If lithium is insufficiently effective, consider adding valproate; if lithium not well tolerated, consider valproate or olanzapine as alternatives. If it has been effective during an episode of mania or bipolar depression, consider quetiapine. Valproate should be used carefully in women of child-bearing age due to the risk of teratogenicity. Before stopping medication, a careful discussion with the patient on how to recognize early signs of relapse and what to do if symptoms recur is necessary.

References

1. Geddes, J. R., Goodwin, G.M., Rendell, J., Azorin, J.M., Cipriani, A., . . . Juszczak, E. (2010). Lithium plus valproate combination therapy versus monotherapy for relapse prevention in bipolar I disorder (BALANCE): A randomised open-label trial. *Lancet, 375*(9712), 385–395.
2. Calabrese, J. R., Shelton, M. D., Rapport, D. J., Youngstrom, E. A., Jackson, K., Bilali, S., . . . & Findling, R. L. (2005). A 20-month, double-blind, maintenance trial of lithium versus divalproex in rapid-cycling bipolar disorder. *American Journal of Psychiatry, 162*(11), 2152–2161.
3. Oquendo, M. A., Galfalvy, H. C., Currier, D., Grunebaum, M. F., Sher, L., Sullivan, G. M., . . . & Mann, J. J. (2011). Treatment of suicide attempters with bipolar disorder: A randomized clinical trial comparing lithium and valproate in the prevention of suicidal behavior. *American Journal of Psychiatry, 168*(10), 1050–1056.
4. Hirschfeld, R. M., Bowden, C. L., Gitlin, M. J., Keck, P. E., Suppes, T., Thase, M. E., . . . Perlis, R. H. (2010). Practice guideline for the treatment of patients with bipolar disorder (2nd ed.). Washington, DC: American Psychiatric Association.

4

Mood Stabilizer Monotherapy versus Adjunctive Antidepressant for Bipolar Depression

The STEP-BD Trial

JOÃO PAULO DE AQUINO AND ROBERT BEECH

> The use of adjunctive, standard antidepressant medication, as compared with the use of mood stabilizers, was not associated with increased efficacy or with increased risk of treatment-emergent affective switch.
>
> —THE STEP-BD INVESTIGATORS[1]

Research Question: Among patients with bipolar disorder receiving mood-stabilizing agents, does adjunctive antidepressant therapy reduce the symptoms of bipolar depression without increasing mania?

Funding: The National Institute of Mental Health; Glaxo Wellcome and SmithKlineBeecham (now GlaxoSmithKline) donated the antidepressant drugs.

Year Study Began: 1999

Year Study Published: 2007

Study Location: Outpatient clinics affiliated with academic medical centers in the United States. All eight study sites had bipolar specialty programs caring for at least 100 active patients and were deemed to be demographically diverse by the STEP-BD lead investigators.

Who Was Studied: Patients aged ≥18 years old who met DSM-IV criteria for a major depressive episode (MDE) associated with DSM-IV diagnosis of bipolar I or bipolar II disorder. The majority of individuals in both treatment groups had experienced one or more MDEs prior to study entry.

Who Was Excluded: Individuals with a history of intolerable side effects or unsatisfactory response to adequate trials of bupropion and paroxetine, substance use disorders requiring current short-term targeted treatment, and prior adjunctive antipsychotic drugs or immediate dose adjustment of a long-term antipsychotic medication.

How Many Participants: 366

Study Overview: See Figure 4.1 for a summary of the study design.

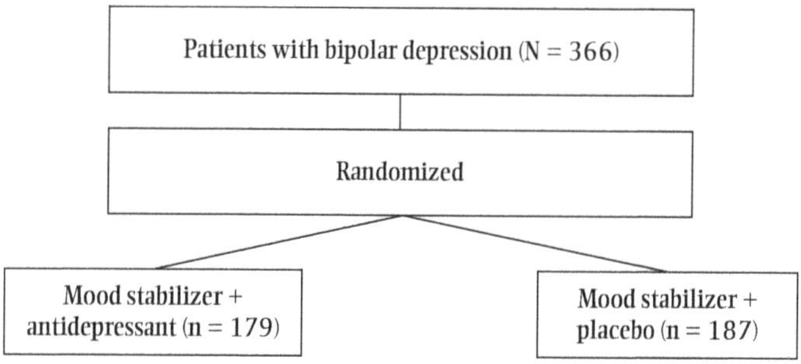

Figure 4.1 Summary of Study Design

Study Intervention: This study was completed in a double-blind fashion. All patients were started on one of the following mood stabilizing regimens: lithium, valproic acid, lithium plus valproic acid, or carbamazepine. The study was later amended to include any FDA-approved anti-mania treatment. Mood stabilizers were titrated to the recommended therapeutic levels.

Individuals randomized to the mood stabilizer plus antidepressant group received either bupropion or paroxetine in addition to a mood stabilizer. These antidepressants were selected by the STEP-BD team of investigators as they were deemed to have a low rate of affective switch to represent the standard of antidepressants commonly prescribed for bipolar depression at the time of the study and due to the fact they have different mechanisms of action and side-effect profiles. Paroxetine was started at 10 mg daily and titrated up to a maximum of 40 mg daily. Bupropion (sustained-release) was started at 150 mg daily and titrated up to a maximum of 375 mg daily.

Individuals randomized to the mood stabilizer plus placebo group received one of the three previously mentioned mood stabilizers plus placebo.

Follow-Up: 26 weeks

Endpoints: Primary outcome: Durable recovery, (≥8 consecutive weeks of euthymia, defined as no more than two depressive or two manic symptoms). Secondary outcomes: Treatment remission (1–7 consecutive weeks of euthymia), treatment-effectiveness response (50% improvement from baseline symptom subscale for depression (SUM-D) score, from the mood modules of the Structured Clinical Interview for DSM-VI (SCID), without meeting criteria for hypomania or mania), treatment-emergent affective switch (hypomania/mania or required clinician intervention for mood intervention), and discontinuation of a study medication because of an adverse event.

RESULTS

- There were no significant differences between the groups in treatment effectiveness; however, there was a nonsignificant trend toward worse outcomes among patients in the mood stabilizer plus antidepressant versus the mood stabilizer plus placebo groups (see Table 4.1).

Table 4.1 Summary of the Effectiveness of Adjunctive Antidepressant Treatment for Bipolar Depression Results

Outcome	**Mood stabilizer + Antidepressant (N = 179) (%)**	**Mood stabilizer + Placebo (N = 187) (%)**	**P value**
Durable recovery (primary outcome)	23.5	27.3	0.40
Transient remission	17.9	21.4	0.40
Treatment-effectiveness response	32.4	38.0	0.27
Treatment-emergent affective switch	10.1	10.7	0.84
Discontinuation of study because of an adverse event	12.3	9.1	0.32

- Although not effective, the antidepressants were well tolerated: Treatment-emergent affective switch occurred in 10% of both the antidepressant/mood stabilizer and placebo/mood stabilizer groups.
- The rates and types of adverse reactions were also similar in the antidepressant and placebo groups (Table 4.1).

Criticisms and Limitations: Since the study had strict eligibility requirements, it may have excluded certain groups of patients, such as those with prior treatment of any of the study antidepressants, limiting the generalizability of the findings. Another potential source of bias is that only patients with good insight and motivation to receive treatment could be involved in the study, due to the requirements for informed consent. As a result, results may not generalize to patients with limited insight or other groups unable or unwilling to consent.

The primary outcome of this study was "durable recovery," defined as 8 consecutive weeks of euthymia; however, longer-term outcomes were not assessed.

Furthermore, some common symptoms of bipolar disorder such as mood instability and impulsivity were not measured.

Other Relevant Studies and Information:

- Similar findings were obtained in a meta-analysis published the next year that included data from seven smaller studies.[2]
- A one-year follow-up of STEP-BD found similar results in subjects treated openly at the same treatment centers. Antidepressant use was associated with somewhat worse outcomes than management of bipolar depression without any standard antidepressants, especially for patients with rapid-cycling bipolar disorder.[3]
- A double-blind controlled trial randomized depressed bipolar patients to quetiapine, paroxetine, or placebo found paroxetine was no better than placebo.[4]
- One randomized double-blind study compared antidepressants with respect to their propensity for causing affective switching. This study found higher switch rates of switching with venlafaxine than with bupropion or sertraline.[5]
- American Psychiatric American (APA) practice guidelines place mood stabilizers as first-line treatment for bipolar depression before an antidepressant adjunct is considered and recommend maintaining treatment with a mood stabilizer to mitigate the risk of

antidepressant-induced mania or increased cycling.[6] To date, the only FDA-approved antidepressants for the depressive phase of bipolar disorder are olanzapine-fluoxetine combination, quetiapine, and lurasidone.

Summary and Implications: In this randomized, multicenter, double-blind, placebo-controlled trial, adding an antidepressant to a mood stabilizer was not effective for treating bipolar depression. Adjunctive antidepressant therapy did not increase affective switching to mania relative to placebo therapy, however. Based on this and other studies, guidelines from the APA recommend mood stabilizers as first-line treatment for bipolar depression and indicate that adjunctive antidepressant therapy should only be considered in refractory cases.

CLINICAL CASE: MOOD STABILIZER MONOTHERAPY VERSUS ADJUNCTIVE ANTIDEPRESSANT IN BIPOLAR DEPRESSION

Case History

A 33-year-old single woman states she has been intermittently depressed for 15 years. Her current symptoms include hypersomnia, increased appetite, craving carbohydrates/sweets, feeling like she is "nailed to the bed in the mornings," and crying spells. She sometimes "prays she will not wake up" and is irritable and anxious. No evidence of psychosis or prior suicide attempts. At times, she can feel more self-confident, "project a different self," and be more impulsive and has decreased need for sleep for approximately 1-week periods. She has a family history of bipolar disorder. She says all antidepressants "work for a while, then stop." Her only current medication is lithium.

Based on the results of the STEP-BD, how should this patient be treated?

Suggested Answer

STEP-BD found that that monotherapy with a mood stabilizer is as effective as dual therapy with a mood stabilizer plus an antidepressant for individuals with bipolar depression.

The clinical picture as previously presented is typical of a patient in the STEP-BD study. Based on these results, the addition of an antidepressant like bupropion or paroxetine would not provide additional benefit. While clinical history and past response to similar treatments remain important factors in treatment decisions,[7] it is important to emphasize there are alternatives to pharmacotherapy, such as psychosocial interventions with reasonable evidence to treat depressive morbidity in bipolar disorder.[8]

References

1. Sachs, G. S., Nierenberg, A. A., Calabrese, J. R., Marangell, L. B., Wisniewski, S. R., Gyulai, L., . . . & Ketter, T. A. (2007). Effectiveness of adjunctive antidepressant treatment for bipolar depression. *New England Journal of Medicine, 356*(17), 1711–1722.
2. Ghaemi, S. N., Wingo, A. P., Filkowski, M. A., & Baldessarini, R. J. (2008). Long-term antidepressant treatment in bipolar disorder: Meta-analyses of benefits and risks. *Acta Psychiatrica Scandinavica, 118*(5), 347–356.
3. Schneck, C. D., Miklowitz, D. J., Miyahara, S., Araga, M., Wisniewski, S., Gyulai, L., . . . Sachs, G. S. (2008). The prospective course of rapid-cycling bipolar disorder: Findings from the STEP-BD. *American Journal of Psychiatry, 165*(3), 370–377.
4. McElroy, S. L., Weisler, R. H., Chang, W., Olausson, B., Paulsson, B., Brecher, M., . . . Young A. H. (2010). A double-blind, placebo-controlled study of quetiapine and paroxetine as monotherapy in adults with bipolar depression (EMBOLDEN II). *Journal of Clinical Psychiatry,* 71(2), 163–174.
5. Leverich, G. S., Altshuler, L. L., Frye, M. A., Suppes, T., McElroy, S. L., Keck, P. E., Jr., . . . Post, R. M. (2006). Risk of switch in mood polarity to hypomania or mania in patients with bipolar depression during acute and continuation trials of venlafaxine, sertraline, and bupropion as adjuncts to mood stabilizers. American *Journal of Psychiatry, 163*(2), 232–239.
6. American Psychiatric Association. (2002). *Practice guideline for the treatment of patients with bipolar disorder (revision).* Washington, DC: Author.
7. Belmaker, R. H. (2007). Treatment of bipolar depression. *New England Journal of Medicine, 356,* 1771–1773.
8. Miklowitz, D. J., Otto, M. W., Frank, E., Reilly-Harrington, N. A., Wisniewski, S. R., Kogan, J. N., . . . Sachs, G. S. (2007). Psychosocial treatments for bipolar depression: A 1-year randomized trial from the Systematic Treatment Enhancement Program. *Archives of General Psychiatry, 64,* 419–426.

5

Suicide Risk in Bipolar Disorder

Comparing Lithium, Divalproex, and Carbamazepine

RACHEL KATZ AND ROBERT BEECH

> *Among patients treated for bipolar disorder, risk of suicide attempt and suicide death is lower during treatment with lithium than during treatment with divalproex.*
>
> —Goodwin et al.[1]

Research Question: Is there a difference in suicide risk for patients with bipolar disorder (BD) who are treated with lithium, divalproex, or carbamazepine?

Funding: Solvay Pharmaceuticals and Best Practice LLC

Year Study Began: 1994

Year Study Published: 2003

Study Location: Two large integrated health plans in Washington and California (Group Health Cooperative and Kaiser Permanente, respectively)

Who Was Studied: Patients 14 years or older with a diagnosis of BD with at least one filled prescription for lithium, divalproex or carbamazepine over a seven-year time period.

Who Was Excluded: Patients with a previous diagnosis of schizophrenia, schizoaffective disorder prior to bipolar diagnosis, cognitive disorder, or dementia.

How Many Participants: 20,638

Study Overview: See Figure 5.1 for a summary of the study design.

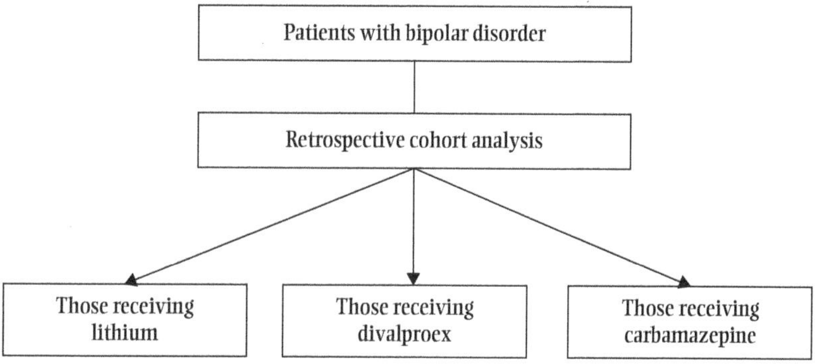

Figure 5.1 Summary of Study Design
NOTE: Only measured at one of the two sites.

Study Intervention: This was a retrospective cohort study comparing outcomes among patients who were prescribed lithium, divalproex, or carbamazepine.

Follow-Up: Mean of 2.9 years

Endpoints: Primary outcomes included suicide attempts (by hospital discharge diagnosis) and death by suicide (by death certificate). Secondary outcomes included suicidal behavior (by emergency department discharge diagnosis, not leading to hospitalization).

RESULTS

- An analysis that adjusted for various confounds including year of BD diagnosis and use of other psychotropic medications found that those prescribed divalproex had a 2.7 (95% CI [1.1, 6.3], $p = 0.03$) times increased risk of death compared to those taking lithium.

- Those taking carbamazepine did not have significant differences in rates of completed suicide compared with lithium ($p = 0.61$), though did have a 2.9 (95% CI [1.9, 4.4], $p < 0.001$) times higher risk of suicide attempts resulting in hospitalization.
- There were 53 total completed suicides in the study (Table 5.1).

Table 5.1 SUMMARY OF KEY FINDINGS

Outcome	**Li**	**VPA**	**CBZ**	**Combo**	**None**
Suicidal Behavior leading to ED visit[a,b]	10.8	31.3*	22.1*	34.3*	15.0*
Suicide attempts resulting in hospitalization[b]	4.2	10.5*	15.5*	12.4*	4.8
Suicidal deaths[b]	0.7	1.7*	1	1.5	1.2

[a]Kaiser Permanente site only.
[b]Event rate per 1000 person-years.
NOTES: Li = lithium. VPA = divalproex. CBZ = carbamazepine. ED = emergency department. *P value vs lithium is statistically significant (<0.05).

Criticisms and Limitations: Since this was not a randomized trial, confounding factors may have influenced the results. For example, patients with significant impulsivity, behavioral dysregulation or substance abuse may have preferentially have been prescribed divalproex or carbamazepine (given lithium's narrow therapeutic index/overdose risk). Furthermore, psychiatrists may avoid prescribing lithium to patients with a history of suicide attempts or gestures, especially those with a history of medication overdose, due to its risk of overdose. This may have excluded the highest risk patients from the lithium cohort and skewed the results in favor of lithium.

Since this analysis was based on administrative data, it was not possible to assess the accuracy of bipolar diagnoses, the frequency or type of mood episodes (depression, mania or mixed) or the severity of suicidal behavior.

Additionally, there was no confirmation that study patients were actually took what they were prescribed.

Finally, accuracy of the number of suicide deaths was solely dependent on coroner diagnoses, which may underestimate the rate of suicide, especially in the context of drug overdose.[2] Forensic psychiatric autopsy of all deaths (regardless of cause) in the cohort may have provided a more accurate estimate of completed suicide.

Other Relevant Studies and Information:

- A previous small study suggested that those randomized to lithium had antisuicidal effects compared to those that received carbamazepine or amitriptyline.[3]
- Another study found that lithium had an independent antisuicidal effect, independent from its mood stabilizing properties, in both unipolar and bipolar mood disorders.[4]
- A large recent study further supports lithium's antisuicidal and anti-self-injury effects are more powerful than other agents used for mood stabilization, including divalproex, carbamazepine, olanzapine, or quetiapine.[5]
- Yet another study that randomized those with BD and previous suicide attempts to lithium or divalproex found no difference between groups, though the sample size was small and there were many confounders.[6]
- American Psychiatric Association (APA) guidelines suggest there is "strong and consistent evidence" that long-term maintenance treatment with lithium, both for unipolar depression and BD, is associated with "major reductions in risk of both suicide and suicide attempts."[7]

Summary and Implications: This landmark study suggests that lithium therapy for BD is associated with a lower risk of suicide vs divalproex and carbamazepine. However, since this was not a randomized trial, confounding factors may have influenced the results, and thus the findings are not definitive. Nevertheless, based on this and other studies, the APA guidelines on treating suicidal behavior recommend considering lithium for suicidality prophylaxis preferentially to divalproex and carbamazepine among patients requiring mood stabilization.

CLINICAL CASE: CHOOSING A FIRST MOOD STABILIZER

A 22-year-old woman presents to the hospital with her first manic episode. She has symptoms of euphoria, grandiosity, decreased need for sleep, and delusions about being the Queen of England. Her psychiatric history is notable for two previous depressive episodes and two previous suicide attempts. Based on the results of this study, which would be the best mood stabilizer for treatment of acute mania, mania prophylaxis and prevention of further suicidal behavior?

Suggested Answer

This study investigated the effect of lithium, divalproex, and carbamazepine on suicidality. Based on this and other studies, the APA recommended that psychiatrists consider the effect of lithium in reducing suicidal behavior in patients with BD. The APA also warns about the dangers of lithium overdose in these same recommendations.

The patient in the vignette has BD and is at increased risk for suicide especially considering her history of previous attempts. Based on the results of this study, lithium should be considered as a first-line mood stabilizer and would be indicated for treatment of acute mania and mania prophylaxis. Along with these indications, it would likely decrease the patient's risk of future suicidal behavior and suicidal attempts more than divalproex or carbamazepine. The decision to start lithium over another mood stabilizer should be made carefully after weighing the risks and benefits in accordance with the patient's preferences.

References

1. Goodwin, F. K., Fireman, B., Simon, G. E., Hunkeler, E.M., Lee, J., Revicki, D. (2003). Suicide risk in bipolar disorder during treatment with lithium and divalproex. *JAMA, 290*(11), 1467–1473.
2. Hayes, J. F. Pitman, A., Marston, L., Walters, K., Geddes, J. R., King, M., & Osborn, D. P. (2016). Self-harm, unintentional injury, and suicide in bipolar disorder during maintenance mood stabilizer treatment: A UK population-based electronic health records study, *JAMA Psychiatry, 73*, 630–637.
3. Thies-Flechtner, K., Müller-Oerlinghausen, B., Seibert, W., Walther, A., & Greil, W. (1996). Effect of prophylactic treatment on suicide risk in patients with major affective disorders: Data from a randomized prospective trial. *Pharmacopsychiatry, 29*(3), 103–107.
4. Ahrens, B., & Müller-Oerlinghausen, B. (2001). Does lithium exert an independent antisuicidal effect? *Pharmacopsychiatry, 34*(4), 132–136.
5. Cipriani, A., Hawton, K., Stockton, & Geddes, J. R. (2013). Lithium in the prevention of suicide in mood disorders: Updated systematic review and meta-analysis. *British Journal of Medicine, 346*, f3646.
6. Oquendo, M. A., Galfalvy, H. C., Currier, D., Grunebaum, M. F., Sher, L., Sullivan, G. M., . . . Mann, J. J. (2011). Treatment of suicide attempters with bipolar disorder: A randomized clinical trial comparing lithium and valproate in the prevention of suicidal behavior. *American Journal of Psychiatry, 168*(10), 1050–1056.
7. Jacobs, D. G., Baldessarini, R. J., Conwell, Y., Fawcett, J. A., Horton, L., Meltzer, H., . . . Simon, R. I. (2010). *Assessment and treatment of patients with suicidal behaviors.* APA Practice Guideline. Washington, DC: American Psychiatric Association.

6

The Long-Term Natural History of Bipolar I Disorder

ZACHARY ENGLER AND ROBERT BEECH

> Although BP-I is traditionally described in terms of episodes of major depressive episodes and mania, we found that subthreshold, minor depressive/dysthymic, and hypomanic symptoms were the modal expressions of BP-I during its prospective course.
>
> —JUDD ET AL.[1]

Research Question: What is the natural progression of symptoms in patients with bipolar I disorder (BD-I)? Overall, how long do people with BD-I spend with depressive, manic, or other affective symptoms versus periods of euthymia?

Funding: National Institute of Mental Health and Roehr Fund of the University of California, San Diego

Year Study Began: 1978

Year Study Published: 2002

Study Location: Five academic centers in the United States: University of California–San Diego, Columbia University, Brown University, Cornell University, and Washington University.

Who Was Studied: Patients with a history of depressive as well as manic episodes were selected from the National Institute of Mental Health Collaborative Depression Study (NIMH-CDS). These individuals were recruited to the NIMH-CDS during inpatient psychiatric admission, were white, spoke English, had an IQ >70, and had no evidence of organic mental disorder or terminal medical illness.

Who Was Excluded: People with a diagnosis of schizophrenia or schizoaffective disorder as well as those who showed evidence of organic neurological disorder or terminal medical illness. Patients with bipolar II disorder were not included in this study.

How Many Patients: 146

Study Overview: See Figure 6.1 for a summary of the study design.

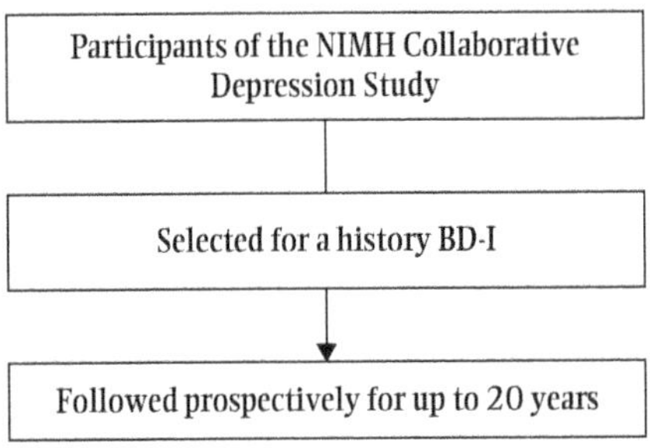

Figure 6.1 Summary of Study Design
NOTES: NIMH = National Institute of Mental Health. BD-I = bipolar I disorder.

Study Intervention: People who met criteria were identified from the participants in the NIMH-CDS. Of those, nine patients dropped out within two years and two patients had poor quality data and thus were eliminated.

The remaining 146 people were followed up every six months for the first five years and then yearly for up to a total of 20 years using the Longitudinal Interval Follow-up Evaluation (LIFE). This evaluation used "chronological memory prompts" to obtain information on weekly changes in mood symptoms and severity. Researchers used the information acquired during the interview along with a detailed review of the medical record to determine a final score.

The patient's subjective level of illness was rated on a weekly basis using the LIFE Psychiatric Status Rating (PSR) scale.[2] Interviewers assigned a rating regarding the accuracy of the participant's self-report based on their clinical impression, and those with a rating of "poor" or worse were not included in the analysis.

Based on the PSR score, affective conditions were assigned to level of severity. Diagnoses included major depression, mania, minor depression/dysthymia, hypomania, atypical depression (DSM-IV), adjustment disorder with depressed mood (DSM-III), and cyclothymic personality (Research Diagnostic Criteria).

Follow-Up: The study followed up with patients for up to 20 years. However, the mean follow-up was for 12.8 years due to participants dropping out.

Endpoints: Primary: weekly measure of affective symptom severity based on PSR, proportion of weeks spent at each level of symptom severity, and polarity (mania or depression). Secondary: chronicity, defined as proportion of weeks with symptoms reaching mania or depression, and proportion of weeks with any affective symptoms.

RESULTS

- Patients' symptoms status changed an average of six times per year.
- Patients' polarity changed on average of more than three times per year.
- Predictors of more chronic illness included longer intake episodes, having only depressive or cycling symptoms, and comorbid substance abuse disorder (Tables 6.1 and 6.2).

Table 6.1 Time Spent with Diagnoses as Part of Natural Course of BD-I Study

Outcome	**Total**	**Major Depression**	**Mania**	**Subsyndromal symptoms**	**Minor depression/ dysthymia/ hypomania**
% of weeks (SD)	47.3 (34)	8.9 (12.5)	2.3 (4.0)	14.8 (18.7)	20.2 (21.0)

NOTE: BD-I = bipolar I disorder.

Table 6.2 Time Spent with Symptoms as Part of Natural Course of BD-I Study

Outcome	Pure depressive symptoms	Pure mania symptoms	Cycling/mixed affective symptoms
% of weeks (SD)	31.9 (29.9)	9.3 (15.6)	5.9 (14.2)

NOTE: BD-I = bipolar I disorder.

Criticisms and Limitations: Given the homogeneity of the participants, the generalizability of the findings are limited.

In addition, since the study utilized patients' subjective memory of their mood symptoms at six month intervals, recall bias may have influenced the results.

Other Relevant Studies and Information:

- Other studies found similar phenomenology of chronic illness that was weighted toward depression for those with bipolar II disorder,[3] and chronic dysthymia in those with major depressive disorder.[4]
- Other research on bipolar disorder, including the BALANCE study (see Chapter 3), suggests that the likelihood of an affective episode (mania or depression) relapse and self-harm decreases with medication maintenance therapy,[5,6,7] especially with lithium.[8]
- The STEP-BD study[9] (see Chapter 4) and others[10] provide further evidence for high relapse rates in BD-I.

Summary and Implications: This important observational, naturalistic study of BD-I followed a cohort of subjects from the NIMH-CDS over a course of 20 years. The data show that people with BD-I go through a spectrum of affective symptoms from manic to depressive and affective states in between. Levels of severity fluctuate over time even within the same patient. The illness is predominated by depressive and subsyndromal manic and depressive states, and patients oscillate between manic and depressive states multiple times throughout the year on average.

CLINICAL CASE: NATURAL COURSE OF BD-I

Case History

A 38-year-old man with BD-I—currently depressed—was admitted to the inpatient psychiatric unit with symptoms of severe depression. He has a history of depression since age 16 and had a manic episode earlier this year when he gambled away money that he was supposed to use toward a down payment on his family's new house. The patient's family is in consultation with the psychiatrist and asks what they can expect over the course of his life. Using data from this naturalistic follow-up study of BD-I, how should the psychiatrist psychoeducate the patient and family?

Suggested Answer

The naturalistic follow-up study of the NIMH-CDS provides evidence that patients with bipolar disorder, on average, have chronic affective symptoms about half of their lives. These symptoms can range from depression to mania, though most of the time do not meet criteria for a discrete manic or depressive episode.

The patient in the vignette has a history of BD-I. Although we as psychiatrists cannot predict his disease progression, it is often important to provide psychoeducation to patients and families using data from naturalistic studies such as this. On average, people with BD-I lead a life with chronic affective symptoms. More often, they will be depressed rather than manic, though polarity can switch several times per year.

References

1. Judd, L. L, Akiskal, H. S., Schettler, P. J., Endicott, J., Maser, J., Solomon, D. A., . . . Keller, M. B. (2002). *Archives of General Psychiatry, 59*(6), 530–537.
2. Judd, L. L., Akiskal, H. S., Schettler, P. J., Coryell, W., Endicott, J., Maser, J. D., . . . Keller, M. B. (2003). A prospective investigation of the natural history of the long-term weekly symptomatic status of bipolar II disorder. *Archives of General Psychiatry, 60*(3), 261–269.
3. Winokur, G., Coryell, W., Keller, M., Endicott, J., & Akiskal, H. (1993). A prospective follow-up of patients with bipolar and primary unipolar affective disorder. *Archives of General Psychiatry, 50*(6), 457–465.
4. Judd, L. L., Akiskal, H. S., Maser, J. D., Zeller, P. J., Endicott, J., Coryell, W., . . . Rice, J. A. (1998). A prospective 12-year study of subsyndromal and syndromal depressive symptoms in unipolar major depressive disorders. *Archives of General Psychiatry, 55*(8), 694–700.
5. Fountoulakis, K. N., Kasper, S., Andreassen, O., Blier, P., Okasha, A., Severus, E., . . . Vieta, E. (2012). Efficacy of pharmacotherapy in bipolar disorder: A report by the WPA section on pharmacopsychiatry. *European Archives of Psychiatry and Clinical Neuroscience, 262*(Suppl 1), 1–48.
6. Geddes, J. R., Goodwin, G. M., Rendell, J., Azorin, J. M., Cipriani, A., Ostacher, M. J., . . . Juszczak, E. (2010). Lithium plus valproate combination therapy versus monotherapy for relapse prevention in bipolar I disorder (BALANCE): A randomised open-label trial. *Lancet, 375*, 385–395.

7. Hayes, J. F., Pitman, A., Marston, L., Walters, K., Geddes, J. R., King, M., & Osborn, D. P. (2016). Self-harm, unintentional injury, and suicide in bipolar disorder during maintenance Mood Stabilizer Treatment: A UK population-based electronic health records study. *JAMA Psychiatry, 73*, 630–637
8. Geddes, J. R., Burgess, S., Hawton, K., Jamison, K., & Goodwin, G. M. (2004). Long-term lithium therapy for bipolar disorder: Systematic review and meta-analysis of randomized controlled trials. *American Journal of Psychiatry, 161*, 217–222.
9. Perlis, R. H., Ostacher, M. J., Patel, J. K., Marangell, L. B., Zhang, H., Wisniewski, S. R., . . . Reilly-Harrington, N. A. (2006). Predictors of recurrence in bipolar disorder: Primary outcomes from the Systematic Treatment Enhancement Program for Bipolar Disorder (STEP-BD). *American Journal of Psychiatry, 163*(2), 217–224.
10. Gitlin, M. J., Swendsen, J., Heller, T. L., & Hammen, C. (1995). Relapse and impairment in bipolar disorder. *American Journal of Psychiatry, 152*(11), 1635–1640.

SECTION 3

Child and Adolescent Disorders

7

The Multimodal Treatment Study of Children with Attention Deficit/Hyperactivity Disorder (MTA)

MICHAEL H. BLOCH

> For ADHD symptoms, our carefully crafted medication management was superior to behavioral treatment and to routine community care.
>
> —The MTA Cooperative Group[1]

Research Question: What is the most effective long-term management strategy in children with attention-deficit/hyperactivity disorder (ADHD): (a) medication management; (b) behavioral treatment; (c) a combination of medication management and behavioral treatment; or (d) routine community care?[1]

Funding: The National Institute of Mental Health and the Department of Education

Year Study Began: 1992

Year Study Published: 1999

Study Location: Eight clinical research sites in the United States and Canada

Who Was Studied: Children between the ages of 7 and 9.9 years meeting DSM-IV criteria for ADHD combined type (the most common type of ADHD, in which children have symptoms of both hyperactivity and inattention). The diagnosis of ADHD was confirmed by study researchers based on parental reports and, for borderline cases, teacher reports. Children were recruited from mental health facilities, pediatricians, advertisements, and school notices.

Who Was Excluded: Children who could not fully participate in assessments and/or treatments.

How Many Participants: 579

Study Overview: See Figure 7.1 for a summary of the study design.

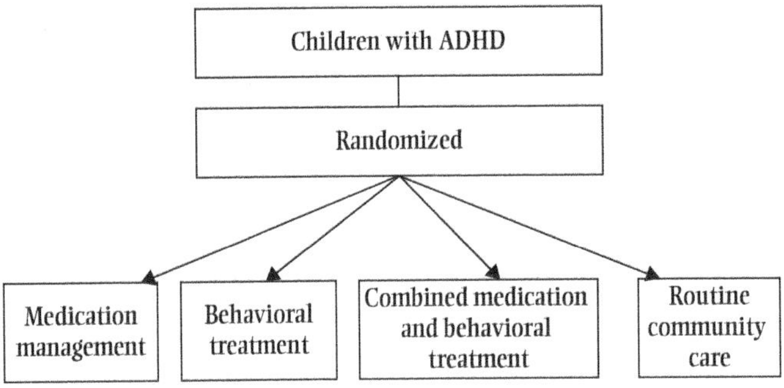

Figure 7.1 Summary of Study Design
NOTE: ADHD = attention deficit/hyperactivity disorder.

Study Intervention:

Arm 1: Medication management—Children in this group first received 28 days of methylphenidate at blinded random daily doses to determine the appropriate dose (based on parent and teacher ratings). Children who did not respond adequately were given alternative medications such as dextroamphetamine. Subsequently, children met monthly with a pharmacotherapist who adjusted the medications using a standardized protocol based on input from parents and teachers.

Arm 2: Behavioral treatment—Parents and children in this group participated in "parent training, child-focused treatment, and a school-based intervention." The parent training consisted of 27 group and eight individual sessions per family led by a doctoral-level psychotherapist. The sessions initially occurred weekly but were tapered over time. The child-focused treatment consisted of an eight-week full-time summer program that promoted the development of social skills and appropriate classroom behavior and involved group activities. The school-based intervention involved 10 to 16 individual consultation sessions with each teacher conducted by the same psychotherapist. Teachers were taught how to promote appropriate behavior in the classroom. In addition, children were assisted daily by a classroom aide working under the psychologist's supervision for 12 weeks.

Arm 3: Combined treatment—Parents and children in this group received both medication management and behavioral treatment. Information was "regularly shared" between the counselors and the pharmacotherapists so that medication changes and behavioral treatment interventions could be coordinated.

Arm 4: Community care—Children in this group were referred to community providers and treated according to routine standards. The vast majority of children in this group received psychostimulant treatment.

Follow-Up: 14 months

Endpoints: The authors assessed six major outcome domains:

- ADHD symptoms based on parent and teacher ratings on a standardized instrument called SNAP,[2] and
- Five other outcome domains including:
  - Oppositional/aggressive symptoms based on parent and teacher SNAP ratings
  - Social skills based on parent and teacher ratings on the standardized Social Skills Rating System (SSRS)[3]
  - Internalizing symptoms (anxiety and depression) based on parent and teacher ratings on the SSRS as well as children's own ratings on the Multidimensional Anxiety Scale for Children[4]
  - Parent–child relations based on a parent–child relationship questionnaire
  - Academic achievement based on reading, math, and spelling scores on the Wechsler Individual Achievement Test[5]

RESULTS

- At the end of the study period, 87% of children in the medication management and combined treatment groups were receiving medications, and of these children 84% were receiving methylphenidate while 12% were receiving dextroamphetamine.
- 49.8% of children receiving medications experienced mild side effects, 11.4% experienced moderate side effects, and 2.9% experienced severe side effects (based on parental report).

Table 7.1 SUMMARY OF MTA'S KEY FINDINGS

Treatment Comparison	Outcome
Medication management vs. behavioral treatment	• Medication management was superior with respect to parent and teacher ratings of inattention and teacher ratings of hyperactivity/impulsivity.
Combined treatment vs. medication management	• There were no significant differences for any of the primary outcome domains. In secondary analyses of global outcomes, however, combined treatment offered slight advantages over medication management alone, particularly among children with complex presentations of ADHD. • Children in the combined treatment group also required lower average daily medication doses than those in the medication management group (31.2 mg vs. 37.7 mg).
Combined treatment vs. behavioral treatment	• Combined treatment was superior with respect to parent and teacher ratings of inattention and parent ratings of hyperactivity/impulsivity, parent ratings of oppositional/aggressive symptoms, and reading scores.
Community care vs. other study treatments	• Medication management and combined treatment were generally superior to community care for ADHD symptoms and for some of the other outcome domains. Although children generally received the same medication (methylphenidate) in both the medication management and community care arms. The medication management arm was thought to be more effective because children received a higher dose of the methylphenidate (>50% higher) in the medication management group suggesting that community physicians are under dosing stimulants in clinical practice. • Behavioral treatment and community care were similar for ADHD symptoms, however behavioral treatment was superior to community care for parent–child relations.

- 67.4% of children in the community care group received medications at some point during the study.
- ADHD symptoms improved considerably among children in all four arms during the study period; however, as noted in the following discussion, children receiving medication management and combined treatment had better outcomes than children receiving community treatment or the behavioral treatment (Table 7.1).

Criticisms and Limitations: The MTA was instrumental in demonstrating the superiority of medications (psychostimulants) compared to behavioral treatments for the core symptoms of ADHD. However, concomitant behavioral treatments may be beneficial when children have additional comorbidities (especially anxiety and oppositional defiant disorder symptoms). The medication management and behavioral treatment strategies used in this trial were time-intensive and might not be practical in some real-world settings.

Other Relevant Studies and Information: After the MTA trial was completed, study children returned to their usual community care team for ongoing treatment. The cohort has been followed for well over a decade into adulthood and continues to inform us about the long-term clinical course of ADHD.

- These long-term outcome studies from the MTA cohort suggest that long-term psychostimulant use is associated with modest height reduction (1 cm at adulthood).[6]
  - These studies also suggest that while the hyperactivity/impulsivity symptoms of ADHD may improve during adolescence and early adulthood, the inattention symptoms often persist.[7]
  - Despite over half of children experiencing impairment from their ADHD symptoms in adulthood, fewer than 10% remained on medication.[7]
- Other studies have also demonstrated the benefits of stimulant medications in children with ADHD.[8,9,10]
- Guidelines from the American Academy of Pediatrics for children with ADHD recommend[11]:
  - medications and/or behavioral treatment for children <12 depending on family preference.
  - medications with or without behavioral therapy as first-line treatment for children 12 to 18 (behavioral therapy can be used instead if the child and family do not want medications).

Summary and Implications: For children with ADHD, carefully controlled medication management was superior to behavioral treatment and to routine community care during the 14-month study period. Children receiving combined medication and behavioral treatment had similar outcomes as those receiving medications alone; however, these children required lower medication doses to control their symptoms. Despite its limitations, the MTA trial is frequently cited as evidence that carefully controlled medications are superior to behavioral treatment for children with ADHD. Nevertheless, behavioral therapy may be an appropriate and efficacious therapy when the child and family prefer this approach.

CLINICAL CASE: MANAGEMENT OF ADHD

Case History

A 6-year-old boy is diagnosed with ADHD based on reports from his teachers and parents that he has a short attention span and is hyperactive, sometimes disrupting classroom activities. His school performance has been adequate; however, both his teachers and parents believe he would perform better if his attention span improved.

Based on the results of the MTA trial, should this boy be treated for his ADHD with medications, behavioral therapy, or both?

Suggested Answer

The MTA trial suggests that symptoms of ADHD are better controlled with medications than with behavioral therapy. If there is significant comorbid symptomatology like anxiety or oppositional defiant disorder symptoms than specific complementary therapies may be helpful for managing those symptoms.

References

1. The MTA Cooperative Group. (1999). A 14-month randomized clinical trial of treatment strategies for attention-deficit/hyperactivity disorder. *Archives of General Psychiatry, 56*(12), 1073–1086.
2. Swanson, J. M. (1992). *School-based assessments and interventions for ADD students.* Irvine, CA: KC Publications.
3. Gresham, F. M., & Elliott, S. N. *Social Skills Rating System: Automated System for Scoring and Interpreting Standardized Test* [computer program]. Version 1. Circle Pines, MN: American Guidance Systems, 1989.

4. March, J. S., Parker, J. D., Sullivan, K., Stallings, P., & Conners, C. K. (1997). The Multidimensional Anxiety Scale for Children (MASC): Factor structure, reliability, and validity. *Journal of the American Academy of Child and Adolescent Psychiatry, 36*(4), 554–565.
5. Psychological Corporation. (1992). *Wechsler Individual Achievement Test: Manual.* San Antonio, TX: Author.
6. Swanson, J. M., Arnold, L. E., Molina, B. S. G., Sibley, M. H., Hechtman, L. T., Hinshaw, S. P., . . . MTA Cooperative Group. (2017). Young adult outcomes in the follow-up of the multimodal treatment study of attention-deficit/hyperactivity disorder: Symptom persistence, source discrepancy, and height suppression. *Journal of Child Psychology and Psychiatry, 58*(6), 663–678.
7. Sibley, M. H., Swanson, J. M., Arnold, L. E., Hechtman, L. T., Owens, E. B., Stehli, A., . . . MTA Cooperative Group. (2017). Defining ADHD symptom persistence in adulthood: Optimizing sensitivity and specificity. *Journal of Child Psychology and Psychiatry, 58*(6), 655–662.
8. Schachter, H. M., Pham, B., King, J., Langford, S., & Moher, D. (2001). How efficacious and safe is short-acting methylphenidate for the treatment of attention-deficit disorder in children and adolescents? A meta-analysis. *Canadian Medical Association Journal, 165*(11), 1475–1488.
9. Biederman, J., Krishnan, S., Zhang, Y., McGough, J. J., & Findling, R. L. (2007). Efficacy and tolerability of lisdexamfetamine dimesylate (NRP-104) in children with attention-deficit/hyperactivity disorder: A phase III, multicenter, randomized, double-blind, forced-dose, parallel-group study. *Clinical Therapeutics, 29*(3), 450–463.
10. Wigal, S., Swanson, J., Feifel, D., Sangal, R. B. . . . Conners, C. K. (2004). A double-blind, placebo-controlled trial of dexmethylphenidate hydrochloride and d,l-threo-methylphenidate hydrochloride in children with attention-deficit/hyperactivity disorder. *Journal of the American Academy of Child and Adolescent Psychiatry, 43*(11), 1406–1414.
11. Subcommittee on Attention-Deficit/Hyperactivity Disorder, Steering Committee on Quality Improvement and Management. (2011). ADHD: Clinical practice guideline for the diagnosis, evaluation, and treatment of attention-deficit/hyperactivity disorder in children and adolescents. *Pediatrics, 128*(5), 1007.

8

Adolescents with SSRI-Resistant Depression

The TORDIA Trial

AMALIA LONDONO TOBON AND HANNA E. STEVENS

> For adolescents with depression not responding to an adequate initial treatment with an SSRI, the combination of cognitive behavioral therapy and a switch to another antidepressant resulted in a higher rate of clinical response than did a medication switch alone . . . A switch to another SSRI was just as efficacious as a switch to venlafaxine and resulted in fewer adverse effects.
>
> —THE TORDIA INVESTIGATORS[1]

Research Question: Should adolescents with selective serotonin reuptake inhibitor (SSRI) resistant depression be switched to another SSRI or to venlafaxine with or without cognitive behavioral therapy (CBT)?

Funding: National Institute of Mental Health

Year Study Began: 2000

Year Study Published: 2008

Study Location: Six academic and community clinics in the United States

Who Was Studied: 12 to 18 year old adolescents in treatment for major depressive disorder based on DSM-IV criteria, Children's Depression Rating Scale–Revised (CDRS-R) score ≥40, and Clinical Global Impressions-Severity (CGI-S) subscale ≥4 (moderate severity or worse). Participants had SSRI-resistant depression, defined as persistent depression after a dose of fluoxetine 40 mg or an equivalent SSRI for eight weeks or more.

Who Was Excluded: Patients with two or more SSRI trials or history of non-response to venlafaxine or CBT. Also excluded were those currently receiving CBT or diagnosed with bipolar disorder, psychosis, pervasive developmental disorders, eating disorder, substance use disorders, or hypertension. Pregnant, breastfeeding, and other females having unprotected sex were excluded.

How Many Participants: 334

Study Overview: See Figure 8.1 for a summary of the study design.

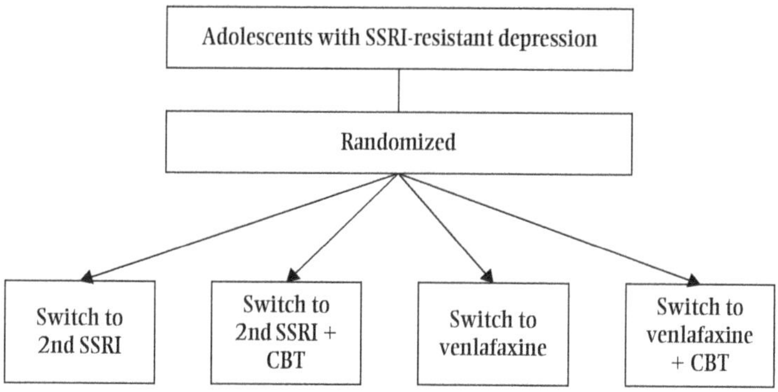

Figure 8.1 Summary of Study Design
NOTES: SSRI = selective serotonin reuptake inhibitor. CBT = cognitive behavioral therapy.

Study Interventions: First, the current SSRI was tapered over two weeks (if fluoxetine, discontinuation was immediate). Then, patients were randomized to one of four interventions: (a) switch to another SSRI; (b) switch to venlafaxine; (c) switch to another SSRI + CBT; or (d) switch to venlafaxine + CBT. SSRIs were started at 10 mg per day of fluoxetine or equivalent for one week, and were increased to 20 mg for weeks two to six. Participants were started on low doses of SSRIs or venlafaxine, which were titrated as needed per protocol. The CBT groups received twelve weekly sessions (60–90 minutes) by at least a master's degree level therapist, covering cognitive restructuring, behavior activation, emotion regulation, social skills, problem solving, and parent–child communication sessions. Assessments were made at baseline, six weeks, and twelve weeks.

Follow-Up: Twelve weeks

Endpoints: Primary outcomes: (1) "adequate clinical response" defined as (a) Clinical Global Impressions–Improvement (CGI-I) ≤2; (b) CDRS-R score decrease by at least 50%; (c) endpoint CDRS-R <40; and (2) changes in CDRS-R scores. Secondary outcomes: Beck Depression Inventory, the Suicide Ideation Questionnaire-Jr, and Children's Global Adjustment Scale. Other outcomes included side effects to medications.

RESULTS

- CBT plus a switch to either medication regimen showed a higher response rate than a medication switch alone (Table 8.1).
- There was no difference in response rate between venlafaxine and a second SSRI.
- There were no differential treatment effects on CDRS-R scores with switch to either medication and/or CBT. In addition, change in self-ratings of depressive symptoms, suicidal ideation, or the rate of harm-related or any other adverse events all showed no significant differences between groups.

Table 8.1 Summary of TORDIA's Key Findings

Outcome	**Switch to 2nd SSRI**	**Switch to Venlafaxine**	**P value**	**No CBT**	**CBT**	**P value**
Response Rate	47%	48.2%	0.83	40.5%	54.8%	0.009
CGI-I score ≤2	51.2%	55.4%	0.44	47.6%	59%	0.04
Change in CDRS-R ≥50%	56%	51.8%	0.45	47%	60.8%	0.01
Baseline CDRS-R Score (SD)	59.8 (10.6)	57.8 (10.1)	–	58.4 (9.7)	59.2 (11.0)	–
Week 12 CDRS-R Score (SD)	37.9 (13.7)	37.0 (13.1)	–	38.1 (12.9)	36.9 (13.9)	–

NOTES: TORDIA = Treatment of Resistant Depression in Adolescents. SSRI = selective serotonin reuptake inhibitor. CBT = cognitive behavioral therapy. CGI-I = Clinical Global Impressions–Improvement. CDRS-R = Children's Depression Rating Scale–Revised.

- There was a greater increase in medically related side effects in venlafaxine than SSRI treatment including increases in diastolic blood pressure and pulse and more frequent occurrence of skin problems.

Criticisms and Limitations: The patient population in this trial consisted primarily of White females with a mean age of 16 years, limiting the generalizability. Combined treatment participants had greater contact and attention from research staff, which was not accounted for in analyses. There was no CBT-only arm, preventing a comparison of CBT in isolation with continued pharmacotherapy. Lastly, blinding was compromised in some of the patients receiving CBT.

Other Relevant Studies and Information:

- Few studies of treatment-resistant depression exist in adolescents.
- Other studies in depressed adolescents comparing cognitive, family, and supportive psychotherapies have demonstrated that CBT is the most efficacious of these options.[2]
- The American Academy of Child and Adolescent Psychiatry practice parameters for the treatment of children and adolescents with depression suggest that failure of SSRI response be followed by CBT and a switch to a second SSRI.[3]

Summary and Implications: Adolescent depression is a common, recurring, impairing condition, and more than 40% of adolescent patients do not respond to a first antidepressant trial.[4] Findings from this trial suggest that among patients not responsive to initial first-line therapy, combination treatment with CBT along with a different antidepressant results in a higher rate of clinical response than a medication switch alone. In this study, patients who were switched to SSRIs had fewer adverse effects compared to those switched to venlafaxine.

CLINICAL CASE: SSRI-RESISTANT DEPRESSION

Case History

A 15-year-old girl presents has ongoing depressive symptoms despite citalopram 40 mg treatment for the past eight weeks. She continues to have increased sleep, anhedonia, and decreased school attendance. Based on the Treatment of Resistant Depression in Adolescents (TORDIA) study, how should this patient be treated?

Suggested Answer

This patient is typical of those included in the TORDIA trial, as she has SSRI-resistant depression. Clinical guidelines and the TORDIA trial suggest that in such patients, combination treatment of another SSRI or venlafaxine and CBT has a superior response rate to a medication switch alone. Prior to making a change, the clinician should carefully assess whether the patient is being adherent with treatment, as lower adherence, determined by pill-count remainder, was related to a lower response rate.[5]

The TORDIA trial did not address augmenting treatment with CBT, which could be an option before switching medication. In TORDIA, SSRIs showed better tolerability than venlafaxine. Other treatment strategies such as augmentation with a second antidepressant or other medication, strategies that are commonly used in adults, were not studied in this trial and had not been studied in youth at the time of this trial. Therapies other than CBT were also not studied in TORDIA. Therefore, appropriate clinical judgment may be useful to determine whether an alternative therapy such as family or supportive therapy may be helpful.

References

1. Brent, D., Emslie, G., Clarke, G., Wagner, K. D., Asarnow, J. R., Keller, M., . . . Birmaher, B. (2008). Switching to another SSRI or to venlafaxine with or without cognitive behavioral therapy for adolescents with SSRI-resistant depression: The TORDIA randomized controlled trial. *JAMA, 299*(8), 901–913.
2. Brent, D. A., Holder, D., Kolko, D., Birmaher, B., Baugher, M., Roth, C., . . . Johnson, B. A. (1997). A clinical psychotherapy trial for adolescent depression comparing cognitive, family, and supportive therapy. *Archives of General Psychiatry, 54*(9), 877–885.
3. Birmaher, B., Brent, D., & AACAP Work Group on Quality Issues. (2007). Practice parameter for the assessment and treatment of children and adolescents with depressive disorders. *Journal of the American Academy of Child & Adolescent Psychiatry, 46*(11), 1503–1526.
4. Brent, D., Emslie, G., Clarke, G., Wagner, K. D., Asarnow, J. R., Keller, M., . . . Birmaher, B. (2008). Switching to another SSRI or to venlafaxine with or without cognitive behavioral therapy for adolescents with SSRI-resistant depression: The TORDIA randomized controlled trial. *JAMA, 299*(8), 901–913.
5. Woldu, H., Porta, G., Goldstein, T., Sakolsky, D., Perel, J., Emslie, G., . . . Brent, D. (2011). Pharmacokinetically and clinician-determined adherence to an antidepressant regimen and clinical outcome in the TORDIA trial. *Journal of the American Academy of Child & Adolescent Psychiatry 50*(5), 490–498.

9

Treatment of Early-Onset Schizophrenia Spectrum Disorders (TEOSS) Study

J. COREY WILLIAMS AND HANNA E. STEVENS

> The results of this study do not support the widely held assumption that risperidone and olanzapine . . . are superior to an advantageous first-generation antipsychotic for the treatment of early-onset schizophrenia and schizoaffective disorder.
>
> —TEOSS Investigators[1]

Research Question: Are second generation antipsychotics (SGA) superior to first generation antipsychotics (FGA) in the treatment of early-onset schizophrenia spectrum disorders?

Funding: National Institute of Mental Health

Year Study Began: 2002

Year Study Published: 2008

Study Locations: Four academic centers in the United States; outpatient and inpatient settings

Who Was Studied: Children and adolescents 8 to 19 years old with a diagnosis of schizophrenia, schizoaffective disorder, or schizophreniform disorder and current positive psychotic symptoms of at least moderate intensity.

Who Was Excluded: Patients with a history of mental retardation, experiencing a major depressive episode, or with active substance abuse were excluded. Also, patients who did not tolerate any study medication in the past, those with a prior trial of a study medication, and those at imminent risk of harming themselves were excluded.

How Many Participants: 116

Study Overview: See Figure 9.1 for a summary of the study design.

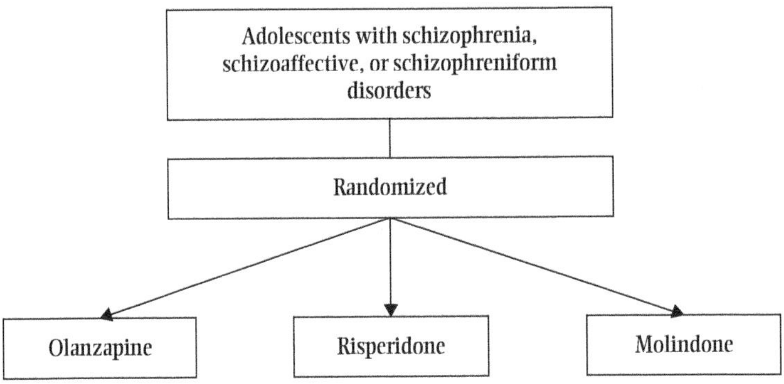

Figure 9.1 Summary of Study Design

Study Intervention: Eligible subjects were randomly assigned to receive either molindone (10–140 mg), olanzapine (2.5–20 mg), or risperidone (0.5–6 mg) treatment for eight weeks. The protocol permitted clinician judgment for dose adjustments; however, typically patients were started on the lowest dose and increased to the middle range within 10 to 14 days. Patients receiving molindone received 1 mg daily of benztropine prophylactically, and others received placebo.

Follow-Up: Eight weeks

Endpoints: The primary outcomes: Rate of "response," which was defined as patients with a Clinical Global Impression score of 1 or 2 at the conclusion of the study, who experienced a more than 20% decrease in the Positive and Negative Syndrome Scale (PANSS), and who tolerated eight weeks of treatment;

change from baseline in scores on the PANSS, Brief Psychiatric Rating Scale for Children (BPRS-C), and the Child and Adolescent Functional Assessment Scale (CAFAS). Secondary outcomes: neurological side effects, changes in weight and stature, vital signs, laboratory analyses (i.e., prolactin, lipids, liver enzymes, insulin), electrocardiogram analyses, and adverse events.

RESULTS

- In an intent-to-treat analysis, the rate of response did not differ between groups (Table 9.1).
- All symptom measures (including PANSS, BPRS-C, and CAFAS) showed statistically significant improvements (average declines of 21%–47%) across treatment groups; however, there was no significant between-group differences on any primary endpoints.
- During the first two weeks of treatment, symptom reductions were the most robust with no between-group differences.
- There were no differences in the time to treatment discontinuation due to adverse events or in lack of effectiveness between groups.
- Prolactin levels and constipation were significantly increased in the risperidone group compared to other groups.

Table 9.1 Summary of TEOSS's Key Findings

Outcome	Molindone	Olanzapine	Risperidone	P value
Response rate (CGI was 1 or 2, PANSS >20% decrease, completed 8 weeks of treatment)	50% ± 16	34% ± 16	46% ± 16	Not significant
PANSS decrease (%)	27.0 ± 5.6 (27%)	26.6 ± 6.3 (27%)	23.7 ± 7.3 (23%)	Not significant
BPRS-C decrease (%)	16.3 ± 3.3 (39%)	17.3 ± 4 (41%)	15.4 ± 6.2 (34%)	Not significant
CAFAS decrease (%)	29.3 ± 13.6 (32%)	40.0 ± 18.9 (40%)	47.5 ± 16.2 (47%)	Not significant

NOTES: TEOSS = Treatment of Early-Onset Schizophrenia Spectrum Disorders study. CGI = Clinical Global Impressions scale. PANSS = Positive and Negative Syndrome Scale. BPRS-C = Brief Psychiatric Rating Scale for Children. CAFAS = Child and Adolescent Functional Assessment Scale.

- Over the eight-week period, the olanzapine group showed the highest increase in mean weight and body mass index followed by the risperidone group. The molindone did not show significant changes in body mass index.
- Measures of metabolic syndrome and liver function tests were significantly more elevated in the olanzapine group.
- Participants in the molindone group reported significantly higher rates of drug-induced akathisia despite use of propranolol for that indication in all groups.

Criticisms and Limitations: The study was powered for 168 patients but only enrolled 116, which was sufficient only to detect large differences across the three treatments and limited the ability to identify predictors of response or adverse effects.

There was a fairly heterogeneous patient population including youth across a broad age range with both first-episode and chronic early-onset schizophrenia, youth with schizoaffective disorder, treatment-naïve patients, and antipsychotic-exposed individuals as well as some individuals taking concomitant antidepressant/mood stabilizers. Thus, it is possible that a more in-depth analysis might have identified differences in treatment efficacy in certain subgroups.

Finally, because pharmacotherapy is the standard of care for patients with schizophrenia-spectrum disorders, the study did not have a placebo arm for comparison.

Other Relevant Studies and Information:

- Other studies comparing outcomes among young people with thought disorders receiving FGAs versus SGAs have come to similar conclusions as this one.[2,3]
- The American Academy of Child and Adolescent Psychiatry (AACAP) guidelines recommend FGA as initial therapy for patients with schizophrenia-spectrum disorders, while acknowledging that SGAs are typically the treatment of choice. The guidelines recognize the choice of a particular agent should be based on FDA approval status, side effects, patient and family preferences, clinician familiarity, and cost.[4]

Summary and Implications: This study failed to demonstrate a benefit of the SGAs olanzapine and risperidone versus the FGA molindone in the treatment of children and adolescents with early-onset schizophrenia and schizoaffective disorder. While SGAs are used more commonly as initial therapy for patients with early-onset schizophrenia and schizoaffective disorder, FGAs appear to be similarly efficacious. The choice of antipsychotic in young people should be made on the basis of side effects, preferences, and cost.

CLINICAL CASE: FIRST-GENERATION VERSUS SECOND-GENERATION ANTIPSYCHOTICS IN THE TREATMENT OF EARLY ONSET SCHIZOPHRENIA NAD SCHIZOAFFECTIVE DISORDER

Case History

An 18-year-old African American woman with a past psychiatric history significant for childhood onset schizophrenia (diagnosed at age 13) and multiple inpatient psychiatric hospitalizations for thought disorganization now presenting with worsening visual hallucinations of an animal running around her room and seeing "spirits leave her body." She was trialed on a SGA (olanzapine) but experienced significant sedation and weight gain within two weeks.

Based on the results of the TEOSS trial, how should this patient be treated?

Suggested Answer

The TEOSS trial showed that FGAs may be at least as effective as antipsychotic medication in management of early onset schizophrenia. The medication selection ought to be based on side-effect profile and tolerability rather than efficacy. Less weight gain in particular can be an advantage of using a FGA in some cases. AACAP guidelines support the use of FGAs to treat early onset thought disorders.

The patient in this vignette is typical of patients included in TEOSS. In a young female patient who may need to be on antipsychotic treatment for many years, the choice of olanzapine and risperidone may be suboptimal given the risk of metabolic syndrome and hyperprolactinemia, respectively. Thus, she could reasonably be treated with a FGA such as haloperidol, perphenzine or fluphenazine and be monitored closely for side effects. To reduce the acute risk of extrapyramidal symptoms, it may be useful to add an anticholinergic medication such as benztropine.

References

1. Sikich, L., Frazier, J. A., McClellan, J., Findling, R. L., Vitiello, B., Ritz, L., . . . Lieberman, J. A. (2008). Double-blind comparison of first- and second-generation antipsychotics in early-onsetschizophrenia and schizo-affective disorder: findings from the treatment of early-onsetschizophrenia spectrum disorders (TEOSS) study. *American Journal of Psychiatry, 165*(11), 1420–1431.
2. Sikich, L., Hamer, R. M., Bashford, R. A., Sheitman, B. B., & Lieberman, J. A. (2004). A pilot study of risperidone, olanzapine, and haloperidol in psychotic youth: A double-blind, randomized, 8-week trial. *Neuropsychopharmacology, 29*(1), 133–145.
3. Kumra, S., Frazier, J. A., Jacobsen, L. K., McKenna, K., Gordon, C. T., Lenane, M. C., & Rapoport, J. L. (1996). Childhood-onset schizophrenia: A double-blind clozapine-haloperidol comparison. *Archives of General Psychiatry, 53*(12), 1090–1097.
4. McClellan, J., & Stock, S. (2013). Practice parameter for the assessment and treatment of children and adolescents with schizophrenia. *Journal of the American Academy of Child and Adolescent Psychiatry, 52*(9), 976–990.

10

Cognitive Behavioral Therapy, Sertraline, or a Combination in Childhood Anxiety

CAMS

DAVID SAUNDERS, ANDRES MARTIN, AND JEROME H. TAYLOR

> Both cognitive behavioral therapy and sertraline reduced the severity of anxiety in children with anxiety disorders; a combination of the two therapies had a superior response rate.
>
> —Walkup et al.[1]

Research Question: Is sertraline in combination with cognitive behavioral therapy (CBT) more effective than monotherapy with either treatment alone in children with anxiety disorders? Also, how do these treatments compare with placebo therapy?

Funding: National Institute of Mental Health

Year Study Began: 2002

Year Study Published: 2008

Study Location: Six sites in the United States

Who Was Studied: Children between 7 and 17 years of age with generalized anxiety disorder, separation anxiety disorder, or social phobia (also known as social anxiety disorder).

Who Was Excluded: Children with an IQ less than 80, an unstable medical condition, or school refusal due to anxiety; nonresponders to two adequate trials of selective serotonin reuptake inhibitors (SSRI) or an adequate trial of CBT; patients taking medication for comorbid major depressive, bipolar, psychotic or pervasive development disorders; and pregnant or sexually active girls not using birth control.

How Many Participants: 488

Study Overview: See Figure 10.1 for a summary of the study design.

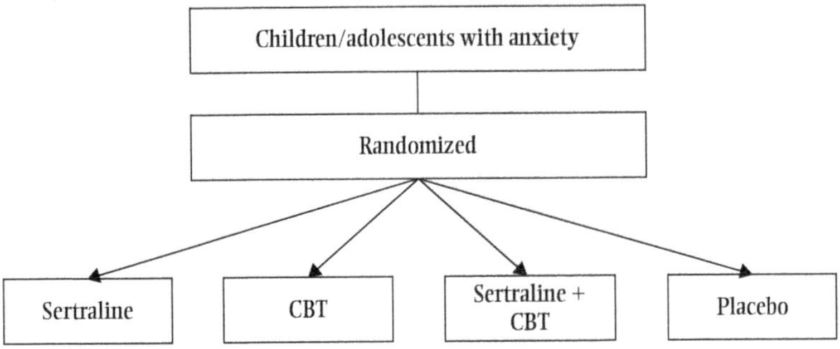

Figure 10.1 Summary of Study Design
NOTE: CBT = cognitive behavioral therapy.

Study Intervention: Patients randomized to receive CBT attended fourteen 60-minute sessions. CBT was based on a modified version of the Coping Cat program,[2] a cognitive-behavioral intervention composed of psychoeducation, exposure tasks, and relaxation techniques. Parents attended weekly check-ins and two parent-only sessions. Therapists were certified in the Coping Cat protocol and received regular supervision.

Patients randomized to receive pharmacotherapy attended eight 30- to 60-minute clinic visits by psychiatrists and nurse practitioners. The sessions included a review of the subjects' anxiety, response to treatment, and adverse events. Sertraline and placebo were titrated up from 25 mg per day at week 1 to 200 mg per day by week 8, based on response and side effects.

Follow-Up: Weeks 4, 8, and 12 after initiation of treatment

Endpoints: Clinical Global Impression-Improvement (CGI-I) scale and the Pediatric Anxiety Rating Scale. Children's Global Assessment Scale was used to rate overall impairment. Assessments were completed by a blinded independent evaluator, who was not the child's clinician.

RESULTS

- Combination therapy was superior to either sertraline alone or cognitive therapy alone on all measures: CGI-I, Pediatric Anxiety Rating Scale, CGI-Severity scale, Children's Global Assessment Scale. Each active treatment was superior to placebo (see Table 10.1).

Table 10.1 Summary of CAMS's Key Findings

Outcome	Sertraline	CBT	Combo	Placebo	Comparisons
Response rate, %	54.9	59.7	80.7	23.7	
Number needed to treat (95% CI)	3.2	2.8	1.7	n/a	
OR vs. placebo	3.9	4.8	13.6		All three treatment groups reached significance
OR vs. sertraline			3.4		Combo but not CBT group reached significance
OR vs. CBT			2.8		Combo but not sertraline group reached significance

NOTES: CAMS = Child/Adolescent Anxiety Multimodal Study. CBT = cognitive behavioral therapy. OR = odds ratio.

- There was no significant difference between sertraline monotherapy and CBT monotherapy on any measures.
- The average number of patients who need to be treated to achieve a favorable response was 1.7 for combination therapy, 2.8 for CBT and 3.2 for sertraline.
- Favorable response (i.e., "much improved" or "very much improved" on the CGI-scale) rates at week 12 were 81% for children in combined treatment, 60% for CBT, 55% for sertraline, and 24% in placebo. Remission rates were 68% with combined treatment, 46% with sertraline, 46% with CBT, and 24% with placebo.[3]

- In youths with severe anxiety (Pediatric Anxiety Rating Scale ≥20, n = 220), combination treatment increased remission (relative risk [RR] 2.93, 95 CI [1.41, 3.91], p = 0.001), while CBT (RR 1.59, 95 CI [0.79, 3.19], p = 0.19) and sertraline (1.34, 95 CI [0.79, 3.19], p = 0.46) did not significantly increase remission relative to placebo.[4]
- The rates of suicidal and homicidal ideation did not significantly differ between the sertraline and placebo groups. There were no suicide or homicidal attempts in any treatment condition in the Child/Adolescent Anxiety Multimodal Study (CAMS; Table 10.1).

Critiques and Limitations: The generalizability of the findings is limited since the sample did not include the most socio-economically disadvantaged children and because the subjects were mostly younger children and those with comorbid attention-deficit/hyperactivity disorder and other anxiety disorders, but excluded children with major depression and bipolar and pervasive developmental disorders, limiting generalizability to these groups.

The observed advantage of combination therapy over CBT alone or sertraline alone could be attributed to additional contact time in the combination group or to expectancy effects on the part of both subjects and clinicians.

Other Relevant Studies and Information:

- Previous trials have shown efficacy from psychotherapy[5,6] and medications[7,8] as monotherapy or treatment of childhood anxiety disorders.
- Based on these data, the American Academy of Child and Adolescent Psychiatry recommends a combination of SSRIs and psychotherapy for the treatment of childhood anxiety disorders.[9]

Summary and Implications: CAMS provides evidence that CBT and sertraline are effective short-term treatments for anxiety disorders in children and adolescents, and their combination is superior to either intervention alone.

CLINICAL CASE: TREATMENT FOR PEDIATRIC ANXIETY DISORDERS

Case History

An eight-year-old boy is brought to your office by his parents because for the past two months, they have noticed that he has been following them around the house from room to room, refusing to bathe or sleep alone, and having nightmares about getting lost or his parents dying. He tells his parents that he does not like going to school because he is worried they may die and he will never see them again. When he makes it to school, he often complains of headaches, stomachaches or nausea, and frequently gets sent home; he does not have these symptoms on the weekends, when he spends most of his time with his parents. He is now struggling and falling behind his classmates. He has also been invited to multiple sleepover birthday parties but refused to go because he does not want to be apart from his parents.

Based on the results of CAMS, how should the patient be treated?

Suggested Answer

This boy's presentation suggests a diagnosis of separation anxiety disorder. The results from CAMS suggest that the use of sertraline and CBT in combination are more effective than either intervention alone in the treatment of children with anxiety disorders. Based on the results of this and other studies, we recommend using SSRI in combination with CBT for the treatment of childhood anxiety.

This anxious child would fit inclusion criteria for CAMS, and since his illness is affecting his school and social functioning, treatment with CBT and an SSRI like sertraline would be indicated. While treatment with sertraline alone or CBT alone would likely reduce his symptoms, combination therapy with both interventions is better than either alone.

References

1. Walkup, J. T., Albano, A. M., Piacentini, J. C., Birmaher, B. J. Compton, S. N., Sherrill, J., . . . Kendall, P. C. (2008). *New England Journal of Medicine*, 359(26), 2753–2766.
2. Kendall, P. C., & Hedtke, K. A. (2006). *Cognitive-behavioral therapy for anxious children: Therapist manual.* Ardmore, PA: Workbook.
3. Ginsburg, G. S., Kendall, P. C., Sakolsky, D., Compton, S. N., Piacentini, J., Albano, A. M., . . . Keeton, C. P. (2011). Remission after acute treatment in children and adolescents with anxiety disorders: findings from the CAMS. *Journal of Consulting and Clinical Psychology*, 79(6), 806–813.
4. Taylor, J. H., Lebowitz, E. R., Jakubovski, E., Coughlin, C. G., Silverman, W. K., & Bloch, M. H. (in press). Monotherapy insufficient in severe anxiety? Predictors and moderators in the Child/Adolescent Anxiety Multimodal Study (CAMS). *Journal of Clinical Child & Adolescent Psychology*. https://doi.org/10.1080/15374416.2017.1371028
5. Beidel, D. C., Turner, S. M., Sallee, F. R., Ammerman, R. T., Crosby, L. A., & Pathak, S. (2007). SET-C versus fluoxetine in the treatment of childhood social phobia. *Journal of the American Academy of Child and Adolescent Psychiatry*, 46(12), 1622–1632.

6. Manassis, K., Mendlowitz, S. L., Scapillato, D., Avery, D., Fiksenbaum, L., Freire, M., . . . Owens, M. (2002). Group and individual cognitive-behavioral therapy for childhood anxiety disorders: A randomized trial. *Journal of the American Academy of Child & Adolescent Psychiatry, 41*(12), 1423–1430.
7. Strawn, J.R., Welge, J.A., Wehry, A.M., Keeshin, B., & Rynn, M.A. (2015). Efficacy and tolerability of antidepressants in pediatric anxiety disorders: A systematic review and meta-analysis. *Depression and Anxiety*, 32(3), 149–157.
8. Birmaher, B., Axelson, D. A., Monk, K., Kalas, C., Clark, D. B., Ehmann, M., . . . Brent, D. A. (2003). Fluoxetine for the treatment of childhood anxiety disorders. *Journal of the American Academy of Child & Adolescent Psychiatry*, 42(4), 415–423.
9. Connolly, S. D., & Bernstein, G. A. (2007). Practice parameter for the assessment and treatment of children and adolescents with anxiety disorders. *Journal of the American Academy of Child & Adolescent Psychiatry*, 46(2), 267–283.

11

Predictors of Suicidal Events

The Treatment of Adolescent Suicide Attempters (TASA) Study

MICHAEL MAKSIMOWSKI AND ZHEALA QAYYUM

> Youths with depression and a history of a suicide attempt are at high risk for recurrent suicidal behavior. Important treatment targets include suicidal ideation, family cohesion, and sequelae of previous abuse.
>
> —The TASA Investigators[1]

Research Question: What are the predictors of suicidal events and attempts in adolescents with a history of suicide attempts and depression?

Funding: National Institute of Mental Health

Year Study Began: Unknown

Year Study Published: 2009

Study Location: Duke University Medical Center, Johns Hopkins University, New York State Psychiatric Institute, University of Pittsburgh, and University of Texas Southwestern Medical Center

Who Was Studied: Adolescents 12 to 18 years old with a major unipolar mood disorder who had made a recent suicide attempt within 90 days of intake and had at least moderate symptoms of depression based on a Children's Depression Ratings Scale score ≥36. Suicidal events were defined using the Columbia Classification Algorithm of Suicide Assessment and included completed or attempted suicide, suicidal ideation, or acts that were in preparation of imminent.

Who Was Excluded: Patients with substance dependence, bipolar disorder, psychosis, or a developmental disorder.

How Many Participants: 124

Study Overview: See Figure 11.1 for a summary of the study design.

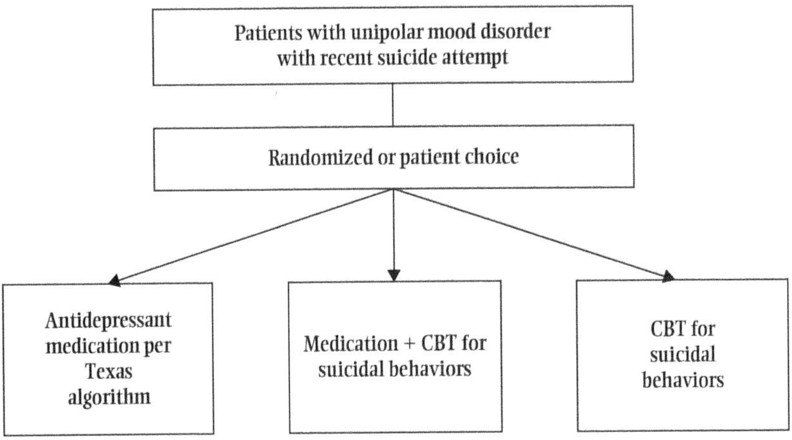

Figure 11.1 Summary of Study Design
NOTE: CBT = cognitive behavioral therapy.

Study Intervention: Patients were initially randomized into one of three treatment groups: psychotherapy, medication, or a combination of these two treatments. There was no placebo, so all medications were given as open label. Patients were later given a choice of treatment group to improve recruitment. Treatment lasted for six months in all groups.

Psychotherapy consisted of a modified version of cognitive behavioral therapy for suicidal behavior (CBT-SB) for adults who have attempted suicide, drawing from protocols from the Treatment of Adolescent Depression Study, treatment of selective serotonin reuptake inhibitor (SSRI) resistant depression in adolescents, and dialectical behavioral therapy. The adult protocol was extensively modified to fit the developmental and clinical needs of adolescents. Psychotherapy was delivered over approximately 12 sessions and included an analysis of suicidal events, the development of a safety plan, skill building, psychoeducation, family treatment, and relapse prevention.[2]

Medication management utilized the Texas Medication Algorithm, which suggests initial treatment with citalopram, fluoxetine, or sertraline. If the symptoms do not respond, the algorithm supports switching to an alternative SSRI. If there is still no response, the algorithm suggests switching to venlafaxine, duloxetine, mirtazapine, or bupropion.[3]

Follow-Up: Six months

Endpoints: Primary outcome: A suicidal event, assessed using the Suicide Severity Rating Scale. A suicidal event was defined as completed suicide, attempted suicide, preparatory acts towards imminent suicidal behavior, or suicidal ideation.

RESULTS

- A total of 24 of the 124 participants had a suicidal event and 15 of these 24 participants had a repeat suicidal event; 40% of these events and attempts occurred within four weeks of intake.
- There were no significant differences in suicidal events based on age, sex, race/ethnicity, or education.
- Those who experienced a suicidal event had a higher level of suicidal ideation at intake, greater number of suicidal attempts with lower lethality, higher self-reported depression and hopelessness, greater number of borderline traits, and greater severity of anxiety.
- A history of physical or sexual abuse was associated with higher risk and earlier onset of a suicidal event, while higher self-rated family adaptability and cohesion were protective against a suicidal event.
- Because of small sample size and because the majority of participants chose their treatment rather than being randomized, intervention efficacy among the three groups was not assessed (Table 11.1).

Table 11.1 Summary of Primary Outcomes

Outcome	Odds ratio	No suicidal events during study	Suicidal events during study	P value
Number of prior suicide attempts		1.8	3.8	0.007
Beck Inventory of Depression score		20.7	32.4	0.001
Suicidal Ideation		5.4	10.0	0.01
Family Adaptability and Cohesion Evaluation Scale		48.7	41.1	0.006
Hopelessness		8.8	12.6	0.008
Multidimensional Anxiety Scale for Children		44.3	55.3	0.009
History of sexual abuse	18.2 (2.5–130.6)			
Family income	2.6 (1.03–6.8)			
Lethality of previous attempts	0.5 (0.3–0.9)			

Criticisms and Limitations: This study was initially a randomized trial to investigate treatment for adolescents with recent suicide attempts. However, due to recruitment issues, the more meaningful and clinically useful finding turned out to be identifying predictors of suicidality in young people. The trial did not assess for outcome differences between groups due to nonrandomization. Participant size, suicidal events, and suicidal attempts were small, limiting conclusions. There were also site variations in race and rate of suicidal events that were difficult to interpret but could have possibly been related to differences in implementation of treatment or baseline differences in participants.

Other Relevant Studies and Information:

- Hazard ratios for suicidal event and attempt from this study compare favorably with those reported in previous studies,[4,5] suggesting that interventions implemented in this study may be helpful in reducing risk for recurrent suicidal behavior.
- In contrast to a previous study,[6] higher income and White race were associated with earlier time to a suicidal event. This finding was explained by the fact that those with lower income were more likely to be lost to follow-up.

- In contrast to previous studies,[7,8] there was a positive association between lower lethality of suicide attempts and recurrent suicidal behavior.
- Predictors of suicidal events in the TASA study that were consistent with adult predictors of suicidal behavior[9] include those with a history of depression, anxiety, borderline personality traits, and abuse.
- Adult predictors of suicide[9] that were not found as adolescent predictors of suicide in the TASA study include White race, males, and those living in inner cities.

Summary and Implications: The TASA study was designed originally to test treatments for those who had recently attempted suicide. However, due to recruitment issues, this analysis was not possible. Still, the TASA study showed that those with more severe depression, higher family income, greater number and lower lethality of previous suicide attempts, and a history of sexual abuse were strongly associated with subsequent suicidal events. Because suicidal events and attempts tended to cluster at the beginning of intervention, safety planning and therapeutic contact should be emphasized at the beginning of treatment.

CLINICAL CASE: ASSESSING SUICIDAL RISK IN AN ADOLESCENT

Case History

A 15-year-old boy with a history of depression presents for an intake appointment at an outpatient psychiatry clinic. He was recently hospitalized for a suicide attempt.

Based on the results of the TASA study, what information can be obtained to assess suicide risk in this adolescent? What treatment should this adolescent receive?

Suggested Answer

TASA found several risk factors that were positively correlated with a recurrent suicidal event. A history of depression, a previous suicide attempt, a lack of family cohesion and adaptability, and a history of abuse were all found to increase the risk of a suicidal event. After ensuring immediate safety, the patient in this vignette should be screened for these risk factors to help assess his risk of a suicidal event in the future and to identify important treatment targets Additionally, intervention(s) (medication, therapy, or both) should be started as soon as possible. If the risk of repeat suicidal event is high, initial treatment should be intense, given the risk of a suicidal event occurring early in intervention.

References

1. Brent, D., Greenhill, L., Compton, S., Emslie, G., Wells, K., Walkup, J., . . . Turner, J. B. (2009). The Treatment of Adolescent Suicide Attempters (TASA) study: Predictors of suicidal events in an open treatment trial. *Journal of the American Academy of Child and Adolescent Psychiatry, 48*(10): 987–996.
2. Stanley, B., Brown, G., Brent, D., Wells, K., Poling, K., Curry, J., . . . Hughes, J. (2009). Cognitive Behavior Therapy for Suicide Prevention (CBT-SP): Treatment model, feasibility and acceptability. *Journal of the American Academy of Child and Adolescent Psychiatry, 48*(10): 1005–1013.
3. Hughes, C. W., Emslie, G. J., Crismon, M. L. Posner, K., Birmaher, B., Ryan, N., . . . The Texas Consensus Conference Panel on Medication Treatment of Childhood Major Depressive Disorder. (2007). Texas Children's Medication Algorithm Project: Update from Texas consensus conference panel on medication treatment of childhood major depressive disorder. *Journal of the American Academy of Child and Adolescent Psychiatry, 46*(6), 667–686.
4. Brent, D. A., Kolko, D. J., Wartella, M. E., Boylan, M.B., Moritz, G., Baugher, M., & Zelenak, J. P. (1993). Adolescent psychiatric inpatients' risk of suicide attempt at 6-month follow-up. *Journal of the American Academy of Child and Adolescent Psychiatry, 32*(1), 95–105.
5. Goldston, D. B., Daniel, S. S., Reboussin, D. M., Reboussin, B. A., Frazier, P. H., & Kelley, A. E. (1999). Suicide attempts among formerly hospitalized adolescents: a prospective naturalistic study of risk during the first 5 years after discharge. *Journal of the American Academy of Child and Adolescent Psychiatry, 38*(6), 660–671.
6. Hawton, K., Harriss, L., Hodder, K., Simkin, S., & Gunnell, D. (2001). The influence of the economic and social environment on deliberate self-harm and suicide: an ecological and person-based study. *Psychological Medicine, 31*(5), 827–836.
7. Miranda, R., Scott, M., Hicks, R., Wilcox, H. C., Harris Munfakh, J. L., & Shaffer D. (2008). Suicide attempt characteristics, diagnoses, and future attempts: Comparing multiple attempters to single attempters and ideators. *Journal of the American Academy of Child and Adolescent Psychiatry, 47*(1), 32–40.
8. Baca-Garcia, E., Diaz-Sastre, C., Basurte, E., Prieto, R., Ceverino, A., Saiz-Ruiz, J., & de Leon, J. (2001). A prospective study of the paradoxical relationship between impulsivity and lethality of suicide attempts. *Journal of Clinical Psychiatry, 62*(7), 560–564.
9. Sadock, B. J., & Sadock, V. A. *Kaplan and Sadock's synopsis of psychiatry* (9th ed.). Philadelphia: Lippincott Williams & Wilkins, 2007, pp. 897–907.

12

Cognitive Behavior Therapy, Sertraline, and Their Combination for Children and Adolescents with OCD

FALISHA GILMAN AND ZHEALA QAYYUM

> Children and adolescents with OCD should begin treatment with the combination of CBT plus a selective serotonin reuptake inhibitor or CBT alone.
>
> —POTS INVESTIGATORS[1]

Research Question: To assess and compare the efficacy of sertraline, cognitive behavioral treatment (CBT), and their combination, in the initial treatment of children and adolescents with clinically significant obsessive-compulsive disorder (OCD).

Funding: National Institute for Mental Health (NIMH)

Year Study Began: 1997

Year Study Published: 2002

Study Location: Duke University, University of Pennsylvania, and Brown University

Who Was Studied: Outpatients 7 to 17 years old with a DSM-IV diagnosis of OCD, Children's Yale–Brown Obsessive Compulsive Scale (CY-BOCS) total score ≥16, NIMH Global Severity Score >7, IQ >80, and who have been off of anti-OCD medications prior to initiation of the study. Patients with attention-deficit/hyperactivity disorder (ADHD) who had been stably medicated with psychostimulants for 3 consecutive months were included.

Who Was Excluded: Patients with major depression or bipolar illness, a primary diagnosis of Tourette disorder, pervasive developmental disorders, psychosis, simultaneous treatment with psychotropic medication or psychotherapy outside the study, a history of two or more unsuccessful trials of a selective serotonin reuptake inhibitor (SSRI) or CBT for OCD, intolerance of sertraline, pregnancy, and children previously treated who had complete or near complete remission of symptoms.

How Many Participants: 112

Study Overview: See Figure 12.1 for a summary of the study design.

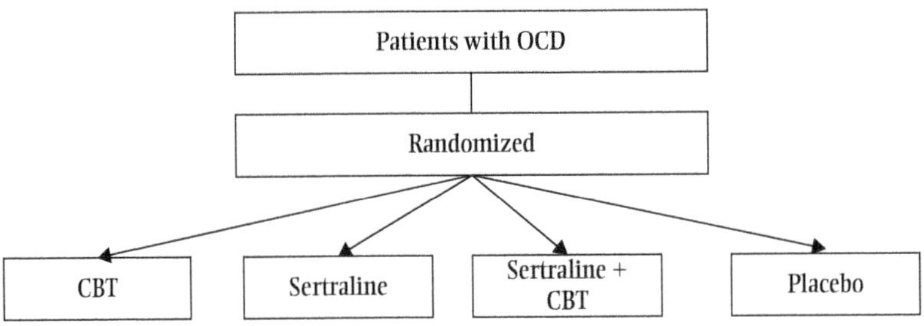

Figure 12.1 Summary of Study Design
NOTES: OCD = obsessive-compulsive disorder. CBT = cognitive behavioral therapy.

Study Intervention: Patients assigned to treatment with sertraline or placebo were clinically monitored by one child and adolescent psychiatrist (CAP) who oversaw medication titration and provided general support to cope with OCD symptoms. The CAP saw patients weekly for the first 6 weeks during titration of sertraline from 25 mg to 200 mg. After reaching maximum dose, adjustments were only made if there was an adverse drug event. For the remaining 6 weeks, patients met every other week with the CAP, totaling nine visits over 12 weeks. Psychotherapy specific for OCD was not allowed in groups receiving sertraline or placebo alone.

CBT consisted of two visits during the first two weeks of the intervention, followed by 10 one-hour long sessions every week. Therapeutic interventions included psychoeducation, self and parental monitoring of OCD symptoms, exposure and response prevention, and developing cognitive based strategies to resist OCD symptoms.

Patients with combination of CBT and sertraline medication management (placebo or sertraline) started interventions simultaneously. To decrease inconvenience and increase compliance, medication and therapy appointments were scheduled to be around the same time. Protocols were conducted independently, so changes in one protocol did not alter the other protocol.

Patients were assessed by the same independent masked evaluator.

Follow-Up: 12 weeks

Endpoints: Change in CY-BOCS score over 12 weeks; "rate of clinical remission," defined as a CY-BOCS score ≤10

RESULTS

- Combined sertraline and CBT treatment was statistically superior to all of the other groups for the CY-BOCS outcome measure, though was not statistically superior to the CBT group for the remission rate measure.
- The sertraline and CBT monotherapy groups were not significantly different from each other on either measure.
- On the remission rate measure, sertraline alone did not differ from placebo; however, CBT alone was superior to placebo.
- All three active treatments were well tolerated (Table 12.1).

Table 12.1 Summary of the POTS Key Findings at 12 Weeks

Outcome	**CBT**	**P value**	**Sertraline**	**P value**	**CBT + Sertraline**	**P value**	**Placebo**
Mean CY-BOCS	14.0	0.003	16.5	0.007	11.2	0.001	21.5
Rate of clinical remission (95% CI)	39.3% [24%, 58%]		21.4% [10%, 40%]		53.6% [36%, 70%]		3.6% [0%, 19%]

Notes: POTS = Pediatric OCD Treatment Study. CBT = cognitive behavioural therapy. CY-BOCS = Children's Yale–Brown Obsessive Compulsive Scale. P values are as compared to placebo.

Criticisms and Limitations: The impact of CBT without medication was statistically greater at the University of Pennsylvania than Duke, but there was no site effect for combined treatment. The presence of site differences raises concern about the generalizability of the CBT intervention. In particular, this study did not grade the patient's symptoms (mild, moderate, severe), which may have led to a differences in the patient populations having different responses to the CBT intervention. The site could also be explained by system factors (e.g., location of sessions, payment source, culture of clinical practice), as well as differences in therapist characteristics (i.e., specialized training, supervision, compensation). This questions the transportability of these evidenced-based treatments when implemented in community practices where expertise in CBT for OCD is limited.[2]

OCD in children commonly co-occurs with other psychiatric illnesses including Tourette disorder, bipolar illness, major depressive disorder, and persistent depressive disorder.[3] Although patients with ADHD on stimulant medication were included in this study, patients with comorbid psychiatric disorders and those prescribed other psychotropic medications were excluded. Therefore, results of this study may not apply to children and adolescents with OCD and additional comorbidities.

Other Relevant Studies and Information:

- A follow-up Pediatric OCD Treatment Study (POTS) investigated CBT +/− sertraline in patients with comorbid diagnoses. The analysis showed that for patients who had a partial response to a SSRI alone, there is additional benefit to adding full CBT to improve patients' quality of life, anxiety not attributed to OCD, hyperactivity, and inattention, but not depression.[4]
- Based on the results of this and other studies, the American Academy of Child and Adolescent Psychiatry recommends OCD-focused CBT for the treatment of mild to moderate cases of OCD. For moderate to severe cases, medications (including SSRIs) are warranted in addition to CBT.[5]

Summary and Implications: The Pediatric OCD Treatment Study found that in children and adolescents with OCD, CBT alone or CBT plus an SSRI should be first line treatment. Sertraline is not as efficacious as CBT alone or in combination. Existing CBT protocols are efficacious; however, few children are provided this evidence-based treatment in practice.

CLINICAL CASE: TREATMENT OF OCD IN A CHILD OR ADOLESCENT

Case History

A 10-year-old boy in fifth grade is referred to a child psychiatrist by his teacher. The patient describes checking that doors are locked in his family's home every night and obsessing about things being clean, such as his food and hands. He also experiences ruminating thoughts about his parents dying to the point of not being able to go to school. The psychiatrist makes the diagnosis of OCD. No comorbid psychiatric illnesses were diagnosed.

Based on the results of the POTS, how should this patient be treated?

Suggested Answer

The POTS found that for children or adolescents diagnosed with OCD, OCD-specific CBT or the combination of sertraline and CBT were both effective first-line treatment options. This and other studies support recent American Academy of Child and Adolescent Psychiatry guidelines to consider therapy for mild to moderate cases of pediatric OCD and the combination of an SSRI and CBT for moderate to severe cases.

The boy in this case is typical of a patient included in the POTS. Therefore, the psychiatrist should consider treatment with CBT or CBT plus an SSRI such as sertraline. The psychiatrist should provide psychoeducation to the parents and child about OCD and have a detailed conversation about the risks and benefits of the various types of psychotherapy and medication interventions before initiating treatment.

References

1. Pediatric OCD Treatment Study (POTS) Team. (2004). Cognitive-behavior therapy, sertraline, and their combination for children and adolescents with obsessive-compulsive disorder: The Pediatric OCD Treatment Study (POTS) randomized controlled trial. *JAMA, 292*(16), 1969–1976.
2. Schoenwald, S. K., & Hoagwood, K. (2001). Effectiveness, transportability, and dissemination of interventions: What matters when? *Psychiatric Services, 52*(9), 1190–1197.
3. Boileau, B. (2011). A review of obsessive-compulsive disorder in children and adolescents. *Dialogues in Clinical Neuroscience, 13*(4), 401–411.

4. Conelea, C. A., Selles, R. R., Benito, K. G., Walther, M. M., Machan, J. T., Garcia, A. M., . . . Freeman, J. B. (2017). Secondary outcomes from the pediatric obsessive compulsive disorder treatment study II. *Journal of Psychiatric Research, 92*, 94–100.
5. Mancuso, E., Faro, A., Joshi, G., & Geller, D. A. (2010). Treatment of pediatric obsessive-compulsive disorder: A review. *Journal of Child and Adolescent Psychopharmacology, 20*(4), 299–308.

13

Initial Treatment of Bipolar I Disorder in Children and Adolescents

The TEAM Trial

STEPHANIE NG AND ANDRES MARTIN

> *Risperidone was more efficacious than lithium or divalproex sodium for the initial treatment of childhood mania but had potentially serious metabolic effects.*
>
> —THE TEAM INVESTIGATORS[1]

Research Question: In medication-naïve children and adolescents with bipolar I disorder who have had a recent manic or mixed phase episode, should risperidone, lithium, or divalproex sodium be used for initial treatment? Also, for partial responders or nonresponders to the first medication, which agent should be added on, or switched to?

Funding: National Institute of Mental Health

Year Study Began: 2003

Year Study Published: 2012

Study Location: Five academic outpatient clinics in the United States

Who Was Studied: Children/adolescents (6–15 years old) with a DSM-IV diagnosis of bipolar I disorder, currently in a manic or mixed episode, who were clinically impaired and in good physical health. Patients with co-occurring attention-deficit/hyperactivity disorder (ADHD; on a stable medication regimen), oppositional defiant disorder, and conduct disorders were also included, as were participants with suicidal ideation, as long as there was no imminent risk.

Who Was Excluded: Those with IQ <70, history of schizophrenia, pervasive developmental disorder or major medical or neurological disease, substance use dependence or recent abuse, pregnancy or the possibility of pregnancy, or nursing. Medications associated with psychiatric symptoms were not permitted with the exception of stimulants. Those who had been previously exposed to risperidone, lithium, or divalproex were also excluded.

How Many Participants: 279

Study Overview: See Figure 13.1 for a summary of the study design.

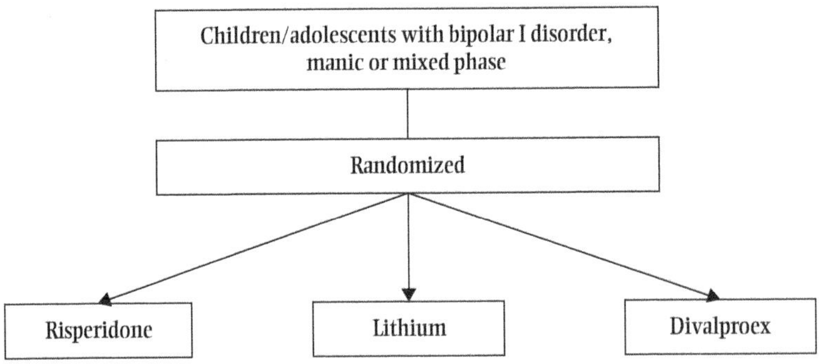

Figure 13.1 Summary of Study Design

Study Intervention: Subjects meeting criteria for DSM-IV mania based onthe Washington University in St. Louis Kiddie Schedule for Affective Disorders and Schizophrenia, a semi-structured interview tool. Before being randomized, participants were stratified by age group (6–12 years and 13–15 years) and by whether they had mixed mania, psychosis, or daily rapid cycling.

Subjects were randomly assigned to risperidone, lithium, or divalproex. Medications could be increased weekly in a prespecified weight-based titration schedule if there was inadequate response (based on Clinical Global Impressions for Bipolar Illness Improvement–Mania [CGI-BP-IM] scales) and if the current dosage was tolerated. Risperidone could be titrated up to a maximum dose of 4 to 6 mg, while lithium could be titrated up to a serum level of 1.1 to 1.3 mEq/L and divalproex up to a level of 111 to 125 μg/L.

Of note, patients, family members, and treating clinicians were not blinded to their assignments, although independent evaluators who did the baseline and endpoint assessments were.

Follow-Up: Eight weeks

Endpoints: Primary outcome: clinical improvement as rated by the CGI-BP-IM scale. Secondary outcome was a measure of mania symptom severity per the Kiddie Schedule for Affective Disorders and Schizophrenia–Mania Rating Scale (KMRS).

RESULTS

- Effect size was 0.85 (95% CI [0.54, 1.15]) for risperidone vs lithium and 1.03 (95% CI [0.73, 1.33]) for risperidone versus divalproex.
- Discontinuation rate was higher for lithium than for risperidone ($p = 0.011$), but otherwise there were no significant differences in discontinuation rates among medications.
- Risperidone was associated with greater likelihood of increased weight gain ($p < 0.001$ compared to lithium and divalproex sodium), body mass index ($p < 0.001$ compared to lithium and divalproex sodium), and prolactin level ($p < 0.001$ compared to lithium and divalproex sodium).
- For children with bipolar I disorder who were partial responders or nonresponders to an initial anti-manic medication trial, switching to risperidone was found to be more useful than lithium or divalproex[2] (Table 13.1).

Table 13.1 SUMMARY OF TEAM'S KEY FINDINGS

Outcome	Risperidone (P value vs. lithium; P value vs. divalproex sodium)	Lithium (P value vs. divalproex sodium)	Divalproex	P value
CGI-BP-IM (% with ratings of 1 or 2)	68.5% (<0.001, <0.001)	35.6% (0.20)	24.0%	<0.001, <0.001, 0.20
KMRS	16.4 (<0.001, <0.001)	26.2 (0.46)	27.6	<0.001, <0.001, 0.46

NOTES: CGI-BP-IM = Clinical Global Impressions for Bipolar Illness Improvement–Mania. KMRS = Kiddie Schedule for Affective Disorders and Schizophrenia–Mania Rating Scale. P values correspond to comparisons of risperidone versus lithium, risperidone versus divalproex, and lithium versus divalproex, respectively.

Criticisms and Limitations: There was no placebo or nonpharmacologic control group in this study.

The generalizability of this study to nonpsychotic bipolar disorder is limited, as the majority of participants (77%) had psychosis. The generalizability to other studies about childhood bipolar disorders may also be limited since there are no valid diagnostic biological measures, and the validity of a childhood diagnosis is still to be determined. Furthermore, 4,959 out of the 5,671 patients screened were not eligible, indicating a very specific subset who were studied.

Other Relevant Studies and Information:

- A follow-up analysis of the TEAM study suggests that the magnitude of the effect size in the risperidone group was influenced by site-related characteristics, presence of ADHD, and obesity.[3]
- Other studies in adult patients with acute mania have found that antipsychotics are more efficacious than mood stabilizers as monotherapy.[4]
- Practice parameters from the American Academy of Child and Adolescent Psychiatry (AACAP) recommend consideration of an antipsychotic and/or mood stabilizer in the acute treatment of mania.[5] However, these guidelines were last updated before the publication of this trial and are based on data from adult patients with mania.

Summary and Implications: The TEAM study was the first randomized control trial to compare mood stabilizers with antipsychotics in children and adolescents. The study found that in acute initial treatment of pediatric mania, risperidone was more effective than lithium or divalproex sodium, but had significant metabolic effects (weight gain, BMI increase, hyperprolactinemia). Guidelines from the AACAP, written prior to publication of this study, recommend consideration of a mood stabilizer and/or antipsychotic for acute mania.

CLINICAL CASE: TREATMENT OF ACUTE MANIA IN CHILDHOOD

Case History

A 10-year-old boy is brought in after his parents and teachers noticed a shift in his behavior over the past month. He had taken his parents' credit cards and ordered hundreds of dollars' worth of shoes and been observed laughing loudly and talking to himself even when nobody was around. In class, his teachers have noticed that he sometimes talks so fast that nobody can understand him and is constantly moving around. He is given a diagnosis of acute mania with psychotic features.

Suggested Answer

Based on the TEAM trial, risperidone would be expected to be more effective than mood stabilizers as an initial treatment for the treatment of acute mania in bipolar disorder in children (especially given the suggestion of psychotic symptoms). However, risperidone was also associated with metabolic side effects including weight gain.

The patient in the vignette is typical of one that would be included in the TEAM study. Based on the results of this study, risperidone should be considered as a first-line agent. However, the child and family should be informed about the potential weight gain and endocrine changes in the long-term to guide their clinical decisions.

References

1. Geller, B., Luby, J. L., Joshi, P., Wagner, K. D., Emslie, G., Walkup, J. T., . . . Lavori, P. (2012). A randomized controlled trial of risperidone, lithium, or divalproex sodium for initial treatment of bipolar I disorder, manic or mixed phase, in children and adolescents. *Archives of General Psychiatry, 69*(5), 515–528.
2. Vitiello, B., Riddle, M. A., Yenokyan, G., Axelson, D. A., Wagner, K. D., Joshi, P., . . . Tillman, R. (2012). Treatment moderators and predictors of outcome in the Treatment of Early Age Mania (TEAM) study. *Journal of the American Academy of Child and Adolescent Psychiatry, 51*(9), 867–878.
3. Walkup, J. T., Wagner, K. D., Miller, L., Yenokyan, G., Luby, J. L., Joshi, P. T., . . . Riddle, M. A. (2015). Treatment of early-age mania: Outcomes for partial and nonresponders to initial treatment. *Journal of the American Academy of Child and Adolescent Psychiatry, 54*(12), 1008–1019.
4. Cipriani, A., Barbui, C., Salanti, G., Rendell, J., Brown, R., Stockton, S., . . . Geddes, J. R. (2011). Comparative effectiveness and acceptability of antimanic drugs in acute mania: A multiple-treatments meta-analysis. *Lancet, 378*(9799), 1306–1315.
5. McClellan, J., Kowatch, R., & Findling, R. L. (2007). Practice parameter for the assessment and treatment of children and adolescents with bipolar disorder. *Journal of the American Academy of Child & Adolescent Psychiatry, 46*(1), 107–125.

14

The Treatment for Adolescents with Depression Study (TADS)

ZACHARY ENGLER AND ZHEALA QAYYUM

Because accelerating symptom reduction by using medication is an important clinical outcome in psychiatry, as it is in other areas of medicine, use of fluoxetine should be made widely available, not discouraged.

—The TADS Team[1]

Research Question: Among adolescents with depression, is fluoxetine and cognitive behavioral therapy (CBT) efficacious, and, if so, how does the efficacy of these treatments compare with each other and in combination?

Funding: National Institute of Mental Health. Fluoxetine and matching placebo were provided by Eli Lilly.

Year Study Began: 2000

Year Study Published: 2007

Study Location: Thirteen academic centers in the United States

Who Was Studied: Adolescents 12 to 17 years old with a DSM-IV diagnosis of major depressive disorder not on an antidepressant prior to the start of the study. Participants had moderate to severe symptoms of depression at the time of enrollment. The sample included those with suicidal ideation.

Who Was Excluded: Patients with bipolar or thought disorders, severe conduct disorder, pervasive developmental disorder, and substance abuse; those who had failed at least two prior selective serotonin reuptake inhibitor (SSRI) trials or one failed CBT trial; and those who were suicidal or homicidal.

How Many Participants: 439

Study Overview: See Figure 14.1 for a summary of the study design.

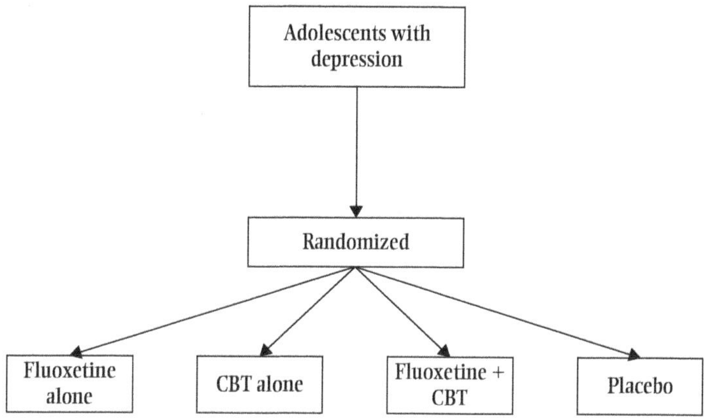

Figure 14.1 Summary of Study Design
NOTE: CBT = cognitive behavioral therapy.

Study Intervention: Participants randomized to receive fluoxetine were started on fluoxetine 10 mg daily, which was titrated to a maximum of 40 mg daily by the twelfth week and up to 60 mg daily by the eighteenth week.[2] A flexible dosing schedule was used based on the result of the clinician-rated Clinical Global Impressions (CGI) score. Of note, after week 12, subjects were told whether they were assigned to placebo or fluoxetine.

Participants randomized to receive CBT were given 15 sessions of therapy lasting 50 to 60 minutes each over the course of 12 weeks. The CBT course required six weeks of psychoeducation and six weeks of flexible tailored treatment topics to address the relevant social skill deficit. Parent-only psychoeducation sessions and parent–adolescent sessions were also completed if needed.

In the CBT and fluoxetine group only, prescribers consulted therapists to decide on dose adjustment when there was a partial response.

Follow-Up: 6, 12, 18, 24, and 36 weeks

Endpoints: Children's Depression Rating Scale–Revised (CDRS-R), and the Clinical Global Impressions–Improvement scale (CGI-I). Response rate was defined as the percentage of subjects whose CGI score indicated the patient was "much or very much improved."

RESULTS

- At week 12, combination treatment was most efficacious followed by the fluoxetine only group (Table 14.1).

Table 14.1 SUMMARY OF TADS KEY FINDINGS

Outcome	**Fluoxetine**	**CBT**	**Fluoxetine + CBT (combo)**	**Placebo[a]**	**Statistically Significant Comparisons**
CDRS-R scores at week 12	35.98 ± 8.15	40.33 ± 9.07	33.65 ± 8.62	41.47	Combo vs CBT and fluoxetine vs CBT
Week 18	32.64 ± 7.86	36.73 ± 8.53	30.86 ± 8.03		Combo vs CBT and fluoxetine vs CBT
Week 36	28.44 ± 7.53	28.49 ± 8.77	27.62 ± 8.00		None
CGI-I % of response rates at week 12	62 ± 7%	48 ± 8%	73 ± 6%	35%	Combo vs CBT
Week 18	69 ± 6%	65 ± 7%	85 ± 4%		Combo vs CBT and combo vs fluoxetine
Week 36	81 ± 4%	81 ± 5%	86 ± 4%		none

NOTES: TADS = Treatment for Adolescents with Depression Study. CBT = cognitive behavioral therapy. CDRS-R = Children's Depression Rating Scale-Revised. CGI-I = Clinical Global Impressions–Improvement.

[a]Placebo results were taken from a different paper from this study,[11] reported here for reference. Placebo was not continued after week 12.

- By week 18, combination group remained significantly more efficacious; however, there was no longer a significant difference between the two monotherapy groups
- By week 24 there was no statistical difference among all three groups with regard to treatment of depression.
- Suicidality:
    - o There were no completed suicides in any patients in the study.
    - o Suicidal thinking significantly decreased in all treatment groups, though combination group had the greatest reduction.

Criticisms and Limitations: The study became open label after week 12, and there was no placebo group after week 12. This is standard, however, for studies involving vulnerable child/adolescent groups. In addition, subjects in the fluoxetine/CBT group spent more time with providers, which could have biased the findings in favor of this study arm.

Finally, most of the population in the study was moderately to severely depressed (90%+), and these results may not be generalizable to other patients with depression.

Other Relevant Studies and Information:

- Several other smaller randomized controlled trials have studied monotherapy of adolescent depression with pharmacology[3–7] and psychotherapy[8,9] and, similar to this study, have found that either treatment alone can be effective for adolescent depression.
- Based on this and other studies of depression therapy in adolescents, the American Academy of Child and Adolescent Psychiatry[10] and American Academy of Pediatrics[11] recommend that those with moderate or severe depression should be treated with CBT and antidepressants. Those with mild depression should be treated with psychotherapy alone.

Summary and Implications: Among adolescents with moderate to severe depression, combination therapy with fluoxetine and CBT is superior to placebo as well to both fluoxetine and CBT monotherapy. Combination therapy also results in faster improvement of symptoms. Based on the results of this and other studies, guidelines currently recommend using an antidepressant (SSRI) and psychotherapy (CBT) in combination in the treatment of children and adolescents with moderate to severe depression. For those with mild depression, guidelines favor psychotherapy alone.

CLINICAL CASE: THE TREATMENT FOR ADOLESCENTS WITH DEPRESSION STUDY (TADS)

Case History

A 15-year-old boy with a history of attention-deficit/hyperactivity disorder presents to an outpatient psychiatrist complaining of depressed mood. The patient endorses poor sleep, poor appetite, decreased concentration, psychomotor slowing, and suicidal ideation without plan or intent for the last two weeks. His history is negative for mania and psychosis.

Based on the results of TADS, what is the appropriate management for this teen?

Suggested Answer

The TADS found that starting an antidepressant in combination with psychotherapy was an effective treatment for moderate to severely depressed teens. Use of both treatments provided the most speedy response time for adolescents with depression.

The patient described is typical of one treated in the TADS. This adolescent should therefore be started on an antidepressant such as fluoxetine along with a referral for CBT. The clinician should pay special attention to response and titrate the medication according to efficacy and side-effect profile while maintaining a collaborative relationship with the psychotherapist.

References

1. Treatment for Adolescents with Depression Study Team. (2007). The Treatment for Adolescents with Depression Study (TADS): Long-term effectiveness and safety outcomes. *Archives of General Psychiatry, 64*(10), 1132–1143.
2. Treatment for Adolescents with Depression Study Team. (2003). Treatment for Adolescents with Depression Study (TADS): Rationale, design, and methods. *Journal of the American Academy of Child & Adolescent Psychiatry, 42*(5), 531–542.
3. Keller, M. B., Ryan, N. D., Strober, M., Klein, R. G., Kutcher, S. P., Birmaher, B., . . . McCafferty, J. P. (2001). Efficacy of paroxetine in the treatment of adolescent major depression: A randomized, controlled trial. *Journal of the American Academy of Child and Adolescent Psychiatry, 40*(7), 762–772.
4. Emslie, G. J., Rush, A. J., Weinberg, W. A., Kowatch, R. A., Hughes, C. W., Carmody, T., & Rintelmann, J. (1997). A double-blind, randomized, placebo-controlled trial of fluoxetine in children and adolescents with depression. *Archives of General Psychiatry,* 54(11), 1031–1037.
5. Wagner, K. D., Robb, A. S., Findling, R. L., Jin, J., Gutierrez, M. M., & Heydorn, W. E. (2004). A randomized, placebo-controlled trial of citalopram for the treatment of

major depression in children and adolescents. *American Journal of Psychiatry, 161*(6), 1079–1083.

6. Wagner, K. D., Jonas, J., Findling, R. L., Ventura, D., & Saikali, K. (2006). A double-blind, randomized, placebo-controlled trial of escitalopram in the treatment of pediatric depression. *Journal of the American Academy of Child and Adolescent Psychiatry,* 45(3), 280–288.
7. Wagner, K. D., Ambrosini, P., Rynn, M., Wohlberg, C., Yang, R., Greenbaum, M. S., . . . Deas, D. (2003). Efficacy of sertraline in the treatment of children and adolescents with major depressive disorder: two randomized controlled trials. *JAMA, 290*(8), 1033–1041
8. Mufson, L., Dorta, K. P., Wickramaratne, P., Nomura, Y., Olfson, M., & Weissman, M. M. (2004). A randomized effectiveness trial of interpersonal psychotherapy for depressed adolescents. *Archives of General Psychiatry, 61*(6), 577–584.
9. Harrington, R., Whittaker, J., Shoebridge, P., & Campbell, F. (1998). Systematic review of efficacy of cognitive behaviour therapies in childhood and adolescent depressive disorder. *BMJ, 316*(7144), 1559–1563.
10. Birmaher, B., & Brent, D. J. (2007). Practice parameter for the assessment and treatment of children and adolescents with depressive disorders. *Journal of the American Academy of Child and Adolescent Psychiatry,* 46(11), 1503–1526.
11. Cheung, A. H., Zuckerbrot, R. A., Jensen, P. S., Ghalib, K., Laraque, D., & Stein, R. E. (2007). Guidelines for adolescent depression in primary care (GLAD-PC): II.: Treatment and ongoing management. *Pediatrics, 120*(5), e1313–e1326.
12. March, J., Silva, S., Petrycki, S., Curry, J., Wells, K., Fairbank, J., . . . Severe, J. (2004). Fluoxetine, cognitive-behavioral therapy, and their combination for adolescents with depression: Treatment for Adolescents with Depression Study (TADS) randomized controlled trial. *JAMA, 292*(7), 807–820.

SECTION 4

Cognitive Disorders: Delirium/ Dementia

15

Effectiveness of Atypical Antipsychotic Drugs in Patients with Alzheimer's Disease

CATIE-AD

ADAM P. MECCA AND RAJESH R. TAMPI

> Adverse effects offset advantages in the efficacy of atypical antipsychotic drugs for the treatment of psychosis, aggression, or agitation in patients with Alzheimer's disease.
>
> —The CATIE-AD Investigators[1]

Research Question: Are atypical antipsychotics an effective treatment for psychosis, aggression, or agitation in outpatients with Alzheimer's disease (AD)?

Funding: The National Institute of Mental Health

Year Study Began: 2001

Year Study Published: 2006

Study Location: 42 outpatient sites in the United States

Who Was Studied: Adults who met criteria for dementia of the Alzheimer's type (DSM-IV) or probable AD (National Institute of Neurological and

Communicative Disorders and Stroke and the Alzheimer's Disease and Related Disorders Association [NINCDS-ADRDA]). In addition, participants had a Mini-Mental State Examination (MMSE) between 5 and 26, were ambulatory, and lived at home or in an assisted-living facility. Participants had delusions, hallucinations, aggression, or agitation that developed after the onset of dementia and disrupted function enough to justify treatment with medications.

Who Was Excluded: Individuals with a primary psychotic disorder, delirium, or non-Alzheimer's dementia, as well as those with psychosis, aggression, or agitation due to another medical condition, medication, or substance abuse

How Many Participants: 421

Study Overview: See Figure 15.1 for a summary of the study design.

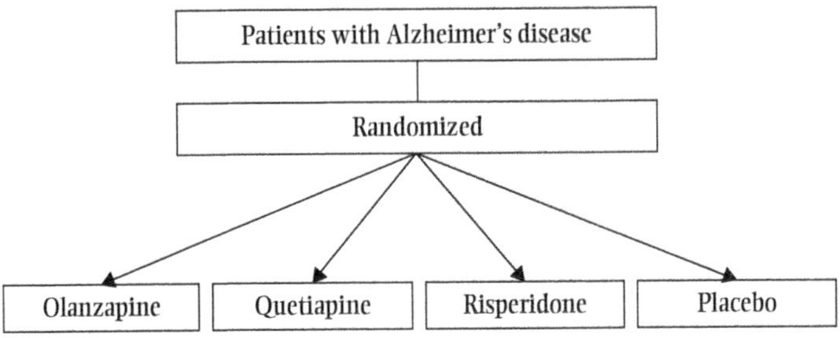

Figure 15.1 Summary of Study Design

Study Intervention: In phase 1 of this randomized, double-blind study, participants were assigned to olanzapine, quetiapine, risperidone, or placebo at starting doses determined by study physicians. After two weeks on the starting dose, adjustments were made, or the medication could be discontinued based on clinical judgment. Medications were dispensed in identical-appearing small and large capsules containing, respectively, a low and high dose of olanzapine (2.5 mg or 5.0 mg), quetiapine (25 mg or 5.0 mg), risperidone (0.5 mg or 1.0 mg), or placebo. Patients with an adequate response to study medication continued treatment for 36 weeks.

In phase 2 of the study, which is out of the scope of this chapter, participants who discontinued treatment during phase 1 were randomly assigned to receive one of the antipsychotic medications that they did not receive during phase 1, or citalopram. These results have not been reported.

In addition to increasing study medication for difficult symptoms, physicians could prescribe a benzodiazepine, oral haloperidol, or parenteral haloperidol. All patients were given equivalent access to psychoeducation.

Follow-Up: 36 weeks for phase 1

Endpoints: Primary outcome: Time to discontinuation of treatment for any reason during phase Secondary outcomes: Minimal or greater improvement on the Clinical Global Impression of Change (CGIC) scale at week 12 of phase 1, time to discontinuation of treatment because of lack of efficacy, time to discontinuation of treatment because of adverse events, intolerability, or death.

RESULTS

- Median time to discontinuation for any reason was not significantly different between olanzapine, quetiapine, risperidone, and placebo.
- Improvement on the CGIC at week 12 was not significantly different between treatment groups.
- Median time to discontinuation because of lack of efficacy was longer with olanzapine and risperidone but not quetiapine when compared to placebo.
- Risk of discontinuation due to adverse events, intolerance of medication, or death was significantly higher in patients on olanzapine, quetiapine, and risperidone when compared to placebo.
- Overall 82% of patients discontinued their initially assigned medication during the 36-week follow-up period. There were no significant differences between groups for serious adverse events including stroke or death.
- Extrapyramidal symptoms were significantly more common in the olanzapine and risperidone groups but not the quetiapine group when compared to placebo group.
- Sedation was significantly more common in all three antipsychotic groups when compared to placebo group.
- Cognitive disturbance and psychotic symptoms were significantly more common with olanzapine but not other antipsychotics compared to placebo (Tables 15.1 and 15.2).

Table 15.1 SUMMARY OF NINCDS-ADRDA CRITERIA FOR PROBABLE AD DEMENTIA

Dementia established by clinical exam, cognitive screening, or neuropsychological testing
Deficits in two or more cognitive domains
Progressive worsening of cognitive function
No disturbance of consciousness
Onset between age 40 and 90
Absence of another disease that could account for the progressive deficits

NOTES: NINCDS-ADRDA = National Institute of Neurological and Communicative Disorders and Stroke and the Alzheimer's Disease and Related Disorders Association. AD = Alzheimer's disease.
SOURCE: McKhann et al.[11]

Table 15.2 SUMMARY OF CATIE-AD PHASE 1 KEY FINDINGS

Outcome	**Olanzapine**	**Quetiapine**	**Risperidone**	**Placebo**	**P Value**
Mean initial/final dose (mg/day)	3.2/5.5	34.1/56.5	0.7/1.0	–	–
Time to discontinuation – all cause (weeks)	8.1	5.3	7.4	8.0	0.52
Treatment response based on CGIC (% patients)	32%	26%	29%	21%	0.22
Time to discontinuation – lack of efficacy (weeks)	22.1	9.1	26.7	9.0	0.002
Risk of discontinuation due to adverse events (HR)	4.32	3.58	3.62	1.0	0.009

NOTES: CATIE-AD = Clinical Antipsychotic Trials of Intervention Effectiveness–Alzheimer's Disease study. CGIC = Clinical Global Impression of Change. HR = hazard ratio compared to placebo group.

Criticisms and Limitations: The trial included patients with probable AD dementia but excluded those with other causes of dementia included mixed etiology. Therefore, the results may only be applicable to patients with AD.

Patients in this study had a large range of disease stages (MMSE range between 5 and 26 for inclusion). This likely adds variability to the results since medications may have differential effectiveness depending on disease severity.

The study did not detect an increased risk of serious adverse events with antipsychotic use, but the sample size may be too small to detect a difference for these outcomes since the event rates are relatively low.

Other Relevant Studies and Information:

- Antipsychotic use is associated with increased risk of death in patients with dementia[2] (see Chapter 16).
- A population based cohort study in nursing homes suggests that quetiapine may carry slightly less risk of mortality and cerebrovascular events when compared to olanzapine, aripiprazole, ziprasidone, and risperidone. Haloperidol appears to have twice the risk of mortality and cerebrovascular events when compared to risperidone.[3]
- One discontinuation study showed that patients with AD who responded to treatment with risperidone for agitation or psychosis are at increased risk of relapse when medication is stopped.[4]
- This is contrasted by evidence from another study that reports no detriment to cognition or neuropsychiatric symptoms with antipsychotic discontinuation.[5]
- Citalopram has been shown to significantly improve symptoms of agitation in AD in a randomized control trial, but its use may be limited by QTc prolongation and increased cardiovascular risk at higher doses.[6]
- The effect of citalopram is thought to extend to escitalopram and this is being studied in an ongoing randomized controlled trial.[7]
- After ruling out an otherwise treatable cause for behavioral or perceptual disturbances and patients are not responsive to redirection, the American Psychiatric Association (APA) clinical guidelines,[8] American Association for Geriatric Psychiatry (AAGP),[9] and American Geriatric Society (AGS)[10] recommend the judicious use of antipsychotics to treat psychosis, agitation, and other behavioral symptoms in those with dementia.

Summary and Implications: The CATIE-AD trial showed that among patients with psychosis, agitation, or aggression due to AD, the efficacy of atypical antipsychotics is questionable, and their use comes with considerable risks of side effects and adverse events. The trial did suggest that the efficacy of olanzapine and risperidone may be slightly greater than quetiapine. The use of atypical antipsychotics to manage behavioral symptoms among patients with AD should be reserved for patients who have not adequately responded to nonpharmacological methods or lower risk medications and are in danger of harm due to continued neuropsychiatric symptoms.

CLINICAL CASE: ATYPICAL ANTIPSYCHOTIC USE FOR AGITATION IN DEMENTIA DUE TO ALZHEIMER'S DISEASE

Case History

A 75-year-old woman with diabetes, hypertension, and dementia due to AD (recent MMSE was 21) comes to clinic for an urgent appointment. Her husband explains that despite a trial on escitalopram to 10 mg daily for agitation that was initiated 8 weeks ago, his wife is getting increasingly upset in the late afternoon. She became aggressive toward him, swinging her arms, and then fell backwards but luckily onto her bed and did not sustain any injuries. She is still sleeping well at night, and her gait is otherwise stable. He is worried that she may get hurt during one of these episodes and asks if there is a stronger medication to help calm her down.

Based on the results of the Clinical Antipsychotic Trials of Intervention Effectiveness–Alzheimer's Disease (CATIE-AD), how should this patient be treated?

Suggested Answer

CATIE-AD showed that there is substantial rate of discontinuation with the use of atypical antipsychotics used to treat psychotic symptoms, aggression, or agitation due to AD. This was largely due to adverse events and side effects. The secondary outcomes of time to discontinuation due to lack of efficacy favored olanzapine and risperidone over quetiapine and placebo.

The patient in this vignette is typical of patients included in CATIE-AD and has the additional history of trialing a selective serotonin reuptake inhibitor (SSRI) for agitation that was unsuccessful. There are considerable risks of side effects with atypical antipsychotics, but there is also significant risk to the patient's well-being due to continued agitation. Published guidelines by the APA, AAGP, and AGS suggest that if education about behavioral interventions and non-antipsychotic medications like SSRIs are not effective, the use of atypical antipsychotics like aripiprazole, olanzapine, quetiapine, or risperidone may be warranted despite the risks. This treatment decision should be undertaken in collaboration with the patient and the caregivers so that the risks and benefits of treatment can be further evaluated.

References

1. Schneider, L. S., Tariot, P. N., Dagerman, K. S., Davis, S. M., Hsiao, J. K., Ismail, M. S., . . . Lieberman, J. A. (2006). Effectiveness of atypical antipsychotic drugs in patients with Alzheimer's disease. *New England Journal of Medicine, 355*, 1525–1538.
2. Schneider, L.S., Dagerman, K.S., & Insel, P. (2005). Risk of death with atypical antipsychotic drug treatment for dementia: Meta-analysis of randomized placebo-controlled trials. *JAMA, 294*(15), 1934–1943.
3. Huybrechts, K. F., Gerhard, T., Crystal, S., Olfson, M., Avorn, J., Levin, R., . . . Schneeweiss, S. (2012). Differential risk of death in older residents in nursing homes prescribed specific antipsychotic drugs: Population based cohort study. *BMJ, 344*, e977.
4. Devanand, D. P., Mintzer, J., Schultz, S. K., Andrews, H. F., Sultzer, D. L., de la Pena, D., . . . Levin, B. (2012). Relapse risk after discontinuation of risperidone in Alzheimer's disease. *New England Journal of Medicine, 367*(16), 1497–1507.
5. Ballard, C., Lana, M. M., Theodoulou, M., Douglas, S., McShane, R., Kossakowski, K., . . . Juszczak, E. (2009). A randomized, blinded, placebo-controlled trial in Dementia Patients Continuing or Stopping Neuroleptics (The DART-AD Trial). *Lancet Neurology, 8*(2), 151–157.
6. Porsteinsson, A. P., Drye, L. T., Pollock, B. G., Devanand, D. P., Frangakis, C, Ismail, Z., . . . Lyketsos, C. G. (2014). Effect of citalopram on agitation in Alzheimer disease: The CitAD randomized clinical trial. *JAMA, 311*(7), 682–691.
7. Leibovici, A. (2012). *Escitalopram treatment of patients with agitated dementia.* Retrieved from https://clinicaltrials.gov/ct2/show/NCT00260624.
8. Reus, V. I., Fochtmann, L. J., Eyler, A. E., Hilty, D. M., Horvitz-Lennon, M., Jibson, M. D., . . . Yager, J. (2016). The American Psychiatric Association practice guideline on the use of antipsychotics to treat agitation or psychosis in patients with dementia. *American Journal of Psychiatry, 173*(5), 543–546.
9. Lyketsos, C. G., Colenda, C. C., Beck, C., Blank, K., Doraiswamy, M. P., Kalunian, D. A., & Yaffe, K. (2006). Position statement of the American Association for Geriatric Psychiatry regarding principles of care for patients with dementia resulting from Alzheimer disease. *American Journal of Geriatric Psychiatry, 14*(7), 561–572.
10. Reuben, D. B., Herr, K. A., Pacala, J. T., Potter, J. F., Semla, T. P., & American Geriatrics Society. (2016). Dementia. In idem, *Geriatrics at your fingertip* (18th ed.). New York: American Geriatrics Society.
11. McKhann, G., Drachman, D., Folstein, M., Katzman, R., Price, D., & Stadlan, E. M. (1984). Clinical diagnosis of Alzheimer's disease: Report of the NINCDS-ADRDA work group under the auspices of Department of Health and Human Services Task Force on Alzheimer's disease. *Neurology, 34*(7), 939–944.

16

Risk of Death with Atypical Antipsychotic Medications for Dementia

ADAM P. MECCA AND RAJESH R. TAMPI

> Atypical antipsychotic drugs may be associated with a small increased risk of death compared with placebo. This risk should be considered within the context of medical need.
>
> —SCHNEIDER ET AL.[1]

Research Question: Does the use of atypical antipsychotics to treat psychosis, aggression, or agitation increase the risk of death in patients with dementia?

Funding: Alzheimer's Disease Centers of California and the National Institute on Aging

Year Study Began: Included studies reported between 2000 and 2005

Year Study Published: 2005

Study Location: Various clinical sites internationally

Who Was Studied: Adults with dementia due to Alzheimer's disease, cerebrovascular disease, mixed etiology, or an unspecified etiology (as defined by DSM-IV)

that were outpatients (4 studies), or cared for in nursing homes (11 studies). Studies included in this meta-analysis were randomized, double-blinded, and placebo-controlled.

Who Was Excluded: Studies were excluded if they were not randomized or placebo-controlled, did not include patients with dementia, utilized intra-muscular administration, or had inadequate data on randomization, dropouts, and deaths.

How Many Participants: 4,528

Study Overview: This was a meta-analysis of 15 individual double-blind placebo-controlled randomized trials of atypical antipsychotics among patients with dementia (Figure 16.1).

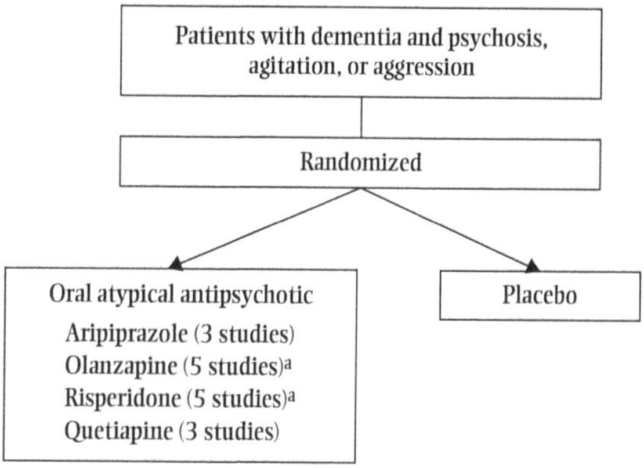

Figure 16.1 Example of a Typical Study Included in the Meta-Analysis
[a]One study was overlapping.

Study Intervention: The design varied for each study included, however an example of a typical study that was included in the meta-analysis is in Figure 16.1. Studies in the meta-analysis involved the medications aripriprazole, olanzapine, risperidone, and quetiapine.

Follow-Up: Three aripiprazole studies (10 weeks), five olanzapine studies (6–26 weeks), five risperidone studies (8–12 weeks), three quetiapine studies (10–26 weeks).

Endpoints: Primary outcomes: risk of dropout and risk of death based on exposure to medication. Secondary outcomes: differential risk of death due to individual drugs, severity of disease, sample selection, or diagnosis.

RESULTS

- Patients randomized to an atypical antipsychotic had equal risk of dropout when compared to those on placebo.
- Atypical antipsychotic use was associated with increased risk of death (see Table 16.1), and the number needed to harm was 100 (95% CI [53, 1000])

Table 16.1 SUMMARY OF PRIMARY OUTCOMES

Outcome	Atypical antipsychotic	Placebo	P value
Incidence of death (%)	3.5	2.3	Not reported
Death (odds ratio)	1.54 (1.06–2.23)		0.02
Death (risk difference)	0.01 (0.004–0.02)		0.01
Dropout (odds ratio)	1.07 (0.88–1.47)		0.50

NOTE: Odds ratios and risk differences are reported with 95% confidence intervals.

- There was no evidence for selection or publication bias (this study included both unpublished and published studies).
- There were no significant differences in risks based on the individual medication used, disease severity, indication for antipsychotic, or treatment setting (Table 16.1).

Criticisms and Limitations: Like all meta-analyses, heterogeneity in study design including dose and patient characteristics may have confounded the findings.

The majority of patients included had dementia due to Alzheimer's disease and psychotic symptoms. Although patients with other causes of dementia were included in some trials, these findings may not be applicable to all patients with dementia. In addition, it was not possible to investigate specific causes of death based on available information. Finally, the length of follow-up is limited, and it is unclear if risk of death is highest early in treatment or increases with length of exposure.

Other Relevant Studies and Information:

- The FDA issued an advisory that use of atypical antipsychotics for behavioral disorders in elderly patients with dementia results in approximately 1.6 to 1.7 fold increase in mortality.[2]
- One study found that quetiapine may carry the least risk among antipsychotics with slightly less risk of mortality and cerebrovascular events than olanzapine, aripiprazole, ziprasidone, and risperidone. Haloperidol has twice the risk of risperidone.[3]

- In patients with psychosis, agitation, or aggression due to Alzheimer's disease, the efficacy of atypical antipsychotics is questionable, and their use comes with considerable risks of side effects and adverse events.[4,5,6]
- A discontinuation study showed that patients with dementia due to Alzheimer's disease who responded to treatment with risperidone for agitation or psychosis are at increased risk of relapse when medication is stopped.[7]
- This is contrasted by evidence from another study that reports no detriment to cognition or neuropsychiatric symptoms with antipsychotic discontinuation.[8]
- The American Psychiatric Association (APA) Clinical Guidelines,[9] American Association for Geriatric Psychiatry (AAGP),[10] and American Geriatric Society (AGS)[11] recommend the judicious use of antipsychotics to treat psychosis, agitation, and other behavioral symptoms in those with dementia. These medications should only be used after ruling out other treatable causes of the symptoms, and after initial attempts to manage the behavior using nonpharmacological therapies.

Summary and Implications: This meta-analysis found that treatment with atypical antipsychotics for psychosis, agitation, or aggression due to dementia is associated with increased risk of death. Treatment with atypical antipsychotics may be appropriate but generally should only be used among patients who cannot be managed with nonpharmacological methods or lower risk medications and are in danger of harm due to continued neuropsychiatric symptoms.

CLINICAL CASE: RISK OF DEATH DUE TO ATYPICAL ANTIPSYCHOTIC USE FOR PSYCHOTIC SYMPTOMS IN PATIENTS WITH DEMENTIA

Case History

An 80-year-old man with hypertension and dementia attributed to his Alzheimer's disease (recent Mini-Mental State Examination was 17) resides in a nursing home. Although he is typically oriented to his living situation, he has become increasingly concerned that people are coming into his room and stealing things at night. This has been going in for the last two months and started when he returned to the nursing home after a hospitalization for his most recent stroke. On multiple occasions over the last three weeks, he confronted several other residents and a nurse, accusing them of entering his room at night. Last week, he became so upset that he grabbed another resident during a confrontation. He is already on escitalopram, which was started about one year ago for anxiety that was also attributed to Alzheimer's disease.

Based on the results of the described meta-analysis, how should this patient be treated?

Suggested Answer

In the meta-analysis described, Schneider et al.[1] showed that there is significant risk of using an atypical antipsychotic to treat psychotic symptoms in patients with dementia. The patient in this vignette is typical of some patients included in that study. There are considerable risks of side effects, cardiovascular events, and death with atypical antipsychotics, but there is also considerable distress and risks associated with this patient's ongoing paranoid delusions and aggression. Published guidelines by the APA, AAGP, and AGS suggest that if education about behavioral interventions and non-antipsychotic medications like selective serotonin reuptake inhibitors are not effective, use of atypical antipsychotics like aripiprazole, olanzapine, quetiapine, or risperidone may be warranted despite the risk. This treatment decision should be undertaken in collaboration with the patient and caregiver so that the risks and benefits can be explored.

References

1. Schneider, L. S., Dagerman, K., & Insel, P. S. (2005). Risk of death with atypical antipsychotic drug treatment for dementia: Meta-analysis of randomized placebo-controlled trials. *JAMA, 294*(15), 1934–1943.
2. Administration UFaD. (2005). *FDA public health advisory: Deaths with antipsychotics in elderly patients with behavioral disturbances.* Washington, DC: Food and Drug Administration.
3. Huybrechts, K. F., Gerhard, T., Crystal S., Olfson, M., Avorn, J., Levin, R. . . . Schneeweiss, S. (2012). Differential risk of death in older residents in nursing homes prescribed specific antipsychotic drugs: Population based cohort study. *BMJ, 344*, e977.
4. Schneider L. S., Tariot P. N., Dagerman K. S., Davis, S. M., Hsiao, J. K., Ismail, M. S., . . . Lieberman, J. A. (2006). Effectiveness of atypical antipsychotic drugs in patients with Alzheimer's disease. *New England Journal of Medicine, 355*(15), 1525–1538.
5. Tampi, R. R., Tampi, D. J., & Balachandran, S. (2017). Antipsychotics, antidepressants, anticonvulsants, melatonin, and benzodiazepines for behavioral and psychological symptoms of dementia: A systematic review of meta-analyses. *Current Treatment Options in Psychiatry, 4*(1), 55–79.
6. Schneider, L. S., Dagerman, K., & Insel, P. S. (2006). Efficacy and adverse effects of atypical antipsychotics for dementia: Meta-analysis of randomized, placebo-controlled trials. *American Journal of Geriatric Psychiatry, 14*(3), 191–210.

7. Devanand, D. P., Mintzer, J., Schultz, S. K., Andrews, H. F., Sultzer, D. L., de la Pena, D., . . . Levin, B. (2012). Relapse risk after discontinuation of risperidone in Alzheimer's disease. *New England Journal of Medicine, 367*(16), 1497–1507.
8. Douglas, S., McShane, R., Kossakowski, K., . . . Juszczak, E. (2009). A randomized, blinded, placebo-controlled trial in Dementia Patients Continuing or Stopping Neuroleptics (The DART-AD Trial). *Lancet Neurology, 8*(2), 151–157.
9. Hilty, D. M., Horvitz-Lennon, M., Jibson, M. D., . . . Yager, J. (2016). The American Psychiatric Association practice guideline on the use of antipsychotics to treat agitation or psychosis in patients with dementia. *American Journal of Psychiatry, 173*(5), 543–546.
10. Blank, K., Doraiswamy, M. P., Kalunian, D. A., & Yaffe, K. (2006). Position statement of the American Association for Geriatric Psychiatry regarding principles of care for patients with dementia resulting from Alzheimer disease. *American Journal of Geriatric Psychiatry, 14*(7), 561–572.
11. Reuben, D. B., Herr, K. A., Pacala, J. T., Potter, J. F., Semla, T. P., & American Geriatrics Society. (2016). Dementia. In idem, *Geriatrics at your fingertip* (18th ed.). New York: American Geriatrics Society.

17

Treatment of Delirium in Hospitalized AIDS Patients

A Double-Blind Trial of Haloperidol, Chlorpromazine, and Lorazepam

AMANDA SUN AND RAJESH R. TAMPI

> Symptoms of delirium in medically hospitalized AIDS patients may be treated efficaciously with few side effects by using low-dose neuroleptics (haloperidol or chlorpromazine). Lorazepam alone appears to be ineffective and associated with treatment-limited adverse effects.
>
> —BREITBART ET AL.[1]

Research Question: What is the comparative efficacy and tolerability of haloperidol, chlorpromazine, and lorazepam for the treatment of the symptoms of delirium in the medically ill?

Funding: National Institute of Mental Health

Year Study Began: 1991

Year Study Published: 1996

Study Location: Two large inpatient AIDS units at St. Luke's Hospital and Roosevelt Hospital in New York City

Who Was Studied: Medically hospitalized adult patients with AIDS who later developed delirium

Who Was Excluded: Patients with a known hypersensitivity to neuroleptics or benzodiazepines, a history of neuroleptic malignant syndrome, or seizure disorders. Also excluded were those currently on neuroleptics; those being treated with systemic chemotherapy for Kaposi's sarcoma; those with a delirium with a specific treatment (i.e., withdrawal or anticholinergic delirium); those with a history of schizophrenia, schizoaffective, or bipolar disorder; and patients whose life expectancy was less than 24 hours.

How Many Participants: 244 consented and prospectively followed; 30 developed delirium and were treated.

Study Overview: See Figure 17.1 for a summary of the study design.

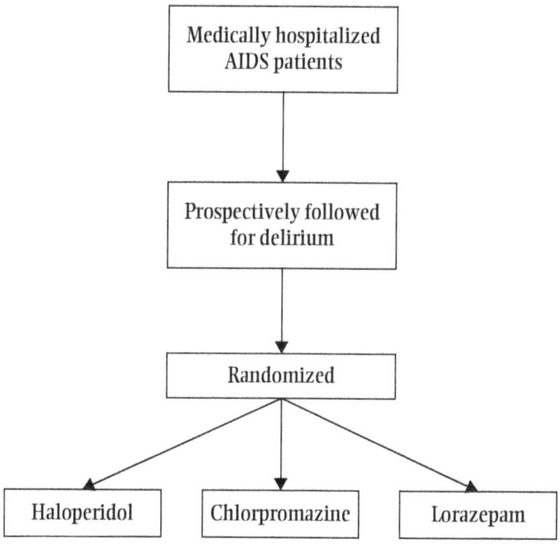

Figure 17.1 Summary of Study Design

Study Intervention: After determining a patient has met criteria for delirium treatment, the patient was randomized to treatment with haloperidol, chlorpromazine, or lorazepam and treated in a double-blind approach. The treatment protocol involved hourly evaluations of each patient with the Delirium Rating Scale (including Mini-Mental State Examination) and the Extrapyramidal Symptom Rating Scale. Subjects randomized to the haloperidol, chlorpromazine, and lorazepam arms were started at 0.25, 10, and 0.50 mg/hour by mouth, respectively. Those requiring intramuscular doses were given half that amount.

If the patient's Delirium Rating Scale score still exceeded 12, the drug dose was increased up to oral dose of 5 mg/hour of haloperidol, 200 mg/hour for chlorpromazine, and 4 mg/hour for lorazepam. After stabilization, the patient would receive a maintenance dose of one-half of the first 24-hour dose requirement in a twice-a-day regimen starting on day 2 and continued for up to six days.

In the middle of the study, it was determined that the patients receiving lorazepam were developing "treatment-limiting adverse side effects," and therefore lorazepam was removed from the study. Those patients were then randomized to haloperidol or chlorpromazine.

Follow-Up: Day 2 after onset of delirium, and end of treatment (up to six days of treatment protocol)

Endpoints: Delirium Rating Scale, Mini-Mental State Examination, Extrapyramidal Symptom Rating Scale, Side Effects and Symptoms Checklist

RESULTS

- Patients receiving low-dose haloperidol and chlorpromazine demonstrated significant improvement in delirium symptoms as determined by the Delirium Rating Scale.
- In contrast, patients exhibited no improvement in delirium symptoms on lorazepam and developed side effects such as oversedation, disinhibition, ataxia, and increased confusion. As a result, this arm of the study had to be terminated early.
- Cognitive functioning significantly improved from baseline to day 2 on chlorpromazine, and there was a trend toward significant improvement on haloperidol but no improvement on lorazepam.
- There was no significant increase in extrapyramidal side effects in the patients receiving antipsychotics in this study (Tables 17.1 and 17.2).

Table 17.1 Summary of Study Key Findings: Delirium Rating Scale Scores

Drug	Baseline	Day 2	P value (baseline to day 2)	End of treatment	P value (day 2 to end of treatment)
Haloperidol	20.45	12.45	0.001	11.64	0.43
Chlorpromazine	20.62	12.08	0.001	11.85	0.81
Lorazepam	18.33	17.33	0.63	17.00	0.81

Table 17.2 Summary of Study Key Findings: Mini-Mental State Scores

Drug	Baseline	Day 2	P value (baseline to day 2)	End of treatment	P value (day 2 to end of treatment)
Haloperidol	13.45	17.27	0.09	17.18	0.96
Chlorpromazine	10.92	18.31	0.001	15.08	0.04
Lorazepam	15.17	12.67	0.40	11.50	0.60

Criticisms and Limitations: This study was limited by its small sample size, which may have reduced the study's ability to detect significant findings and may have contributed to lack of detection of significant side effects. It was also limited to the AIDS population at one institution, therefore limiting generalizability, especially given potentially lower neuroleptic dose requirements to effectively manage delirium symptoms observed in the HIV/AIDS patient population. The study also did not test the use of lorazepam in larger doses, non-oral or intramuscular formulations, or in combination with a neuroleptic. In addition, the researchers did not establish dose requirements in more established delirium with its study design of initiating pharmacotherapy at the onset of delirium.

Other Relevant Studies and Information:

- This was the first randomized controlled trial of neuroleptics for treating the symptoms of delirium, although haloperidol had been used for this purpose for several generations. A follow-up article from the same study also showed that hypoactive and hyperactive delirious patients responded equally well to treatment with antipsychotics.[2]
- For information on interventions for preventing delirium in hospitalized patients, see the Cochrane Database review article[3] on this topic.
- Other more recent randomized controlled trials have investigated the use of other treatments for delirium such as second generation antipsychotics, dexmedetomidine, and nonpharmacological interventions.[4–6]
- Some data has suggested the importance of treating delirium to shorten hospital stays[7] and possibly prevent long term cognitive impairment[8,9]
- For additional information on the use of antipsychotics in the treatment for delirium, see the corresponding systematic review and meta-analysis.[10]
- According to American Psychiatric Association practice guidelines,[11] the pharmacologic agent of choice in most cases of delirium is

an antipsychotic, specifically oral, intramuscular or intravenous haloperidol at an initial dose of 1 to 2 mg every two to four hours as needed or 0.25 to 0.50 mg every four hours as needed for elderly patients, with titration to higher doses if still agitated.

Summary and Implications: In medically ill patients with AIDS, antipsychotics administered at low doses can result in significant reduction in delirium symptoms and improve cognitive status without significant adverse effects. Lorazepam, however, may result in significant adverse effects in delirium. This was the first double-blind, randomized comparison trial to examine optimal medication management of delirium in the medically ill.

CLINICAL CASE: NEUROLEPTICS VERSUS BENZODIAZEPINES IN THE TREATMENT OF DELIRIUM IN THE MEDICALLY ILL

Case History

A 37-year-old man with HIV/AIDS (last CD4 26, VL 46,000), history of opportunistic infections, and poor adherence to his antiretroviral therapy treatment and Bactrim prophylaxis, was brought in by family after developing fevers, shortness of breath, nonproductive cough, and altered mental status. His workup included a chest X-ray that showed widespread pulmonary infiltrates, and the patient was diagnosed with and treated for Pneumocystis pneumonia on the inpatient medical floor. He was also found to have disorientation, impaired cognition, attention deficits, and agitation of fluctuating nature, with onset over the past two days.

Based on this study, how should this patient be treated?

Suggested Answer

It would be appropriate to first treat the underlying causes of delirium in this hospitalized patient, which is most likely the infection. According to the results of this and other reviews on this topic, American Psychiatric Association guidelines support the use of low-dose neuroleptics as the treatment of choice for hospitalized patients with delirium rather than benzodiazepines.

The patient described in the vignette would fit general inclusion criteria in this study. Based on the results, low-dose haloperidol, chlorpromazine, or another neuroleptic is an effective way to treat delirium.

References

1. Breitbart, W., Marotta, R., Platt, M. M., Weisman, H., Derevenco, M., Grau, C., . . . Jacobson, P. (1996). A double-blind trial of haloperidol, chlorpromazine, and lorazepam in the treatment of delirium in hospitalized AIDS patients. *American Journal of Psychiatry, 153*(2), 231–237.
2. Platt, M. M., Breitbart, W., Smith, M., Marotta, R., Weisman, H., & Jacobsen, P. B. (1994). Efficacy of neuroleptics for hypoactive delirium. *Journal of Neuropsychiatry and Clinical Neurosciences, 6*(1), 66–67.
3. Siddiqi, N., Harrison, J. K., Clegg, A., Teale, E. A., Young, J., Taylor, J., & Simpkins, S. A. (2016). Interventions for preventing delirium in hospitalised non-ICU patients. *Cochrane Database of Systematic Reviews*, 3, CD005563.
4. Skrobik, Y., Bergeron, N., Dumont, M., & Gottfried, S. (2004). Olanzapine vs haloperidol: Treating delirium in a critical care setting. *Intensive Care Medicine, 30*(3), 444–449.
5. Reade, M. C., Eastwood, G. M., & Bellomo, R. (2016). Effect of dexmedetomidine added to standard care on ventilator-free time in patients with agitated delirium: A randomized clinical trial. *JAMA, 315*(14), 1460–1468.
6. Abraha, I., Trotta, F., Rimland, J. M., Cruz-Jentoff, A., Lozano-Montoya, I., Soiza, R. L. . . . Cherubini, A. (2015). Efficacy of the non-pharmacological interventions to prevent and treat delirium in older patients: A systematic overview. The SENATOR project ONTOP Series. *PLoS One, 10*(6), e0123090.
7 Ouimet, S., Kavanagh, B. P., Gottfried, S. B., & Skrobik, Y. (2007). Incidence, risk factors and consequences of ICU delirium *Intensive care medicine, 33*(1), 66–73.
8. Girard, T. D., Jackson, J. C., Pandharipande, P. P., Pun, B. T., Thompson, J. L., Shintani, A. K., . . . Ely, E. W. (2010). Delirium as a predictor of long-term cognitive impairment in survivors of critical illness. *Critical Care Medicine, 38*(7), 1513–1520.
9. Pandharipande, P. P., Girard, T. D., Jackson, J. C., Morandi, A., Thompson, J. L., Pun, B. T., . . . Moons, K. G. (2013). Long-term cognitive impairment after critical illness. *New England Journal of Medicine, 369*(14), 1306–1316.
10. Kishi, T., Hirota, T., Matsunaga, S., & Iwata, N. (2016). Antipsychotic medications for the treatment of delirium: A systematic review and meta-analysis of randomized controlled trials. *Journal of Neurology, Neurosurgery, and Psychiatry, 98*(7), 767–774.
11. Trzepacz, P., Breitbart, W., Franklin, J., Levenson, J., Martini, D. R., & Wang, P. (1999). Practice guideline for the treatment of patients with delirium. *American Psychiatric Association, 156*(5 suppl), 1–20.

18

Memantine in Patients with Moderate to Severe Alzheimer's Disease Already Receiving Donepezil

BRANDON M. KITAY AND RAJESH R. TAMPI

> In patients with moderate to severe AD receiving stable doses of donepezil, memantine resulted in significantly better outcomes than placebo on measures of cognition, activities of daily living, global outcome, and behavior and was well tolerated.
>
> —THE MEMANTINE STUDY GROUP[1]

Research Question: In patients with moderate to severe Alzheimer disease (AD) treated with a cholinesterase inhibitor (donepezil), is the addition of a *N*-methyl-D-aspartate (NMDA) receptor inhibitor (memantine) safe and efficacious?

Funding: Forest Laboratories, Inc.

Year Study Began: 2001

Year Study Published: 2004

Study Location: 37 US study sites

Who Was Studied: Adults 50 years old or older with probable AD according to the National Institute of Neurological and Communicative Disorders and Stroke criteria and a Mini-Mental State Exam (MMSE) score of 5 to 14 (moderate to severe cognitive impairment). Participants must have received donepezil for more than six months and at a stable dose for three or more months. A knowledgeable and reliable caregiver was a further requisite for enrollment to ensure trustworthy outcome assessments.

Who Was Excluded: Patients with clinically significant B_{12} or folate deficiency; active pulmonary, gastrointestinal, renal, or hepatic disease; active psychiatric or central nervous system disorders other than AD; radiological imaging suggestive of central nervous system disorders other than probable AD; dementia complicated by other organic disease; Hachinski Ischemia Score >4 suggestive of vascular dementia.

How Many Participants: 404

Study Overview: See Figure 18.1 for a summary of the study design.

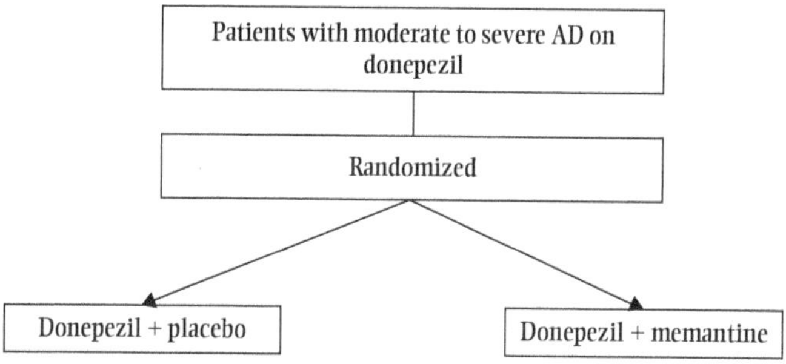

Figure 18.1 Summary of Study Design
NOTE: AD = Alzheimer's disease.

Study Intervention: In this prospective randomized, placebo-controlled trial, patients received either placebo or memantine in addition to their stable dose of donepezil (5–10 mg/day) for 24 weeks.

Patients assigned to receive memantine were titrated by 5 mg/week to a final dose of 20 mg/day (10 mg, twice daily) by week 4. From week 3 to week 8, memantine adjustments were permitted for dose-dependent side effects. Patients who could not tolerate the target dose of 20 mg/day were disenrolled by the end of week 8.

All patients maintained their pretrial dose of donepezil. Patients who changed dose or discontinued donepezil at any point during the course of the study were unenrolled. Patients were permitted to continue all other concomitant medications.

Follow-Up: Primary and secondary outcome measures were obtained at baseline and at the end of 4, 8, 12, 18, and 24 weeks. Patients that were unenrolled prematurely were evaluated during their final visit.

Endpoints: Primary outcomes included the Severe Impairment Battery, a 40-item battery for the evaluation of cognitive dysfunction,[2] and the Modified 19-Item AD Cooperative Study-Activities of Daily Living, an abbreviated assessment of level of independence[3] administered to the patient's caregiver.

Secondary outcomes included a Clinician's Interview-Based Impression of Change Plus Caregiver Input, the Neuropsychiatric Inventory (a caregiver assessment of behavioral symptoms), and the Behavioral Rating Scale for Geriatric Patients (subscales reflect cognitive and functional characteristics associated with increasing need for care).

RESULTS

- More participants in the placebo group discontinued prematurely (12.4%) due to adverse events when compared to the memantine group (7.4%); confusion was the leading adverse event reported (1.5% in placebo vs. 2% in memantine group).
- Statistically significant benefits of memantine over placebo were observed on all primary and secondary outcome measures (Table 18.1), using both observed case (all patients that completed the 24 week trial) and last-observation-carried-forward analyses (Table 18.1).

Table 18.1 Summary of the Study's Key Findings

Outcome	**Donepezil + Placebo**	**Donepezil + Memantine**	**P value**
Severe Impairment Battery	−2.4	+1.0	<0.001
Activities of Daily Living score (ADCS-ADL19)	−3.3	−1.7	0.02
Clinician's assessment of change (CIBIC-Plus)*	+4.64	+4.38	0.03
Neuropsychiatric Inventory[a]	+2.9	−0.5	0.01
Behavioral Rating Scale for Geriatric Patients*	+2.2	+0.6	0.001

[a] Higher scores indicate more impairment or symptoms.

NOTES: ADCS-ADL19 = Modified 19-Item AD Alzheimer Disease Cooperative Study-Activities of Daily Living. CIBIC-Plus = Clinician's Interview-Based Impression of Change Plus Caregiver Input.

Criticisms and Limitations: Although memantine produced statistically significant benefits, the magnitude of the improvements were modest, and the clinical significance uncertain.

Moreover, since patients were only followed for 24 weeks, it is not clear from this analysis whether the addition of memantine to donepezil has persistent long-term benefits.

Several factors also limit generalizability of the results, including the fact that the study population was majority White.

Other Relevant Studies and Information:

- The Donepezil and Memantine in Moderate to Severe Alzheimer's Disease (DOMINO-AD) study was a UK-based, multicenter, double-blind, placebo-controlled, clinical trial spanning 52 weeks that assessed donepezil continuation versus discontinuation, switch from donepezil to memantine, and combinatorial treatment with donepezil and memantine.[4] This study reported no significant benefit from combination therapy, however reanalyses of these data do indicate a benefit with memantine.[5]
- The American Psychiatric Association (APA) has concluded that there may be benefit from memantine in addition to cholinesterase inhibitors in patients with advanced AD and therefore recommends consideration of combinatorial therapy.[6]

Summary and Implications: This was the first published, prospective study to suggest benefits of the adjunctive use of memantine among patients with advanced AD already receiving donepezil with respect to cognitive and functional outcomes. Though the observed benefits were modest, as well as the fact that other studies have raised questions about the efficacy of adjunctive memantine therapy, guidelines from the APA recommend consideration of combination therapy with cholinesterase inhibitors and memantine among patients with advanced AD.

CLINICAL CASE: MEMANTINE TREATMENT IN PATIENTS WITH MODERATE TO SEVERE AD ALREADY RECEIVING DONEPEZIL

Case History

A 76-year-old man with a history of moderate to severe AD, hypertension, and cardiovascular disease presents to an outpatient geriatric psychiatrist for a three-month follow-up visit accompanied by his daughter and primary care taker. At his first evaluation one-year ago, his MMSE was 19 and he required assistance with most instrumental activities of daily living. He was started on donepezil and tolerated titration to 10 mg daily. Over the past several months, his family has noted significant decline in his short-term memory, and he now requires assistance with toileting and dressing. At this visit, his MMSE was 16. His daughter would like to know if there are any additional therapies that might prevent further cognitive and functional decline.

Based on this study, how should the psychiatrist proceed in counseling this patient and caregiver?

Suggested Answer

This study demonstrated that over 24 weeks, patients with moderate to severe AD demonstrated objective preservation in baseline cognition and clinically significant delay in decline of function with the addition of memantine to stable donepezil therapy. This combination was well tolerated with more patients in the memantine group completing the study. Confusion was the most common side effect reported; however, it was often rated as "mild" in severity and duration.

Subsequent studies further suggest that the combination of donepezil and memantine is effective in not only delaying the decline of cognition in this patient population but also improving overall caregiver burden.

Based on this study and most current treatment guidelines, this patient may benefit from a trial of memantine in addition to the standing donepezil. In addition to monitoring for tolerability and side effects, the patient and caregiver should be counseled that cognition and function are likely to continue to decline over the long term.

References

1. Tariot, P. N., Farlow, M. R., Grossberg, G. T., Graham, S. M., McDonald, S., & Gergel, I. (2004). Memantine treatment in patients with moderate to severe Alzheimer disease already receiving donepezil: A randomized controlled trial. *JAMA, 291*(3), 317–324.
2. Schmitt, F. A., Ashford, W., Ernesto C., Saxton, J., Schneider, L. S., Clark, C. M. . . . Thal, L. J. (1997). The severe impairment battery: concurrent validity and the assessment of longitudinal change in Alzheimer's disease: The Alzheimer's Disease Cooperative Study. *Alzheimer Disease and Associated Disorders, 11*(Suppl. 2), S51–S56.
3. Galasko, D., Bennett, D., Sano M., Ernesto, C., Thomas, R., Grundman, M., & Ferris, S. (1997). An inventory to assess activities of daily living for clinical trials in

Alzheimer's disease: The Alzheimer's Disease Cooperative Study. *Alzheimer Disease and Associated Disorders, 11*(Suppl 2), S33–S39.

4. Howard, R., McShane, R., Lindesay, J., Ritchie, C., Baldwin, A., Barber, R., . . . Phillips, P. (2012). Donepezil and memantine for moderate-to-severe Alzheimer's disease. *New England Journal of Medicine, 366*, 893–903.
5. Hendrix, S., Ellison, N., Stanworth, S., Otcheretko, V., & Tariot, P. N. (2015). Post hoc evidence for an additive effect of memantine and donepezil: Consistent findings from DOMINO-AD Study and Memantine Clinical Trial Program. *Journal of Prevention of Alzheimer's Disease, 2*(3), 165–171.
6. Rabins, P. V., Rovner, B. W., Rummans, T., Schneider, L. S., & Tariot, P. N. (2017). Guideline Watch (October 2014): Practice guideline for the treatment of patients with Alzheimer's disease and other dementias. *Focus, 15*(1), 110–128.

SECTION 5

Epidemiology

19

Global Burden of Mental and Substance Use Disorders

STEPHANIE YARNELL AND ELLEN EDENS

> Mental and substance use disorders are notable contributors to the global burden of disease, directly accounting for about 7.4% of disease burden worldwide. These disorders were responsible for more of the global burden than were HIV/AIDS and tuberculosis, diabetes, or transport injuries
>
> —WHITEFORD ET AL.[1]

Research Question: What is the burden of disease attributable to mental and substance use disorders (MSDs)?

Funding:

- Queensland Department of Health
- School of Public Health, The University of Queensland
- National Health and Medical Research Council of Australia
- National Drug and Alcohol Research Centre, University of New South Wales
- Bill & Melinda Gates Foundation
- University of Toronto
- Technische Universität
- Ontario Ministry of Health and Long Term Care
- US National Institute of Alcohol Abuse and Alcoholism

Year Study Began: 2007 (Data obtained 1980–2010)

Year Study Published: 2013

Study Location: 187 countries across 21 world regions

Who Was Studied: The investigators utilized a database from another study, the Global Burden of Diseases, Injuries, and Risk Factors (GBD 2010),[1] which compiled all data on causes of death for persons from 187 countries between 1980 to 2010. Nearly 53 million files were included in the original study. This secondary analysis of GBD 2010[2] examined a subset of registries reporting an International Classification of Diseases (ICD) assigned cause of death related to Mental and Substance Use Disorders (MSDs). The authors attempted to identify a subset of registries representative of the general population with MSDs according *to Diagnostic and Statistical Manual of Mental* Disorders (DSM) or ICD criteria.

Who Was Excluded: Subjects were "excluded for data quality issues such as incompleteness, diagnostic accuracy, missing data, stochastic variations, and probable causes of death."[1]

How Many Participants: Several thousand studies were utilized in the calculation of years lived with disability (YLDs; and subsequently disability-adjusted life years [DALYs]). In total, more than 30,000 subjects were included in the analysis.

Study Overview: See Figure 19.1 for a summary of the study design.

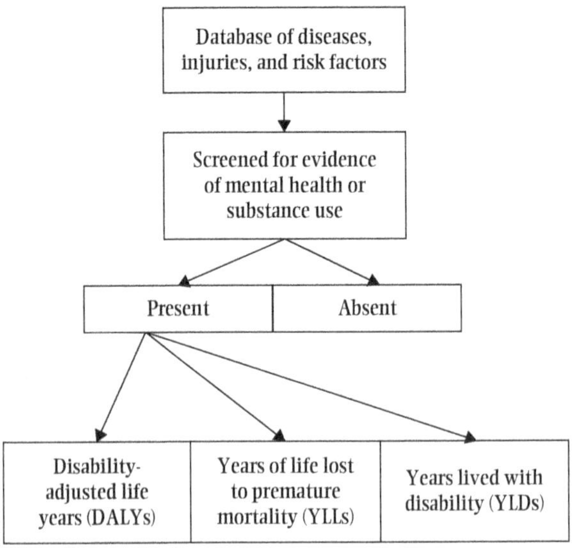

Figure 19.1 Summary of Study Design

Study Intervention: This study was a cross sectional analysis of the GBD 2010 database. The cause of death for each study subject in the dataset was linked with an appropriate ICD code. These codes were then used to estimate annual deaths for the world and 21 regions.

To address psychiatric disorders, investigators reviewed the codes and determined 20 to be associated with MSDs. To determine YLDs, the authors did a separate literature search and meta-analysis for each code. New disability weights for GBD 2010 were derived from 30,000 face-to-face interviews (Bangladesh, Indonesia, Peru, and Tanzania), telephone interviews (United States), and online (an open-access Web-based survey). Years of life lost to premature mortality (YLLs) were calculated using the standard life expectancy as derived from the GBD 2010 standard model life table.

Follow-Up: N/A

Endpoints:

- Calculated YLLs of subjects in the data set: YLLs are calculated by subtracting the age at death from the standard life expectancy for a person at that age. For example, if the standard life expectancy for men in a given country is 75, but a man dies of cancer at 65, this would be 10 years of life lost due to cancer. This value is then multiplied by the number of deaths to give total YLLs.
- Calculated YLDs of subjects in the dataset: YLDs can be described as years lived in less than ideal health as measured by financial cost, mortality, morbidity, or other indicators. It is measured by taking the prevalence of the condition multiplied by the disability weight for that condition. Disability weights reflect the severity of different conditions.
- Calculated DALYs, a measure of the overall burden from these conditions: DALYS are derived from the sum of YLDs and YLLs (DALYs = YLD +YLL), DALYs describe the number of years lost due to ill health, disability, or early death combined, measuring overall disease burden. It was developed in the 1990s as a way of comparing the overall health and life expectancy of different countries. One DALY equals 1 lost year of health life.

RESULTS

- MSDs were the leading cause of YLDs worldwide, accounting for 175.3 million (22.9% of total) YLDs.
- MSDs accounted for 183.9 million (7.4% of total) DALYs worldwide.

- The burden of MSDs increased by 37.6% between 1990 and 2010, primarily driven by population growth and aging (Tables 19.1 and 19.2).

Table 19.1 Global Disease Burden for Mental Health

Outcome	Depressive disorders (%)	Anxiety disorders (%)	Illicit drug use disorders (%)	Alcohol use disorders (%)	Schizophrenia (%)
YLL	N/A	N/A	41.7	44.4	7.1
YLD	42.5	15.3	9.4	7.9	7.4
DALY	40.5	14.6	10.9	9.6	7.4

NOTES: Percentages as a proportion of total mental health disorders. N/A = not calculated.

Table 19.2 Global Disease Burden for Mental Health Compared to Other Diseases

Measure	CVD (%)	DLRIM (%)	Neonatal disorders (%)	Cancer (%)	MSDs (%)
DALYs	11.9	11.4	8.1	7.6	7.4
YLDs	2.8	2.6	1.2	0.6	22.9
YLLs	15.9	15.4	11.2	10.7	0.5

NOTES: Percentages as a proportion of all causes. CVD = cardiovascular, DLRIM = infectious diseases, MSK = musculoskeletal disorders. DALYs = disability adjusted life years. YLDs = years lived with disability. YLLs = years of life lost to premature mortality.

Criticisms and Limitations: The study had several limitations. First, only 85 of the 187 countries from the original data set were included in this analysis, and there was differential reporting in many places in the world, particularly in low- and middle-income countries, as well as for certain disorders such as the childhood mental disorders. Where this was the case, statistical modeling was used to extrapolate results; therefore, the lack of raw data resulted in wide uncertainty around the findings. Second, there may have been a reporting bias, as not all countries and regions define conditions the same way. Third, the study included only 20 mental health conditions and did not include all substance use disorders. Fourth, deaths that were causally linked to MSDs were largely captured under other causes (e.g., deaths in people with MSDs were coded to the physical cause of death, and suicide was coded to the category of injuries). Thus, this analysis may have underestimated the impact of MSDs as a cause of death. Finally, the disability measured in GBD captures only health loss and does not recognize welfare loss, burden of families or communities, or any loss likely to occur in future.

Other Relevant Studies and Information: These results are supported by previously published epidemiological studies showing that MSDs are prevalent, lead to considerably impairment, and are responsible for substantial morbidity throughout the world.[3,4,5,6] Expansion of treatment options for MSDs could be beneficial and cost-effective from both employer and societal perspectives.[7,8,9,10]

Summary and Implications: The purpose was to describe the mortality and morbidity associated with MSDs at the global, regional, and national level over a three-decade period. The results show that MSDs are the leading cause of disability worldwide, responsible for more global health burden than HIV/AIDS, tuberculosis, diabetes, or transport injuries—thereby highlighting their impact as a significant worldwide public health concern. Moreover, the rates of disability due to MSDs are growing and pose a significant challenge for health systems. As life expectancies continue to rise and disease burden continues to shift from death toward disability, the prevention and treatment of MSDs must be recognize as a global public health priority.

CLINICAL CASE: GLOBAL BURDEN OF MENTAL AND SUBSTANCE USE DISORDERS

Case History

A young man comes to an outpatient psychiatrist at the request of his employer. He has only recently immigrated to the United States from a war-torn area of the world. He states he is having difficulty adjusting to his life here and has had multiple "melt downs" at work. He is initially hesitant to speak about his symptoms, believing open discussion of behaviors and feelings compromises his masculinity. What might the psychiatrist say to help the man feel comfortable?

Suggested Answer

Unfortunately, this scenario is common. Many cultures do not condone speaking openly about mental health issues—some even seeing it as a sign of weakness. However, the GBD study—along with many others—highlights the universality of MSDs throughout the world. Normalizing the young man's hesitation in light of cultural circumstances may help to initiate conversation, after which an explanation of the high prevalence of MSDs globally may allow for further assessment and evaluation of the particulars of his case.

References

1. Whiteford, H. A., Degenhardt, L., Rehm, J., Baxter, A. J., Ferrari, A. J., Erskine, H. E., . . . & Burstein, R. (2013). Global burden of disease attributable to mental and substance use disorders: findings from the Global Burden of Disease Study 2010. *The Lancet, 382*(9904), 1575–1586.
2. Lozano, R., Naghavi, M., Foreman, K., Lim, S., Shibuya, K., Aboyans, V., . . . Memish, Z.A. (2013). Global and regional mortality from 235 causes of death for 20 age groups in 1990 and 2010: a systematic analysis for the Global Burden of Disease Study 2010. *The Lancet*, 380.9859, 2095–2128.
3. Kessler, R. C., Aguilar-Gaxiola, S., Alonso, J., Chatterji, S., Lee, S., Ormel, J., . . . Wang, P. S. (2009). The global burden of mental disorders: An update from the WHO World Mental Health (WMH) surveys. *Epidemiologia e psichiatria sociale, 18*(01), 23–33.
4. Ustün, T. B. (1999). The global burden of mental disorders. *American Journal of Public Health, 89*(9), 1315–1318.
5. Üstün, T. B., Ayuso-Mateos, J. L., Chatterji, S., Mathers, C., & Murray, C. J. (2004). Global burden of depressive disorders in the year 2000. *British Journal of Psychiatry, 184*(5), 386–392.
6. Wittchen, H. U., Jacobi, F., Rehm, J., Gustavsson, A., Svensson, M., Jönsson, B., . . . Fratiglioni, L. (2011). The size and burden of mental disorders and other disorders of the brain in Europe 2010. *European Neuropsychopharmacology, 21*(9), 655–679.
7. Kessler, R. C., Aguilar-Gaxiola, S., Alonso, J., Chatterji, S., Lee, S., Ormel, J., . . . Wang, P. S. (2009). The global burden of mental disorders: an update from the WHO World Mental Health (WMH) surveys. *Epidemiologia e psichiatria sociale, 18*(01), 23–33.
8. Ustün, T. B. (1999). The global burden of mental disorders. *American Journal of Public Health, 89*(9), 1315–1318.
9. Üstün, T. B., Ayuso-Mateos, J. L., Chatterji, S., Mathers, C., & Murray, C. J. (2004). Global burden of depressive disorders in the year 2000. *British Journal of Psychiatry, 184*(5), 386–392.
10. Wittchen, H. U., Jacobi, F., Rehm, J., Gustavsson, A., Svensson, M., Jönsson, B., . . . Fratiglioni, L. (2011). The size and burden of mental disorders and other disorders of the brain in Europe 2010. *European Neuropsychopharmacology, 21*(9), 655–679.

20

Prevalence and Severity of Psychiatric Comorbidities

The National Comorbidity Survey Replication (NCS-R)

STEPHANIE YARNELL AND ELLEN EDENS

> Although mental disorders are widespread, serious cases are concentrated among a relatively small proportion of cases with high comorbidity.
>
> —KESSLER ET AL.[1]

Research Question: What is the prevalence and severity of comorbid anxiety, mood, impulse control, and substance use disorders?

Funding: National Institute of Mental Health and the National Institute on Drug Abuse

Year Study Began: 2001

Year Study Published: 2005

Study Location: Household survey based in the United States

Who Was Studied: English speaking adults aged 18 years and older

Who Was Excluded: Non-English speakers, anyone under 18 years of age, institutionalized persons, and homeless individuals (non-household)

How Many Participants: 9,282 in first wave of interviews; 5,692 in second wave

Study Overview: See Figure 20.1 for a summary of the study design.

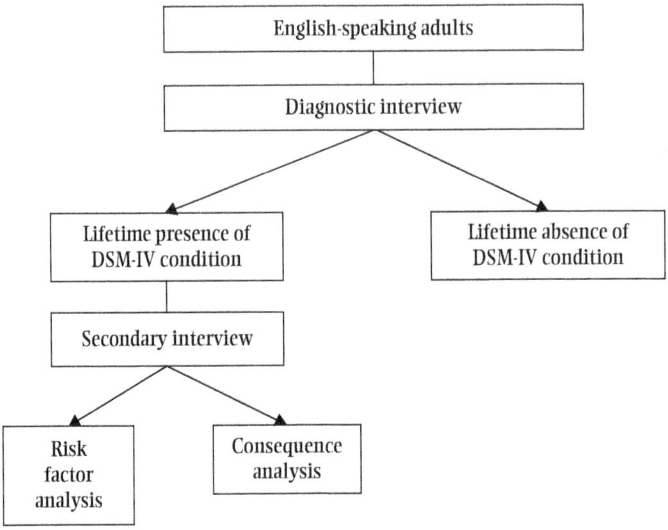

Figure 20.1 Summary of Study Design

Study Design: Participants underwent a structured lay-administered interview using the international World Health Organization–Composite International Diagnostic Interview (WHO-CIDI) evaluating for the presence of DSM-IV anxiety, mood, impulse control, and substance use disorders. While the analysis was limited to adults, participants were screened for childhood diseases through recall-questioning. Mental health issues or comorbidities of late life were not assessed.

If a DSM-IV diagnosis was present, participants were asked to perform dimensional self-ratings to assess risk factors, severity, and perceived impairment. Subsequently, participants were reinterviewed using the Shahan Disability Scale to assess level of functional impairment and severity.

Follow-Up: N/A

Endpoints: Presence of anxiety, mood, impulse control, or substance use disorders by interview

RESULTS

- Of those with diagnosable conditions in the 12 months prior to interview, 55% had a single diagnosis; 45% had two or more co-occurring psychiatric diagnoses.
- The median age of onset for lifetime mental disorder was 14 years. Anxiety (11 years) and impulse control (11 years) disorders present earlier in life; substance use (20 years) and mood (30 years) disorders emerge later. Across diagnoses, three fourths had onset of disease by age 24.
- Approximately one fourth (22.3%) of all 12-month cases were deemed to be severe in nature, while the majority (40.4%) were mild (Table 20.1).

Table 20.1 SUMMARY OF THE NCS-R's KEY FINDINGS

Outcome	**Anxiety Disorders**	**Mood Disorders**	**Impulse Control Disorders**	**Substance Use Disorders**	**Any MH Disorder**
12-month prevalence (SE)	18.1% (0.7)	9.5% (0.4)	8.9% (0.5)	3.8% (0.3)	26.2% (0.3)
Lifetime prevalence (SE)	28.8% (0.9)	20.8% (0.6)	24.8% (1.1)	14.6% (0.6)	46.4% (1.1)

NOTES: NCS-R = National Comorbidity Survey Replication. MH = mental health.

Criticisms and Limitations: The study has several notable limitations regarding inclusion. First, homeless individuals, those in institutions, and non-English speakers were excluded from the analysis, limiting the generalizability of the findings to these populations and ability to make cultural inferences. Moreover, the results may have been impacted by selection bias as the response rate was only 70.9%, and those with mental illness may have been reluctant to participate. Even among those who agreed to be interviewed, a potential reporting bias may exist since mental illness remains stigmatized and unfamiliar to many people and, as a consequence, is commonly underreported.

Additionally, the study only evaluated for a limited number of conditions; it did not include primary psychotic, cognitive, eating, or personality disorders. Finally, interviews were conducted by laypersons ("professional interviewers" from a Social Research Department) and not clinicians trained in the treatment of mental illness, thus introducing the possibility of missed or incorrect diagnoses.

Other Relevant Studies and Information:

- Other relevant studies include the Epidemiological Catchment Area study,[2] the original National Comorbidity Study (NCS),[3] the National Epidemiologic Survey on Alcohol and Related Conditions,[4] and the National Comorbidity Study–Adolescents (NCS-A).
- In 2001 – 2002, respondents of the baseline NCS were reinterviewed (NCS-2) in a follow-up study to evaluate patterns and predictors of mental health and substance use disorders.[5]

Summary and Implications: The NCS (done in the early 1990's) was the first nationally representative mental health epidemiological study to use a structured diagnostic interview to estimate the prevalence and correlates of mental disorders. The NCS-R, completed in 2005, was a replication survey conducted between 2001 and 2003, with analysis of time trends and expanded the assessment of certain diseases. The findings of the NCS-R showed that past year prevalence rates for anxiety, mood, impulse control, or substance use disorders within the United States are high with anxiety and mood disorders being the most common. The lifetime prevalence of mental health disorders including anxiety, mood, impulse control, or substance use disorders within the United States approach 50%, while the 12-month prevalence is approximately 25%.

Additionally, a substantial percentage, 14% of the population, suffer from symptoms in the moderate to severe range. A very substantial minority of people with past-year diagnosis (40%) had another, co-occurring mental health disorder; the severity of disease was strongly correlated with comorbidity. These results suggest that while the majority of cases of anxiety, mood, impulse control, or substance use disorders are mild, they remain highly prevalent in the population. Those suffering from moderate to severe disease are at increased likelihood of having two or more mental health diagnoses compared to those with mild disease.

CLINICAL CASE: PREVALENCE AND SEVERITY OF PSYCHIATRIC COMORBIDITIES

Case History

A 38-year-old mother of two comes into an outpatient psychiatrist's office complaining of severe anxiety. She is afraid to speak with anyone about it and has become very isolative in the wake of these symptoms. Her husband is concerned that she is becoming depressed as a result of impairments brought on by her anxiety. They want to know if this is possible and if there is help available.

Suggested Answer

According to the results of the NCS-R, anxiety is the most common mental disorder in the United States, with approximately 20% of the population meeting DSM-IV criteria for an anxiety disorder in any 12-month period. Co-occurrence of mental illness (i.e., having more than one diagnosable condition at a time) is common. Indeed, approximately 45% of individuals suffer from two or more co-occurring conditions; rates are higher in persons diagnosed with severe impairments. Given this, it is likely she has developed a second diagnosis in the wake of severe anxiety. Anxiety and depression are the two most common mental health disorders, and both are treatable.

References

1. Kessler, R. C., Chiu, W. T., Demler, O., & Walters, E. E. (2005). Prevalence, severity, and comorbidity of twelve-month DSM-IV disorders in the National Comorbidity Survey Replication (NCS-R). *Archives of General Psychiatry, 62*(6), 617–627.
2. Regier, D. A., Myers, J. K., Kramer, M., Robins, L. N., Blazer, D. G., Hough, R. L., . . . Locke, B. Z. (1984). The NIMH Epidemiologic Catchment Area program: Historical context, major objectives, and study population characteristics. *Archives of General Psychiatry, 41*(10), 934–941.
3. Kessler, R. C., McGonagle, K. A., Zhao, S., Nelson, C. B., Hughes, M., Eshleman, S., . . . Kindler, K. S. (1994). Lifetime and 12-month prevalence of DSM-III-R psychiatric disorders in the United States: Results from the National Comorbidity Survey. *Archives of General Psychiatry, 51*(1), 8–19.
4. Grant, B. F., Stinson, F. S., Dawson, D. A., Chou, S. P., Ruan, W. J., & Pickering, R. P. (2003). *Source and accuracy statement: Wave 1 national epidemiologic survey on alcohol and related conditions (NESARC)*. Bethesda, MD: National Institute on Alcohol Abuse and Alcoholism.
5. Kessler, R. (2015). *National Comorbidity Survey: Reinterview (NCS-2), 2001–2002*. Ann Arbor, MI: Inter-university Consortium for Political and Social Research.

SECTION 6

Insomnia

21

Behavioral and/or Pharmacotherapy for Older Patients with Insomnia

ROBERT ROSS AND RAJESH R. TAMPI

> Behavioral and pharmacological approaches are effective for short-term management of insomnia in late life; sleep improvements are better sustained over time with behavioral approaches.
>
> —Morin et al.[1]

Research Question: Should older patients with insomnia be managed with cognitive behavioral therapy (CBT), benzodiazepines, or both?

Funding: The National Institute of Mental Health

Year Study Began: 1996

Year Study Published: 1999

Study Location: Medical College of Virginia/Virginia Commonwealth University

Who Was Studied: Adults with at least six months of sleep onset or maintenance insomnia who were at least 55 years old. Participants also had at least one consequence of insomnia (e.g., daytime fatigue, impaired functioning or mood problems).

Who Was Excluded: Patients with sleep apnea or a comorbid medical condition that interferes with sleep were excluded. Those taking psychotropic medications, suffering from significant psychopathology including major depression, currently in psychotherapy, or cognitive impairment defined as scoring <23 on the Mini-Mental Status Examination were also excluded.

How Many Participants: 78

Study Overview: See Figure 21.1 for a summary of the study design.

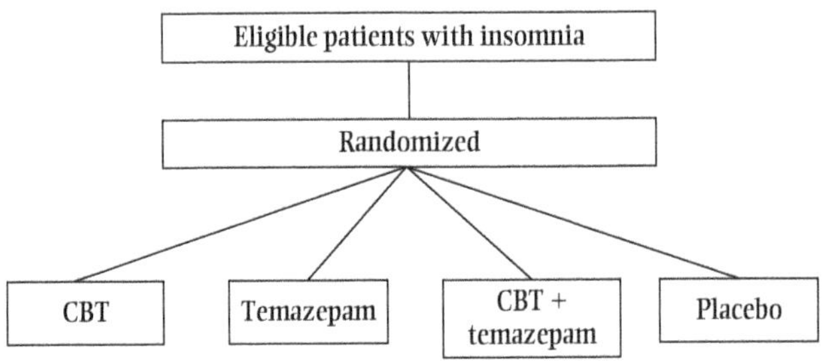

Figure 21.1 Summary of Study Design
NOTE: CBT = cognitive behavioral therapy.

Study Intervention: Patients randomized to CBT groups received CBT in groups of four to six including sleep restriction therapy, stimulus control therapy, cognitive therapy designed to change faulty sleep beliefs, and sleep education. Therapy took place as 90-minute weekly sessions for 8 weeks. Therapists were either postdoctoral fellows in clinical psychology or licensed clinical psychologists with experience treating at least 4 patients using the protocol.

Patients randomized to the temazepam groups received temazepam at an initial nightly dose of 7.5 mg with the option to titrate to maximum dose of 30 mg per night. Patients were to take the medication 1 hour prior to bedtime and use the medication a minimum of two to three nights per week. Patients could use the medication every night if needed. The patients would meet with a physician for 20 minutes per week for medication management consultation. Medication was prescribed by a third-year psychiatry resident.

Patients in the combined group received both CBT and pharmacotherapy. Patients in the placebo group received placebo medication only. No sham CBT was offered.

Follow-Up: Treatment lasted for 8 weeks. After completion of treatment all treated participants were followed up by mail at 3, 12, and 24 months.

Endpoints: Wake after sleep onset, sleep efficiency, total wake time, total sleep time, polysomnography, Sleep Impairment Index

RESULTS

- At the conclusion of eight weeks of treatment, all interventions showed a benefit with respect to the endpoints wake after sleep onset, sleep efficiency, total wake time, and total sleep time.
- All interventions increased the number of patients who met the criteria for normal sleep (sleep efficacy of >85%) after eight weeks of treatment. The number of subjects who had normal sleep in each group were as follows: 55.6% (CBT), 47.1% (pharmacotherapy), 68.8% (combined therapy), and 22.2% (placebo).
- All interventions also yielded a significant decrease in number of patients meeting criteria for insomnia after eight weeks of treatment. The number of subjects who no longer met the diagnostic criteria for insomnia in each group were as follows: 78% (CBT), 56% (pharmacotherapy), 75% (combined therapy), and 14% (placebo).
- At eight weeks, there was a non-significant trend suggesting combined therapy was more effective than CBT or pharmacotherapy alone. For example, wake after sleep percentage improvements were 63.5% (combined), 55% (CBT), 46.5% (pharmacotherapy), and 16.9% (placebo).
- Only the combined treatment group showed improvements on polysomnography at eight weeks ($p < 0.05$) when compared to placebo.
- On the Sleep Impairment Index patients in the CBT and combined groups rated themselves as being less impaired than in the pharmacotherapy ($p = 0.01$) or placebo groups ($p = 0.002$). More patients rated themselves as being more satisfied, less distressed, and with less interference in daytime functioning in the combined and CBT groups when compared to the pharmacotherapy ($p < 0.05$) or placebo ($p < 0.05$) groups.
- At 24-month follow-up, the CBT group had no significant change in total wake time, sleep efficiency, and wake after sleep onset relative to the conclusion of the eight-week intervention.

- At 24-months follow-up, the pharmacologic intervention group scored significantly worse than at the conclusion of the eight-week intervention with respect to total wake time ($p = 0.04$), sleep efficiency ($p = 0.03$), and wake after sleep onset. The combined group also scored worse with respect to all three measures ($p < 0.05$) (Table 21.1).

Table 21.1 Summary of Key Findings

Outcome	CBT	Temazepam	CBT + Temazepam	Placebo
Wake after Sleep Onset at 8 weeks (SD)	22.29 (17.9)	29.48 (19.5)	20.78 (20.2)	51.73 (22.7)
Wake after Sleep Onset at 24 months (SD)	33.06 (41.3)	50.50 (29.5)	39.67 (38.0)	59.93 (48.5)
Sleep efficiency at 8 weeks (SD)	84.80 (7.2)	82.68 (6.4)	84.86 (11.6)	73.49 (11.4)
Sleep efficiency at 24 months (SD)	84.70 (12.2)	75.28 (8.2)	77.87 (19.1)	74.30 (13.7)

NOTE: CBT = cognitive behavioral therapy.

Criticisms and Limitations: The trial assessed only one medication when a number of medications are recommended by the American Academy of Sleep Medicine.[2] Other medications may yield somewhat more lasting benefit or may work better in concert with CBT. The trial was also relatively limited in power, which may have prevented it from detecting a significant benefit from combined CBT and medication therapy.

Importantly, the study excluded those patients with insomnia secondary to medical conditions and adverse medication side effects. It also excluded patients taking psychotropic medications, suffering from serious psychopathology, or suffering from cognitive impairment. The study conclusions may not be generalizable to these groups.

Other Relevant Studies and Information:

- The American College of Physicians recommends CBT for insomnia as first-line treatment. Medication may be added short-term on a case-by-case basis. These recommendations are consistent with and cite this study.[3]

- Another large randomized trial compared CBT to zopiclone with similar results.[4]
- Other studies have demonstrated CBT for treatment of insomnia is effective using internet and video telehealth delivery methods[5,6] and can also provide benefit to those with insomnia and major depression.[7]

Summary and Implications: Insomnia is a common clinical problem, especially in the elderly. This landmark study found that in older adults, benzodiazepine-temazepam, CBT, and a combination of CBT and temazepam are equally effective in the short term for the treatment of insomnia. The benefits of CBT are much more durable than treatment with benzodiazepine or combination therapy. Because CBT is safe and more effective in the long term, it should be the preferred strategy for treating most otherwise healthy older adults with insomnia. However, these findings do not necessarily apply to younger patients and those with serious medical conditions causing insomnia, psychopathology, or cognitive impairment who were not included in the study. The study shows long-term superiority of CBT relative to benzodiazepines but cannot be generalized to other hypnotic agents either alone or in combination with CBT.

CLINICAL CASE: BEHAVIORAL AND/OR PHARMACOTHERAPY FOR OLDER PATIENTS WITH INSOMNIA

Case History

A 67-year-old woman with well-controlled hypertension and obesity reports that she is having trouble sleeping during a routine appointment with her primary care physician (PCP). Screening for psychiatric disorders is unrevealing. Her Sleep Impairment Index is 20. She tells you she has been having this problem for two years. She has tried Benadryl on occasion with some benefit, but she feels it makes her even less alert during the day.

She undergoes polysomnography, which is consistent with insomnia without obstructive sleep apnea or periodic movement syndrome. The PCP calls psychiatry for a "curbside" consult by phone to provide recommendations for the patient. Based on the results of this study, how should this patient be treated?

Suggested Answer

This study showed that behavioral interventions are at least as effective as pharmacologic interventions in the short term and provide much more durable benefit and patient satisfaction. The study found modest short-term benefit, which fell short of statistical significance, for combined therapy of CBT and temazepam and revealed better long-term outcomes for patients receiving CBT alone.

The patient in this vignette is typical of patients included in this study. She meets the definition of insomnia, has been experiencing symptoms for at least 6 months, does not have a medical or psychiatric condition that could explain her insomnia, and is not already frequently using medication to help her sleep. Thus, she should be treated initially with a behavioral intervention (90 minutes per week of CBT).

References

1. Morin, C. M., Colecchi, C., Stone J., Sood, R., & Brink, D. (1999). Behavioral and pharmacological therapies for late-life insomnia: A randomized controlled trial. *JAMA, 281*(11), 991–999.
2. Sateia, M. J., Buysse, D. J., Krystal, A. D., Neubauer, D. N., & Heald, J. L. (2017). Clinical practice guideline for the pharmacologic treatment of chronic insomnia in adults: An American Academy of Sleep Medicine Clinical Practice Guideline. *Journal of Clinical Sleep Medicine, 13*(2), 307–349.
3. Qaseem, A., Kansagara, D., Forciea, M. A., Cooke, M., & Denberg, T. D. (2016). Management of chronic insomnia disorder in adults: A clinical practice guideline from the American College of Physicians. *Annals of Internal Medicine, 165*(2), 125–133.
4. Omvik, S., Pallesen, S., Havik, O. E., Kvale, G., & Nordhus, I. H. (2006). Cognitive behavioral therapy vs zopiclone for treatment of chronic primary insomnia in older adults: a randomized controlled trial. *JAMA, 295*(24), 2851–2858.
5. Ritterband, L. M., Thorndike, F. P., Ingersoll, K. S., Lord, H. R., Gonder-Frederick, L., Frederick, C., . . . Morin, C. M. (2017). Effect of a web-based cognitive behavior therapy for insomnia intervention with 1-year follow-up: a randomized clinical trial *JAMA Psychiatry, 74*(1), 68–75.
6. Gehrman, P., Shah, M. T., Miles, A., Kuna, S., & Godleski, L. (2016). Feasibility of group cognitive-behavioral treatment of insomnia delivered by clinical video telehealth. *Telemedicine and e-Health, 22*(12), 1041–1046.
7. Manber, R., Buysse, D. J., Edinger, J., Krystal, A., Luther, J. F., Wisniewski, S. R., . . . Thase, M. E. (2016). Efficacy of cognitive-behavioral therapy for insomnia combined with antidepressant pharmacotherapy in patients with comorbid depression and insomnia: A randomized controlled trial. *Journal of Clinical Psychiatry, 77*(10), e1316–e1323.

SECTION 7

Major Depressive Disorder

22

Treatment of Depression in Patients with Alcohol or Drug Dependence

A Meta-Analysis

J. COREY WILLIAMS AND GUSTAVO A. ANGARITA AFRICANO

> Drug or alcohol abuse [should] not be a barrier to treatment of depression . . . care is needed in diagnosis either to observe patients during at least a brief period of abstinence prior to diagnosis and treatment of depression or to make efforts to distinguish treatable depression by history.
>
> —NUNES AND LEVIN[1]

Research Question: Are antidepressants efficacious in treatment of combined depression and substance use disorders?

Funding: National Institute on Drug Abuse

Year Study Began: Studies between 1970 and 2003

Year Study Published: 2004

Study Location: Studies included in the meta-analysis were conducted in a variety of academic and community settings, such as Columbia University, University of Miami, and Milan, Italy.

Who Was Studied: Adult patients who met DSM-III, DSM-III-R, or DSM-IV diagnostic criteria for an illicit drug (6 studies) or alcohol-use disorder (8 studies) and a unipolar depressive disorder. Also, prospective, double-blind, placebo-controlled randomized trials of antidepressants versus placebo were included.

Who Was Excluded: Observational studies were excluded from this meta-analysis.

How Many Participants: 848

Study Overview: See Figure 22.1 for a summary of a typical study included.

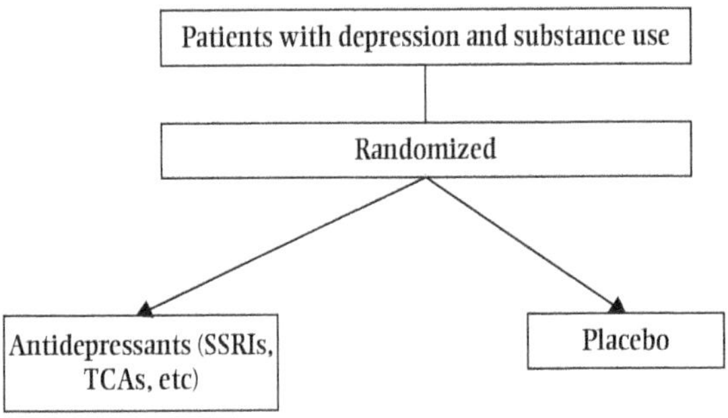

Figure 22.1 Summary of a Typical Study Included
NOTES: SSRI = selective serotonin reuptake inhibitor. TCA = tricyclic antidepressants.

Study Intervention: All patients included in the meta-analysis received antidepressant medications (i.e., selective serotonin reuptake inhibitors (SSRIs), tricyclic antidepressants (TCAs), or other antidepressants) or placebo therapy.

Follow-Up: 6 weeks (1 trial), 8 weeks (1 trial), 12 weeks (10 trials), 14 weeks (1 trial), 24 weeks (1 trial)

Endpoints: Primary outcome: Hamilton Depression Scale (HDS) score. Secondary outcomes: self-reported categorical response measures of substance use (i.e., abstinence or sustained remission) and continuous measures of substance use (i.e., quantity of use).

RESULTS

- Eight studies demonstrated significant benefits of anti-depressant medications while six studies showed no benefit.
- In studies that had a large treatment response for depression (i.e., effect size of >0.5 on the HDS), medication significantly improved substance abuse.
- In studies that had a low rate of placebo response (i.e., <25% improvement in the placebo group), medications improved depressive symptoms to a large degree.
- There was a trend toward greater benefit of medications among patients dependent on alcohol (although only explains 7% of the variance).
- Being inpatient or having at least a week of abstinence had a significant positive effect on the depression outcomes.
- Studies using SSRIs had a smaller pooled effect size compared to studies using TCAs (Tables 22.1 and 22.2)

Table 22.1 Antidepressant Effect on Depression

Outcome	**Studies with a placebo response of <25%**	**Studies with a placebo response >25%**
Pooled antidepressant effect size (Hamilton Depression Scale)	0.68 (0.49 to 0.88)[a]	0.08 (−0.11–0.27)[a]
Pooled sample size	407	420

[a]Larger effect size represents a stronger effect of the antidepressant medication.

Table 22.2 Antidepressant Effect on Substance Abuse

Outcome	**Depression effect size <0.50**	**Depression effect size >0.50**
Pooled medication effect on substance abuse	0.07 (−0.11 to 0.25)[a]	0.56 (0.33 to 0.79)[a]
Pooled sample size	479	306

[a]Larger effect size represents a stronger effect of medication on quantity of substance abuse (mostly self-report).

Criticisms and Limitations: Reviewed studies used mainly self-reported measures of substance abuse, which could introduce recall bias, rather than objective measures of substance use (i.e., urine toxicology).

Like other meta-analyses, studies were not conducted specifically to test the same clinical question, which leads to a heterogeneous study population. For instance, there was significant variability in treatment setting and length of abstinence. Furthermore, the study settings varied considerably (i.e., outpatient, inpatient, methadone programs, etc.). These differences in populations studied and the study settings may also be interpreted as a strength of the study when thinking about external validity.

Other Relevant Studies and Information:

- Other studies have similarly found that depression can be treated effectively in the setting of active substance abuse with modest, if any, effects on the substance use-related outcome.[2,3,4]
- Another systematic review and meta-analysis showed that treatment of depression with antidepressant medications in the setting of alcohol use disorder was associated with large improvements in depression, especially if the depression was independent of the alcohol use. Evidence was less robust for substance-induced depression.[5]
- American Psychiatric Association guidelines recommend that clinicians should address co-occurring psychiatric illness (such as substance abuse) as part of the mood disorders treatment plan. Whenever possible, a period of substance abstinence can help determine whether the depressive episode is related to intoxication or withdrawal-states.[6]

Summary and Implications: This meta-analysis found that antidepressants were effective for the treatment of depression among patients with co-occurring drug/alcohol dependence. This finding suggests that in appropriate circumstances it is beneficial to treat depression among active substance users. Whenever possible, when treating patients with co-occurring depression and drug/alcohol dependence a period of substance abstinence can help determine whether the depressive episode is related to intoxication or withdrawal states. It may also be advisable to start initial therapy with a psychosocial intervention among patients with substance abuse disorders, reserving medications for those with an inadequate response to initial treatment.

CLINICAL CASE: TREATMENT OF DEPRESSION WITH CONCURRENT DRUG DEPENDENCE

Case History

A 28-year-old White man was admitted to the inpatient psychiatry ward for safety because of suicidal ideation and depressed mood. He has a history of cannabis, alcohol, and cocaine use disorders and had been sober for five months. He reported that he relapsed on each of these substances one week ago. He said that his mood has been low for several weeks prior to this and has had trouble sleeping, poor appetite, and low energy. He has never been prescribed an antidepressant.

Based on the results of this meta-analysis, how should this patient be treated?

Suggested Answer

This meta-analysis found that it may be beneficial to treat patients with comorbid mood and substance use disorders with antidepressants. Substance-induced and primary mood disorders are difficult to distinguish clinically, so in some cases an antidepressant may be indicated.

The patient in this vignette is typical of the patients included in the studies used in this meta-analysis. Although this study did not recommend a particular agent, SSRIs and TCAs were a significant moderator of clinical effect along with concurrent psychosocial treatment (i.e., CBT or relapse prevention). It is possible that his depressive disorder may improve in a short time with a period of abstinence. The findings of this study support waiting for at least a week of abstinence in an inpatient or outpatient setting before treating depression, as a period of abstinence was associated with greater antidepressant effect.

References

1. Nunes, E. V., & Levin, F. R. (2004). Treatment of depression in patients with alcohol or other drug dependence: A meta-analysis. *JAMA, 291*(15), 1887–1896.
2. Ciraulo, D. A., & Jaffe, J. H. (1981). Tricyclic antidepressants in the treatment of depression associated with alcoholism. *Journal of Clinical Psychopharmacology, 1*(3), 146–150.
3. Nunes, E. V., Quitkin, F. M., Donovan, S. J., Deliyannides, D., Ocepek-Welikson, K., Koenig, T., . . . Woody, G. (1998). Imipramine treatment of opiate-dependent patients with depressive disorders: a placebo-controlled trial. *Archives of General Psychiatry, 55*, 153–160.

4. Nunes, E., Quitkin, F., Brady, R., & Post-Koenig, T. (1994). Antidepressant treatment in methadone maintenance patients. *Journal of Addictive Diseases, 13*(3), 13–24.
5. Foulds, J. A., Adamson, S. J., Boden, J. M., Williman, J. A., & Mulder, R. T. (2015). Depression in patients with alcohol use disorders: Systematic review and meta-analysis of outcomes for independent and substance-induced disorders. *Journal of Affective Disorders, 185*, 47–59.
6. Gelenberg, A. J. Freeman, M. P., Markowitz, J. C., Rosenbaum, J. F., Thase, M. E., Trivedi, M. H., & Van Rhoads, R. S. (2010). *APA Practice guideline for the treatment of patients with major depressive disorder* (3rd ed.). Washington, DC: American Psychiatric Association, pp. 20–21.

23

Suicidality in Pediatric Patients Treated with Antidepressant Drugs

FDA Meta-Analysis

DAVID SAUNDERS AND MICHAEL H. BLOCH

> The apparent increased risk of drug-induced suicidality may actually represent a greater likelihood of reporting of suicidality events by patients rather than an increased rate of the events themselves. . . . It is important to be clear that the FDA has not contraindicated any of the antidepressant drugs for pediatric use.
>
> —HAMMAD ET AL.[1]

Research Question: Do antidepressants increase suicidality in children and adolescents?

Funding: FDA

Year Study Began: Studies between 1983 and 2001

Year Study Published: 2006

Study Location: Studies included in this meta-analysis were done in various community, academic, and National Institute of Mental Health-supported centers throughout the United States.

Who Was Studied: Pediatric patients between 6 and 18 years of age participating in placebo-controlled trials and being treated with antidepressants for major depressive disorder (16 trials), obsessive-compulsive disorder (4 trials) generalized anxiety disorder (2 trials), attention-deficit/hyperactivity disorder (1 trial), and social anxiety disorder (1 trial).

Who Was Excluded: Patients outside the exposure window of 4 to 16 weeks after initiation of antidepressant treatment.

How Many Participants: 4,582

Study Overview: See Figure 23.1 for a summary of typical studies included in FDA pediatric antidepressant meta-analysis.

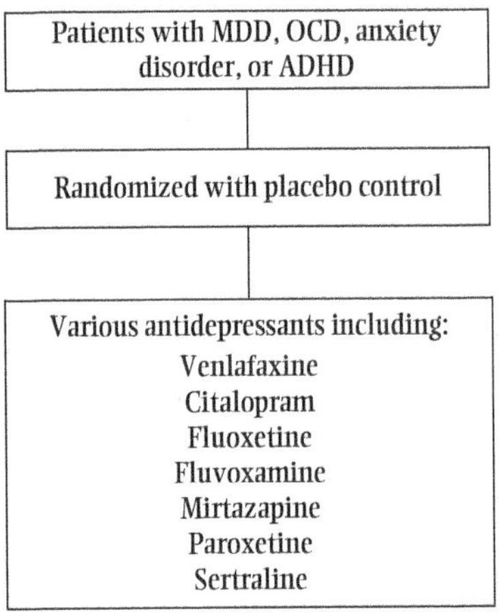

Figure 23.1 Summary of Typical Studies Included in FDA Pediatric Antidepressant Meta-Analysis
NOTES: MMD = major mental disorder. OCD = obsessive-compulsive disorder. ADHD = attention deficit/hyperactivity disorder.

Study Design: A meta-analysis was conducted to obtain overall suicidality risk estimates for selective serotonin reuptake inhibitors (SSRIs) in depression trials as a group, for each drug individually and for all evaluable trials combined (regardless of indication). A total of 23 randomized placebo-controlled studies were included in the meta-analysis.

Follow-Up: 4 to 16 weeks after initiation of antidepressant treatment

Endpoints: The primary outcome was spontaneously reported "suicidal behavior or ideation," a surrogate for suicide attempt, preparatory events toward imminent suicidal behavior, and suicidal ideation. The secondary outcome was "possible suicidal behavior or ideation," including the three previously stated behaviors or ideations plus self-injury with intent unknown and injury events with not enough information to determine whether they represented self-injury or other injury. Finally, the suicide item scores from the depression scales used in the trials were used to assess for worsening of suicidality or the emergence of suicidality based on data collected from all subjects included in the trials.

RESULTS

- There were no completed suicides in any of the trials evaluated.
- The multicenter Treatment of Adolescent Depression Study (TADS) was the only individual trial to demonstrate a statistically significant risk ratio for spontaneously reported suicidality in an antidepressant compared to placebo (4.62; 95% CI [1.02, 20.92]).
- The relative risk of spontaneously reported suicidality for SSRIs compared to placebo was 1.66 (95% CI [1.02, 2.68]) and for all antidepressants was 1.95 (95% CI [1.28, 2.98]).
- For every 100 pediatric patients treated with SSRIs for depression, one to three more patients spontaneously reported suicidal ideation or behavior than would have otherwise occurred on placebo.
- When suicidal ideation was assessed systematically using the individual suicide related items of depression ratings scales (rather than based on spontaneous report), there was a nonsignificant decrease in the risk of worsening suicidal ideation (RR = 0.92, 95% CI [0.72, 1.11]) or emergence of suicidal ideation (RR = 0.93, 95% CI [0.75, 1.15]) on antidepressant agents compared to placebo (Table 23.1).

Table 23.1 Summary of FDA Pediatric Antidepressant Meta-Analysis

Outcome	**SSRIs**	**All antidepressants**
Risk ratio of spontaneous report of suicidal ideation vs. placebo (95% CI)	1.66 (1.02–2.68)	1.95 (1.28–2.98)
Risk ratio of emergence of suicidality as assessed by suicide item score vs. placebo		0.92 (0.76–1.15)
Risk ratio of worsening of suicidality as assessed by suicide item score vs. placebo		0.93 (0.75–1.15)

Notes: FDA = Food and Drug Administration. SSRIs = selective serotonin reuptake inhibitors.

Criticisms and Limitations: There are several reasons that antidepressant medications might increase spontaneously reported suicidality but not increase overall suicidality when assessed systematically with standard questionnaires: (a) Since not all patients who experience suicidal ideation report it to their doctors, antidepressants may decrease other symptoms of anxiety or depression (low energy) that may make patients initially less likely to report suicidal ideation. and (b) patients who experience one side effect in a clinical trial (e.g., headache, sleep problems, sexual dysfunction, gastrointestinal symptoms, which are all more likely on antidepressants) are more likely to be systematically asked and then report other side effects, including suicidal ideation.

Another limitation is that the risk of suicidality beyond 16 weeks was not evaluated.

Furthermore, the study does not compare the 9 different drugs studied and relies on pooling of adverse events from all antidepressants, requiring one to assume that the rate of suicidality is similar in all drugs within the class.

Finally, dose effect was not assessed in this study.

Other Relevant Studies and Information:

- The data from this meta-analysis prompted the FDA to issue a black box warning on antidepressant medication use in pediatric populations, stating that "antidepressants may increase the risk of suicidal thinking and behavior in some children and adolescents." Antidepressant medications were associated with increased risk of suicidal ideation and behavior when these symptoms were reported spontaneously, but not when they were assessed systematically using rating scales.[2]
- Several studies have found a decline in the prescription of SSRIs in young people after the black box warning for pediatric suicidality was issued in 2007.[3,4]
- There was an increase in the overall adolescent suicide rate in United States after the black box warning was issued. It is hypothesized to be related to decreased antidepressant treatment in this population.
- Based on the results of this meta-analysis and subsequent research, the American Academy of Child and Adolescent Psychiatry (AACAP) concludes that the overall risk/benefit ratio for SSRIs is nevertheless favorable as long as careful monitoring is in place.

Summary and Implications: This meta-analysis provided the evidence that led to the FDA placing a black box warning to caution the use of antidepressants in pediatric populations due to the increased risk of spontaneously reported suicidal ideation and behavior on antidepressant medications compared to placebo.

The study did not suggest an increased risk of suicidality with antidepressants when suicidality was assessed using standard questionnaires, however. The FDA also noted that the increased use of SSRIs has coincided with a dramatic decline in adolescent suicide, so the findings should be interpreted with caution.[5]

CLINICAL CASE: SUICIDALITY IN PEDIATRIC PATIENTS TREATED WITH ANTIDEPRESSANT DRUGS

Case History

A 13-year-old girl is brought to your clinic by her parents because she has been sad for the past 6 months. She is having difficulty falling asleep; she is only eating one meal per day because she says that she is not hungry, and she has lost 15 pounds in the last three months; she is struggling in school, saying that she just can't pay attention; she quit track and field and just goes home after school; and she recently asked her best friend if she ever thought about killing herself.

Her parents are concerned that she is depressed and want to know what is the best treatment for adolescent depression. They read online that SSRI use in pediatric populations is associated with an increased risk of suicide.

What do you tell the patient and her parents about SSRI and suicidality?

Suggested Answer

While a recent review of SSRI use in pediatric populations suggests that SSRIs are associated with an increased risk of spontaneously reported suicidal ideation or behavior, there is no evidence that antidepressant use is associated with suicide attempts or completion (or even worsening or emergence of suicidal ideation when assessed systematically). In fact, there is some evidence that antidepressant medications are protective against attempted and completed suicide. In the over 4,500+ children who participated in pediatric antidepressant trials, there were no completed suicides.

Based on the FDA black box warning and AACAP guidelines, if a SSRI is started, the clinician should warn and closely follow the patient weekly for at least four weeks and then biweekly thereafter, with closer monitoring for patients at an increased risk of suicide, such as those with a previous attempt, family history of suicide, a substance use disorder, history of abuse, and so on.[6] This close monitoring of depressed adolescents makes good clinical sense, regardless of whether a new medication is actually prescribed, as suicide is the second-leading cause of death in this age group.

References

1. Hammad, T. A., Laughren, T., & Racoosin, J. (2006). Suicidality in pediatric patients treated with antidepressant drugs. *Archives of General Psychiatry, 63*(3), 332–339.
2. Food and Drug Administration. (2007). *FDA proposes new warnings about suicidal thinking, behavior in young adults who take antidepressant medications*. Washington, DC: Author.
3. Libby, A. M., Orton, H. D., & Valuck, R. J. (2009). Persisting decline in depression treatment after FDA warnings. *Archives of General Psychiatry, 66*(6), 633–639.
4. Lu, C. Y., Zhang, F., Lakoma, M. D., Madden, J. M., Rusinak, D., Penford, R. B., . . . Soumerai, S. B. (2014). Changes in antidepressant use by young people and suicidal behavior after FDA warnings and media coverage: quasi-experimental study. *BMJ, 348*, g3596.
5. Birmhaer, B. D., Brent, D., AACAP Work Group on Quality Issues, Bernet, W., Bukstein, O., Walter, H., . . . Medicus, J. (2007). Practice parameter for the assessment and treatment of children and adolescents with depressive disorders. *Journal of the American Academy of Child and Adolescent Psychiatry, 46*(11), 1503–1526.

24

National Institute of Mental Health (NIMH) Treatment of Depression Collaborative Research Program

JOSEPH J. TAYLOR AND ROBERT OSTROFF

> There was a consistent ordering of treatments at termination, with imipramine plus clinical management generally doing best, placebo plus clinical management worst, and the two psychotherapies in between but generally closer to imipramine plus clinical management.
>
> —Elkin et al.[1]

Research Question: How do cognitive behavioral therapy (CBT), interpersonal therapy (IPT) and imipramine (IMI) compare to one another and to placebo in the treatment of unipolar nonpsychotic depression?

Funding: Cooperative agreement between the NIMH and participating sites

Year Study Began: 1980

Year Study Published: 1989

Study Location: Outpatient psychiatric clinics at three US academic medical centers

Who Was Studied: Patients in an active depressive episode based on Research Diagnostic Criteria (RDC)[2] with a 17-item Hamilton Rating Scale for Depression (HSRD) score >14.

Who Was Excluded: Patients with active suicidal ideation were excluded, as were patients with other diagnoses (e.g., certain personality disorders, active substance abuse or cognitive impairment). Patients with significant neurological or general medical conditions were also excluded.

How Many Participants: 250

Study Overview: See Figure 24.1 for a summary of the study design.

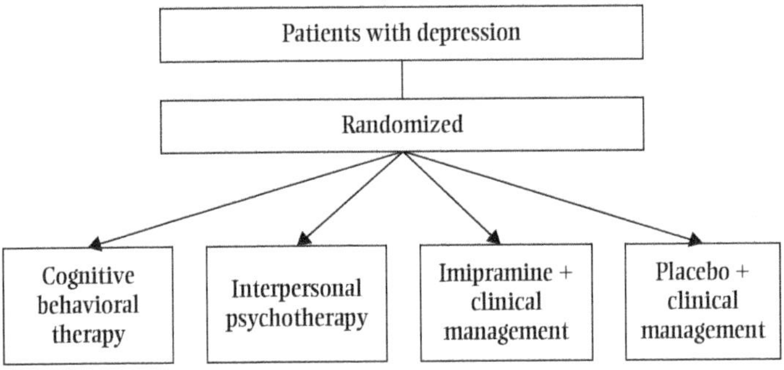

Figure 24.1 Summary of Study Design

Study Intervention: A clinical evaluator screened prospective study participants referred from outpatient clinics and healthcare facilities. After a 7- to 14-day drug washout period, qualified participants were rescreened and asked to provide informed consent. Each participant was randomized to one of four 16-week treatment arms: (a) IPT, (b) CBT, (c) IMI and clinical management (CM; IMI-CM), or (d) placebo–CM (PLA-CM).

A group of therapists (10 psychologists and 18 psychiatrists) with an average of 11 years of experience were responsible for delivering CBT and IPT. All therapists completed a standardized training program. The audiotapes from these training sessions were evaluated via the Collaborative Study Psychotherapy Rating Scale. CBT consisted of weekly one-hour sessions focused on modifying negative automatic thoughts and challenging cognitive distortions. IPT consisted of weekly one-hour sessions focused on identifying interpersonal issues and establishing more adaptive relationships.

IMI and PLA were administered in a double-blind fashion in the context of weekly CM sessions. The average dose of IMI among those who completed the study was 185 mg (averaged over all weeks after the first two weeks of treatment). CM was described as a "minimally supportive therapy" condition designed to standardize clinical care, maximize compliance, and ensure patient safety. These sessions initially lasted 45 to 60 minutes but were subsequently reduced to 20 to 30 minutes as the study progressed.

Follow-Up: Across-treatment assessments were performed at 4, 8, 12, and 16 weeks. Follow-up assessments were performed at 6, 12, and 18 months after treatment.

Endpoints: Four scales were identified *a priori* and measured by independent clinical evaluators: (a) 17-item HSRD, (b) Global Assessment Scale (GAS), (c) Beck Depression Inventory (BDI), and (d) Hopkins Symptom Checklist–90 Total Score (HSCL-90T).

RESULTS

- Patients in all treatment arms had significantly fewer depressive symptoms at the conclusion of the treatment condition (including PLA-CM).
- Relative to the PLA-CM group, the IMI-CM group had statistically superior outcomes. There were no other significant differences in outcomes among the treatment groups but there was a nonsignificant trend favoring the IMI group versus the two psychotherapy groups. (see Table 24.1)

Table 24.1 Summary of NIMH Collaborative Study Findings (Completers)

Outcome	**CBT**	**IPT**	**IMI-CM**	**PLA-CM**
HSRD	19.2→7.6	18.9→6.9	19.2→7.0	19.1→8.8
GAS	52.8→69.4	52.6→70.7	51.6→72.5	53.1→67.6
BDI	26.8→10.2	25.5→7.7	27.1→6.5	28.1→11.0
HSCL-90T	1.38→0.47	1.35→0.48	1.43→0.38*	1.58→0.67

NOTES: Values are reported as pre- and post-study. NIMH = National Institute of Mental Health. CBT = cognitive behavioral therapy. IPT = interpersonal therapy. IMI-CM = Imipramine–clinical management. PLA-CM = placebo–clinical management. HSRD = Hamilton Rating Scale for Depression. GAS = Global Assessment Scale. BDI = Beck Depression Inventory. HSCL-90T = Hopkins Symptom Checklist–90 Total Score.

*Significant difference from PLA-CM ($P < 0.017$, $P < 0.1$ with Bonferroni correction).

Criticisms and Limitations: There are several criticisms and limitations but only a few will be mentioned here. First, participants with comorbid psychiatric disorders, suicidal ideation or general medical or neurological conditions were excluded from the study. These exclusion criteria raise questions about the generalizability of the findings. Second, the results of the study could be confounded by depression severity since those who dropped out of the study were significantly more depressed at intake than those who completed the study. Third, IMI is no longer considered a first-line treatment for depression because of its side-effect profile and thus it is difficult to extrapolate the results of this study onto the modern practice of psychiatry.

Other Relevant Studies and Information:

- The data from this study were subsequently reanalyzed to more robustly address the topic of disease severity in treatment response.[3] These analyses showed that patients with more severe depressive symptoms and a greater impairment in functioning at baseline had a greater response to treatment compared to those that were less severely ill.
- Various studies have evaluated the efficacy of pharmacotherapy versus psychotherapy for depression.[4] Generally speaking, these treatments are equally efficacious for mild to moderate depression although the former may yield a faster response. For patients with more severe depression, pharmacotherapy generally outperforms psychotherapy.[5]
- The American Psychiatric Association (APA) clinical guidelines recommend either pharmacotherapy or psychotherapy for patients to mild to moderate depression, but combined treatment for patients with moderate to severe depression.[6]

Summary and Implications: This study was the first rigorous controlled comparison of psychotherapy and pharmacotherapy, as well as the first comparison of cognitive behavioral therapy and interpersonal therapy, for the treatment of unipolar nonpsychotic depression. All three treatments were associated with significant improvements in depressive symptoms. There was a nonsignificant trend favoring IMI therapy versus psychotherapy, but the former yielded better results in more severely depressed patients. Based on the outcome of this and other studies, APA guidelines recommend the use of either pharmacotherapy or psychotherapy as first-line treatment among patients with mild to moderate depression and combined treatment for patients with severe depression.

CLINICAL CASE: NATIONAL INSTITUTE OF MENTAL HEALTH (NIMH) TREATMENT OF DEPRESSION COLLABORATIVE RESEARCH PROGRAM

Case History

A 37-year-old woman presents to the outpatient clinic with symptoms of anhedonia, lethargy, insomnia, and low concentration. She is diagnosed with major depressive disorder without psychotic features. The patient prefers to avoid medications, explaining that she is "very sensitive to side effects." Based on the results of this study, is psychotherapy equally effective to medications for her condition? If so, which type of therapy is indicated?

Suggested Answer

The NIMH collaborative study on depression found few short-term differences between IMI plus supportive therapy, CBT, IPT, or placebo plus supportive therapy for most patients. For severely depressed patients, however, IMI plus CM works better than either type of therapy.

The patient in the vignette is similar to a patient enrolled in the NIMH collaborative study on depression. It would be reasonable for the patient to choose between CBT or IPT given that she is not severely depressed.

As her clinician, however, you might wish to consider explaining the safety and efficacy data on selective serotonin reuptake inhibitors. Additional changes could subsequently be added to the therapeutic regimen as indicated.

References

1. Elkin, I., Shea, M. T., Watkins, J. T., Imber, S. D., Sotsky, S. M., Collins, J. F., . . . Parloff, M. B. (1989). National Institute of Mental Health Treatment of Depression Collaborative Research Program: General effectiveness of treatments. *Archives of General Psychiatry, 46*(11), 971–982.
2. Spitzer, R., Endicott, J., & Robins, E. (1978). Research diagnostic criteria: Rationale and reliability. *Archives of General Psychiatry, 35*(6), 773–782.
3. Elken, I., Gibbons, R. D., Shea, M. T., Sotsky, S. M., Watkins, J. T., Pilkonis, P. A., & Hedeker, D. (1995), Initial severity and differential treatment outcome in the National Institute of Mental Health Treatment of Depression Collaborative Research Program. *Journal of Consulting and Clinical Psychology, 63*(5), 841–847.
4. Huhn, M., Tardy, M., Spineli, L. M., Kissling, W., Förstl H., & Pitschel-Walz, G. (2014). Efficacy of pharmacotherapy and psychotherapy for adult psychiatric disorders: A systematic overview of meta-analyses. *JAMA Psychiatry, 71*(6), 706–715.

5. Weitz, E. S. Hollon, S. D., Twisk, J., van Straten, A., Huibers, M. J., David, D., . . . Cuijpers, P. (2015). Baseline depression severity as moderator of depression outcomes between cognitive behavioral therapy versus pharmacotherapy: An individual patient data meta-analysis. *JAMA Psychiatry*, 72(11), 1102–1109.
6. Gelenberg, A. J. Freeman, M. P., Markowitz, J. C., Rosenbaum, J. F., Thase, M. E., Trivedi, M. H., & Van Rhoads, R. S. (2010). *APA Practice guideline for the treatment of patients with major depressive disorder* (3rd ed.). Washington, DC: American Psychiatric Association.

25

Efficacy and Safety of Electroconvulsive Therapy in Depressive Disorders

A Systematic Review and Meta-Analysis

JOSEPH J. TAYLOR AND ROBERT OSTROFF

> There is a reasonable evidence base for the use of ECT: it does not rest simply on anecdote, habit and tradition.
>
> —UK ECT Review Group[1]

Research Question: How safe and effective is electroconvulsive therapy (ECT) for patients with a depressive illness?

Funding: UK Secretary of State for Health

Year Study Began: Studies between 1962 and 2003

Year Study Published: 2003

Study Location: University of Oxford

Who Was Studied: Patients with a "depressive illness" who were enrolled in a randomized control trial or observational study of ECT.

Who Was Excluded: Each individual study had unique inclusion and exclusion criteria. The meta-analysis excluded studies if they were improperly randomized, confounded, or deemed to lack quality.

How Many Participants: 73 randomized trials out of 624 reports met criteria for inclusion. Whereas some trials contributed to multiple topic analyses, others were ultimately not included in the quantitative analyses.

Study Overview: The authors searched several scientific and medical databases for randomized controlled trials or observational studies of ECT. Two independent reviewers screened the results before the authors pooled their data to calculate odds ratios and absolute risk differences. Funnel plots were used to assess publication bias.

Study Design: ECT was the primary intervention analyzed. Trials included ECT versus no ECT, ECT versus pharmacotherapy, or comparisons of various forms or doses of ECT. A standardized pooled effect size was calculated to account for various study outcomes.

Follow-Up: Data were collected from a wide range of time points, including short-term effects immediately following ECT to long-term effects years later.

Endpoints: The primary outcome measure was change on a continuous depressive symptom scale at the end of a course of ECT. This change was also examined at six months whenever data were available. Secondary analyses were performed on long-term measures of cognitive function and mortality.

RESULTS

- Based on six trials and 256 patients, real ECT was more effective than sham ECT.
- Based on 18 trials and 1,144 patients, ECT was more effective than pharmacotherapy.
- Based on 22 trials of 1,408 patients, bilateral ECT was more effective than unilateral ECT.
- Three of the four cohort studies analyzing mortality found lower overall mortality in patients receiving ECT versus those not receiving ECT. The 4th study reported no difference (Tables 25.1 and 25.2).

Table 25.1 Summary of Quantitative Analyses

Topic	Trials	Patients
Real vs. sham ECT	6	256
ECT vs. pharmacotherapy	13	760
Bilateral vs. unilateral ECT	22	1,137
Frequency of ECT	6	210
Dose of ECT	6	337
ECT waveform	5	181
Mortality secondary to ECT	4	>1,787[a]
Structural brain changes after ECT	3	83[b]

[a]One study reported patient-years rather than patient numbers.
[b]Excludes healthy control and patients who did not receive ECT.
NOTE: ECT = electroconvulsive therapy.

Table 25.2 Summary of Findings

Topic	Pooled random effects, depressive symptoms (95% CI)
Real vs. sham ECT	−0.908 (−1.270 to −0.537)
ECT vs. pharmacotherapy	−0.802 (−1.290 to −0.289)
Bilateral vs. unilateral ECT	−0.322 (−0.458 to −0.186)
Frequency of ECT	−0.299 (−0.759 to −0.199)
Dose of ECT electrical stimulus	0.575[a] (0.329 to 0.829)
ECT stimulus waveform	0.620[b] (−0.306 to 1.540)

[a]Negative favors lower dose.
[b]Negative favors brief pulse.
NOTES: Table reports standardized effect sizes. Negative values favor electroconvulsive therapy (ECT).

Criticisms and Limitations: This study illustrates the advantages and disadvantages of systematic reviews and meta-analyses. Pooling group data from studies conducted over several decades increases statistical power but also introduces confounders and heterogeneity. The authors discuss the possibility of publication bias in the manuscript and employ statistical techniques to standardize outcome measures across studies. Nevertheless, sources of study heterogeneity remain important to consider.

There were several topics that were not fully explored in the manuscript, including type and severity of depression (e.g., catatonic features, psychotic features, etc.), treatment durability, anesthetic agents, and adjunctive treatments during ECT. Moreover, it is important to remember that existing treatments evolved and new treatments emerged over the decades that are represented in this meta-analysis. These changes make it difficult to use this particular dataset to contextualize ECT in contemporary treatment algorithms.

Other Relevant Studies and Information:

- Since this manuscript was published, various meta-analyses have confirmed the safety and efficacy of ECT[2,3,4,5]
- The American Psychiatric Association (APA)[6] guidelines and Task Force Report on ECT[7] suggest that ECT should be considered for patients with severe depression.

Summary and Implications: The authors of this systematic review and meta-analysis analyzed decades of evidence to assess the safety and efficacy of ECT for depressive symptoms. Their primary analysis showed that ECT is a robust treatment for adults with severe depression. The analysis also showed that ECT is significantly more effective than pharmacotherapy for this population of treatment-refractory patients; that bilateral ECT is moderately more effective than unilateral ECT (despite higher cognitive side effects); and that there may be a correlation between dose of ECT and improvement in depressive symptoms.

CLINICAL CASE: ECT FOR THE TREATMENT OF DEPRESSION

Case History

A 42-year-old man with a history of major depressive disorder is admitted to an inpatient psychiatric unit for neurovegetative symptoms of depression and suicidal ideation with a plan. He has had four adequate trials of antidepressant medications as well as outpatient therapy but has not felt well in over five years. The patient refuses to consider your recommendation of ECT, explaining that he has heard that ECT doesn't work and that it causes "brain damage." How do you respond to the patient?

Suggested Answer

The UK ECT Review Group wrote a systematic review and meta-analysis addressing the topics of ECT safety and efficacy.[1] Their primary analysis showed that ECT is an effective treatment for adults with severe depression. Secondary analyses showed the following: (a) ECT is significantly more effective pharmacotherapy, (b) bilateral ECT is moderately more effective than unilateral ECT (despite higher cognitive side effects), and (c) there may be a correlation between dose of ECT and improvement in depressive symptoms. Modern APA guidelines reflect the findings of this paper and confirm that ECT is efficacious for patients with severe depression. Importantly, the UK ECT Review Group manuscript was published in 2003 and does not include technical advancements in ECT methodology or delivery.

The patient in the vignette is similar to a patient enrolled in one of the many trials included in the UK ECT Review Group manuscript. Based on this systematic review and meta-analysis, your patient is very likely to benefit from ECT. It is critical that psychiatrists combat stigma and base treatment recommendations on empirical data; our confidence in such recommendations is very reassuring to patients. In this case, it would be helpful to educate the patient about ECT using data from systematic reviews and meta-analyses. This conversation would be titrated to the patient's education level and would include a clear summary of risks and benefits. In this patient's case, the evidence clearly favors proceeding with ECT.

References

1. UK ECT Review Group. (2003). Efficacy and safety of electroconvulsive therapy in depressive disorders: A systematic review and meta-analysis. *Lancet, 361*(9360), 799–808.
2. Jelovac, A., Kolshus, E., & McLoughlin, D. M. (2013). Relapse following successful electroconvulsive therapy for major depression: A meta-analysis. *Neuropsychopharmocology, 38*(12), 2467–2474.
3. Semkovska, M., & McLoughlin, D. M. (2010). Objective cognitive performance associated with electroconvulsive therapy for depression: A systematic review and meta-analysis. *Biological Psychiatry, 68*(6) 568–577.
4. Tor, P. C. Bautovich, A, Wang, M. J., Martin, D., Harvey, S. B., & Loo, C. (2015). A systematic review and meta-analysis of brief versus ultrabrief right unilateral electroconvulsive therapy for depression. *Journal of Clinical Psychology, 76*(9), e1092–e1098.
5. Torring, N., Sanghani, S. N., Petrides, G., Kellner, C. H., & Ostergaard, S. D. (2017). The mortality rate of electroconvulsive therapy: A systematic review and pooled analysis. *Acta Psychiatrica Scandinavica, 135*(5), 388–397.

6. Gelenberg, A. J. Freeman, M. P., Markowitz, J. C., Rosenbaum, J. F., Thase, M. E., Trivedi, M. H., & Van Rhoads, R. S. (2010). *APA Practice guideline for the treatment of patients with major depressive disorder* (3rd ed.). Washington, DC: American Psychiatric Association, 20–21.
7. Jaffe, R. (2002). Review of the book *The practice of electroconvulsive therapy: Recommendations for treatment, training, and privileging: A task force report of the American Psychiatric Association, 2nd ed. American Journal of Psychiatry,* 159(2), 331.

26

Initial Severity and Antidepressant Benefits

A Meta-Analysis of Data Submitted to the Food and Drug Administration

MICHAEL MAKSIMOWSKI AND ZHEALA QAYYUM

> Drug–placebo differences in antidepressant efficacy increase as a function of baseline severity, but are relatively small even for severely depressed patients.
>
> —KIRSCH ET AL.[1]

Research Question: What are the drug–placebo differences among antidepressants when both published and unpublished data are analyzed? Does antidepressant efficacy depend on the severity of initial depression scores?

Funding: None

Year Study Began: Included studies from 1985 to 2007

Year Study Published: 2008

Study Location: Various clinical sites internationally

Who Was Studied: Data from all double-blind, placebo-controlled randomized control trials submitted to the FDA for licensing of fluoxetine, venlafaxine, nefazodone, and paroxetine. All patients had been diagnosed with unipolar major depressive disorder using DSM-IV criteria.

Who Was Excluded: Randomized controlled trials that did not have mean improvement scores or improvement data for all trials of the medication

How Many Participants: 5,133

Study Overview: See Figure 26.1 for an example of a typical study included in meta-analysis.

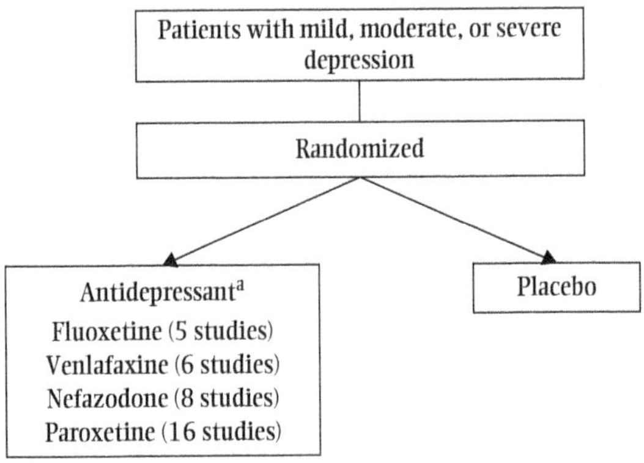

Figure 26.1 Example of a Typical Study Included in the Meta-Analysis
[a]One study was overlapping.

Study Design: The investigators requested from the FDA all publicly releasable information about clinical trials for fluoxetine, venlafaxine, nefazodone, and paroxetine. The studies included in the meta-analysis were not all peer-reviewed or published. A meta-analysis was conducted that included the baseline severity based on the Hamilton Rating Scale for Depression (HRSD).

Depression severity was assessed in all studies using the criteria proposed by the American Psychiatric Association (APA)[2] and adopted by the National Institute for Clinical Excellence (NICE).[3] The HRSD score can range from 0 to 54. Scores between 8 and 13 indicate mild depression, scores between 14 and 18 indicate moderate depression, scores between 19 and 22 indicate severe depression, and scores greater than 22 indicate very severe depression. Baseline depression scores were in the very severe range for all but 1 study. Separate meta-analyses were conducted with and without this study, with no difference in results.

Follow-Up: Follow-up ranged from four to eight weeks among included studies.

Endpoints: Absolute difference in depression between the placebo and treatment groups as well as extent to which drug-related effects are a function of initial depression severity. A clinically significant change in HRSD was defined as a three-point drop based on criteria proposed by NICE.[4]

RESULTS

- HRSD scores were statistically greater in the drug groups versus the placebo groups, but only in patients with very severe depression and not by a three-point difference, which is the criterion for clinical significance used by NICE.
- Patients with mild or moderate depression scores at baseline did not improve significantly with drug compared to placebo.
- The researchers attribute clinical significance between drug and placebo groups for those with very severe depression to a decreased responsiveness to placebo (compared to less depressed patients) rather than an increased responsiveness to the antidepressant.
- Improvements in depression scores among patients in placebo groups were approximately 80% of the improvement observed in the drug groups; the investigators contrasted this finding to the effect of placebo on pain, which is approximately 50% of the response in active treatment groups.[4,5,6] This suggests that among patients with depression who improve following treatment, a relatively small proportion of the improvement may be attributable to the active therapy (Table 26.1).

Table 26.1 Summary of Primary Outcomes

Outcome	Antidepressant	Placebo	P value
HSRD reduction after treatment	9.6	7.8	<0.001

NOTE: HSRD = Hamilton Rating Scale for Depression.

Criticisms and Limitations: This is a meta-analysis, and there were likely differences between studies that were included (e.g., concordant psychotherapy, duration, and dose of treatment). However, the study did test for interactions of these types of variables (assessed as possible moderator variables) and were deemed to have no significant effect on the final results.

Heterogeneity (i.e., variation in results), was low to moderate and moderate for the drug and placebo groups, respectively, with statistically significant differences in heterogeneity between drug and placebo groups. Thus, the mean treatment effects may not accurately describe the results.

Furthermore, findings from this study cannot be generalized to other antidepressants that were not included (e.g., sertraline, citalopram, escitalopram, bupropion, duloxetine).

Finally, 12 randomized controlled trials were not included in the final meta-analysis due to unavailability of the data.

Other Relevant Studies and Information:

- A repeat meta-analysis of antidepressant efficacy data was conducted after this publication by Fountoulakis and Möller.[7] That study reported a higher drug–placebo difference and higher mean improvements in HRSD scores than the study by Kirsch et al. Antidepressant efficacy was not found to relate to depression severity.
- Three of the original authors of the Kirsch et al. study published a response article[8] to Fountoulakis and Möller's paper, arguing that there were methodological flaws in their analysis.
- A previous analysis that did not take into account depression severity found a small, clinically insignificant improvement in depression in those treated with antidepressants versus placebo.[9]
- A study by Hansen and colleagues[10] found second-generation antidepressants (selective serotonin reuptake inhibitors [SSRIs], serotonin–norepinephrine reuptake inhibitors, norepinephrine–dopamine reuptake inhibitors) do not appear to differ substantially in efficacy relative to first-generation antidepressants (e.g., tricyclic antidepressants).

Summary and Implications: This large meta-analysis involving data from both published and unpublished data submitted to the FDA found that fluoxetine, paroxetine, venlafaxine, and nefazodone produce only modest benefits with respect to depression scores that do not meet the clinically significant improvements defined by the NICE criteria. Improvements among the subgroup of most severely depressed patients are, however, larger and do meet the clinically significant improvements defined by NICE. The results also show that patients with depression receiving placebo therapy improve substantially, suggesting that among patients who improve following treatment, a relatively small proportion of the improvement may be attributable to the active therapy. Psychiatrists should consider this finding when prescribing SSRIs while remaining mindful of individual patient presentations and needs.

CLINICAL CASE: PRESCRIBING ANTIDEPRESSANTS

Case History

A 25-year-old woman presents to an outpatient clinic complaining of low mood, anhedonia, weight loss, and insomnia. She has had difficulty getting out of bed in the morning and is in danger of losing her job. She scores a 20 on the HRSD and is diagnosed with major depressive disorder. Informed consent is obtained to start a trial of fluoxetine.

Based on the results from the study by Kirsch and colleagues, describe the efficacy of the medication choice.

Suggested Answer

The study by Kirsch and colleagues found that fluoxetine, paroxetine, venlafaxine, and nefazodone did not produce clinically significant improvements in depression according to NICE criteria except for the most severely depressed patients (i.e., those with a HRSD greater than 28). The patient in the vignette meets criteria for moderate depression, and, on average, we would expect there to be a clinically significant improvement. However, the difference between the observed improvements on a true antidepressant compared to placebo may not be clinically significant.

References

1. Kirsch. I., Deacon. B. J., Huedo-Medina. T. B., Scoboria. A., Moore. T. J., & Johnson. B. T. (2008). Initial severity and antidepressant benefits: A meta-analysis of data submitted to the Food and Drug Administration. *PLoS Medicine, 5*(2), e45.
2. Task Force for the Handbook of Psychiatric Measures. (2000). *Handbook of psychiatric measures*. Washington, DC: American Psychiatric Association.
3. National Institute for Clinical Excellence. (2004). *Depression: Management of depression in primary and secondary care*. Clinical practice guideline no. 23. London: National Institute for Clinical Excellence.
4. Evans, F. J. (1974). The placebo response in pain reduction. *Advances in Neurology, 4*, 289–296.
5. Benedetti, F., Arduino, C., & Amanzio, M. (1999). Somatotopic activation of opioid systems by target-directed expectations of analgesia. *Journal of Neuroscience, 19*, 3639–3648.
6. Evans, F. G. (1985). Expectancy, therapeutic instructions, and the placebo response. In L. White, B. Tursky, & G. E. Schwartz (Eds.), *Placebo: Theory, research and mechanisms* (pp. 215–228). New York: Guilford.

7. Fountoulakis, K. N., & Möller, H. (2011). Efficacy of antidepressants: A re-analysis and re-interpretation of the Kirsch data. *International Journal of Neuropsychopharmacology, 14*(3), 405–412.
8. Huedo-Medina, T. B, Johnson, B. T., & Kirsch, I. (2012). Kirsch et al.'s (2008) calculations are correct: Reconsidering Fountoulakis & Möller's re-analysis of the Kirsch data. *International Journal of Neuropsychopharmacology, 15*(8), 1193–1198.
9. Kirsch, I., Moore, T. J., Scoboria, A., & Nicholls, S. S. (2002). The emperor's new drugs: An analysis of antidepressant medication data submitted to the U.S. Food and Drug Administration. *Prevention & Treatment, 5*(1), art. 23.
10. Hansen, R. A., Gartlehner, G., Lohr, K. N., Gaynes, B. N., & Carey, T. S. (2005). Efficacy and safety of second-generation antidepressants in the treatment of major depressive disorder. *Annals of Internal Medicine, 143*, 415–426.

27

Sequenced Treatment Alternatives to Relieve Depression

*STAR*D*

ERIC LIN AND POCHU HO

> The theoretical cumulative remission rate [for depression] after four acute treatment steps was 67%.
>
> —The STAR*D Investigators[1]

Research Question: What are the outcomes and remission rates for depression? What are the long-term outcomes, especially the relapse rates, for patients receiving sequential depression therapies?

Funding: The National Institute of Mental Health

Year Study Began: 2001

Year Study Published: 2006

Study Location: 41 outpatient sites providing primary or psychiatric care in the United States.

Who Was Studied: Individuals 18 to 75 years old referred by their doctors who were already seeking care for nonpsychotic major depressive disorder (MDD) by DSM-IV criteria and had scores of ≥14 on the Hamilton Rating Scale of Depression 17 (HRSD-17).

Who Was Excluded: Patients with bipolar disorder, psychotic disorders (including depression with psychotic features), anorexia, bulimia, obsessive compulsive disorder, or substance abuse disorders requiring detoxification. Suicidal patients requiring immediate hospitalization. Those who had already attempted an adequate trial of treatments that were utilized in the first two Sequenced Treatment Alternatives to Relieve Depression (STAR*D) treatment steps, or if a STAR*D treatment could not be safely used because of their other health conditions (pregnant or breastfeeding) or medication regimens.

How Many Participants: 3,671

Study Overview: See Figure 27.1 for a summary of the study design. See Figure 27.2 for a summary of the cognitive therapy arm design.

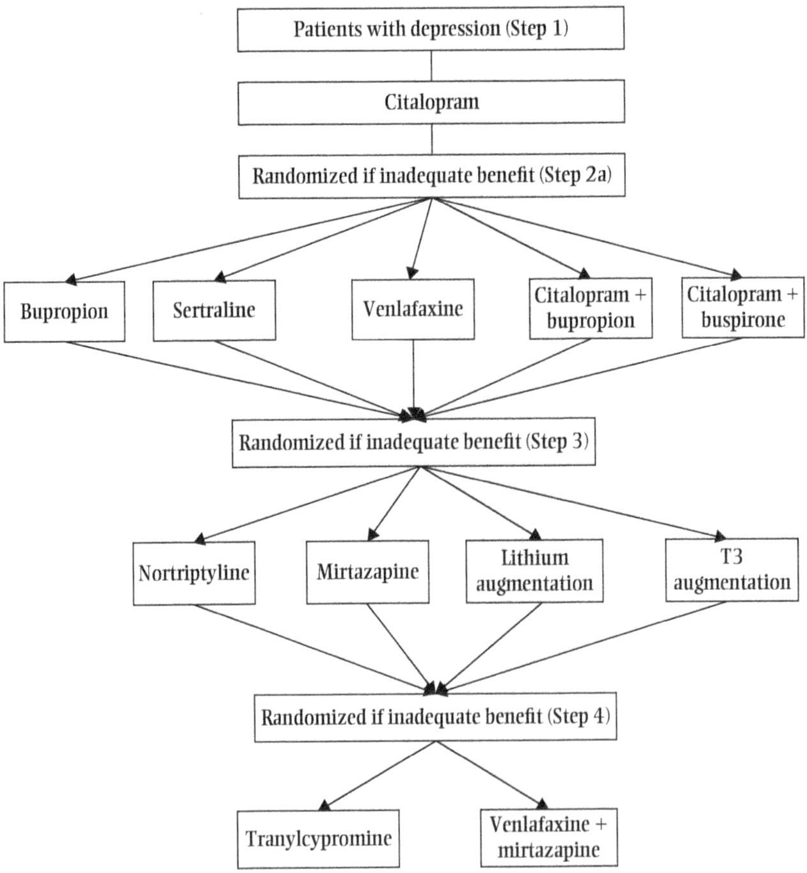

Figure 27.1 Summary of Study Design

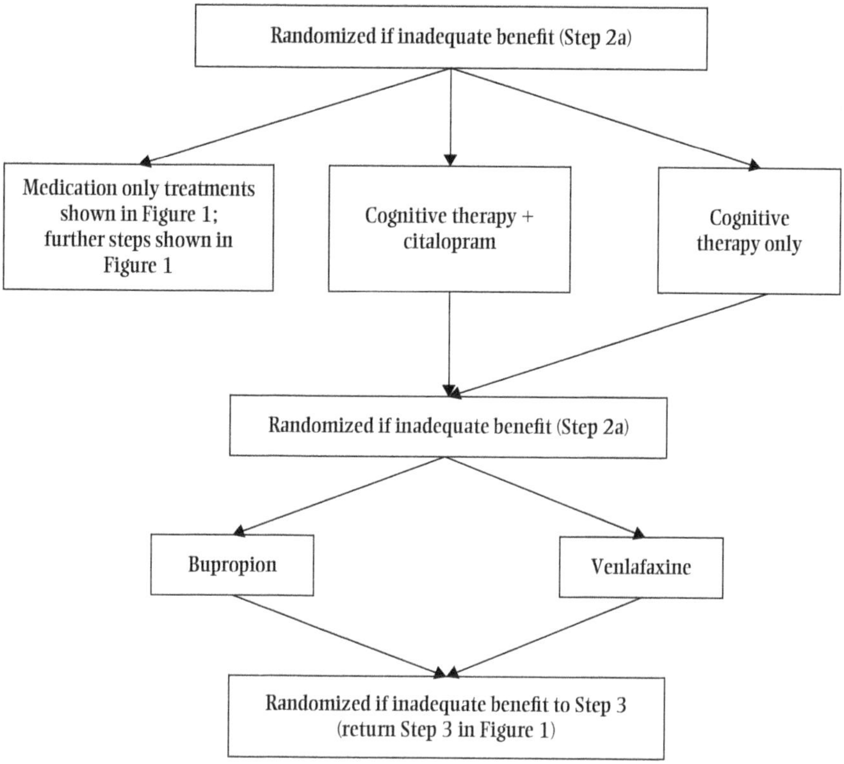

Figure 27.2 Summary of Cognitive Therapy Arm Design

Study Intervention: Participants with depression were treated in stepwise fashion. Patients who improved after any step could exit treatment and were followed for 12 months. During this follow-up phase, subjects could change treatment regimens but were recommended to continue on their final treatment regimen from the STAR*D study. Those who did not remit (defined in the following discussion) continued to the next treatment step and were randomized to subsequent therapies.

All patients in the study started with citalopram treatment as Step 1. Subsequent treatment steps are shown in Figures 27.1 and 27.2.

Dosing was adjusted using measurement-based care methods and were "vigorously" dosed. As an example, citalopram dosing was determined on an individual basis by clinicians, but was guided by a STAR*D treatment manual and clinical research coordinator monitoring and recommendations.

Quick Inventory of Depressive Symptomatology Self-Report (self-rated; QIDS-SR16) and QIDS (clinician rated; QIDS-C) were recommended at weeks 2, 4, 6, 9, and 12 of treatment. The general recommendation was to start citalopram at 20 mg/day and to increase to 40 mg/day by week 4 and 60 mg/day by week 6. Clinicians were permitted to initiate at lower doses, slow titration, stop titration, or switch the medication (and move the patient to the next step) based on clinical judgment.[2]

Follow-Up: 12 months

Endpoints: Primary outcome: "Response rate," defined as a ≥50% reduction on the QIDS-SR16. Other outcomes: "Remission rate," defined as a QIDS-SR16 score of ≤5 (corresponds to HRSD-17 ≤7), time to response/remission, relapse rate defined as a QIDS-SR16 score ≥11 (corresponds to HRSD-17 ≥14) during follow-up, and treatment intolerance/exit.

RESULTS

- Overall, 67% of the patients who started treatment in this study remitted from depression.
- Patients in later treatment steps demonstrated progressively lower remission rates ($p < 0.0001$) (Table 27.1).

Table 27.1 SUMMARY OF STAR*D'S KEY FINDINGS

Outcome	**Step 1** (%)	**Step 2** (%)	**Step 3** (%)	**Step 4** (%)	**Overall** (%)
Remission rate*	36.8	30.6	13.7	13.0	67
Response rate	48.6	28.5	16.8	16.3	75
Intolerance rate	16.3	19.5	25.6	34.1	66
Relapse rate post-treatment	40.1	55.3	64.6	71.1	97

NOTE: STAR*D = Sequenced Treatment Alternatives to Relieve Depression. Pairwise comparisons demonstrated that only Step 1 relapse rate (as monitored during follow-up) was significantly different from the other steps ($P < 0.0001$).

- Patients who entered later treatment steps also had higher relapse rates ($p < 0.0001$).
- Patients who participated in later treatment steps tended to have a higher number of psychiatric and medical diagnoses and tended to have worse illness burden from their depression.
- Substantial numbers of patients exited after each step: 20.9% after Step 1, 29.7% after Step 2, and 42.3% after Step 3. Results reported were from an intent-to-treat analysis.

Criticisms and Limitations: The trial was open label and not placebo-controlled, which is particularly relevant for studies of depression given that there is often a substantial placebo effect in depression studies.

Treatment steps were limited to 12 to 14 weeks each; patients who may have remitted with a longer treatment duration were algorithmically pushed into the next step, which may differ from a more flexible real-world practice strategy.

Treatment options did not include many other common options such as electrocardiogram, psychodynamic therapy, or even some of the newer psychotropic medications.

A lower than expected number of patients received the cognitive therapy treatment option perhaps because of the biases with initial recruitment. Moreover, the study excluded suicidal patients and those with common comorbidities including depression with psychotic features, which limits its generalizability. Other studies suggest that those with these more severe symptoms may respond better to treatment.[3]

Other Relevant Studies and Information:

- Other studies have found similar rates of response to antidepressants as reported in STAR*D.[4,5]
- For patients with unresponsive depression, American Psychiatric Association (APA) guidelines recommend maximizing initial treatments by raising medications to higher doses of medication, switching to other treatment strategies, or augmentation. At the time of its publication, the guidelines stated that there was limited data other than the STAR*D study in recommending a specific switching algorithm.[6]

Summary and Implications: The STAR*D trial was a landmark study exploring the natural history of patients receiving a sequential treatment strategy for depression. It showed that 67% of patients treated according to the sequential management strategy utilized in this study remitted. It also demonstrated that patients with depression who fail multiple treatment trials have lower remission rates and higher relapse rates.

CLINICAL CASE: RATES OF REMISSION AND RELAPSE

Case History

A 37-year-old, medically uncomplicated woman is wondering about her chances of "resolving" her major depressive episode after no response from a six-week trial of citalopram. Notably, she complains of dysphoric mood, anhedonia, insomnia, decreased energy, and poor concentration. Per the STAR*D study, what treatment strategies can she try, and what is her expected chance of remitting with this second treatment?

Suggested Answer

The STAR*D study found that 36.8% of patients remit with citalopram as first-line therapy. Of the patients who required another treatment step (Step 2), another 30.6% responded to either a switch to bupropion, sertraline, or venlafaxine or augmentation with buspirone or bupropion or a switch to cognitive therapy or augmentation with cognitive therapy. Her chance at remission is expected to be 30.6% with the described treatment options since she has already failed citalopram treatment. By the STAR*D follow up statistics, she would have a 55.3% chance of relapsing by the end of 12 months from treatment exit.

The patient in the vignette is typical of one that would be included in the STAR*D trial. Based on the patient's history and preference, the psychiatrist can choose to either augment or switch antidepressants and/or cognitive therapy and should have realistic expectations regarding the likelihood of remission.

References

1. Gaynes, B. N., Rush, A. J., Trivedi, M. H., Wisniewski, S. R., Spencer, D., & Fava, M. (2008). The STAR*D study: Treating depression in the real world. *Cleveland Clinic Journal of Medicine, 75*(1), 57–66.
2. Trivedi, M. H., Rush, A. J., Wisniewski, S. R., Nierenberg, A. A., Warden, D., Ritz, L., . . . Shores-Wilson, K. (2006). Evaluation of outcomes with citalopram for depression using measurement-based care in STAR*D: Implications for clinical practice. *American Journal of Psychiatry, 163*(1), 28–40.
3. Fournier, J. C., DeRubeis, R. J., Hollon, S. D., Dimidjian, S., Amsterdam, J. D., Shelton, R. C., & Fawcett, J. (2010). Antidepressant drug effects and depression severity: A patient-level meta-analysis. *JAMA, 303*(1), 47–53.
4. Fava, M., Dunner, D. L., Greist, J. H., Preskorn, S. H., Trivedi, M. H., Zajecka, J., & Cohen, M. (2001). Efficacy and safety of mirtazapine in major depressive disorder patients after SSRI treatment failure: An open-label trial. *Journal of Clinical Psychiatry, 62*(6), 413–420.
5. Thase, M. E., A Entsuah, A. R., & Rudolph, R. L. (2001). Remission rates during treatment with venlafaxine or selective serotonin reuptake inhibitors. *British Journal of Psychiatry, 178*(3), 234–241.
6. Gelenberg, A. J. Freeman, M. P., Markowitz, J. C., Rosenbaum, J. F., Thase, M. E., Trivedi, M. H., & Van Rhoads, R. S. (2010). *APA Practice guideline for the treatment of patients with major depressive disorder* (3rd ed.). Washington, DC: American Psychiatric Association

28

Cognitive Therapy versus Medication in the Treatment of Moderate to Severe Depression

DANIEL BARRON AND ROBERT OSTROFF

> Cognitive therapy can be as effective as medications for the initial treatment of moderate to severe major depression, but this degree of effectiveness may depend on a high level of therapist experience or expertise.
>
> —DeRubeis et al.[1]

Research Question: Is paroxetine or cognitive therapy (CT) more effective in treating patients with moderate to severe major depressive disorder (MDD)?

Funding: National Institute of Mental Health (NIMH) and GlaxoSmithKline.

Year Study Began: Not specified

Year Study Published: 2005

Study Location: University of Pennsylvania

Who Was Studied: Patients 18 and 70 years old with a DSM-IV diagnosis of MDD with modified 17-item Hamilton Depression Rating Scale (HDRS) scores of ≥20 at the screening and baseline visits, consistent with "moderate to severe" depression.

Who Was Excluded: Patients with a history of bipolar disorder; substance abuse or dependence; history of psychosis; another axis I diagnosis requiring treatment with higher priority than depression; antisocial, borderline, or schizotypal personality disorder; an inability to take a study medication for medial reasons; and an unsuccessful trial of paroxetine in the past year.

How Many Participants: 240

Study Overview: See Figure 28.1 for a summary of the study design.

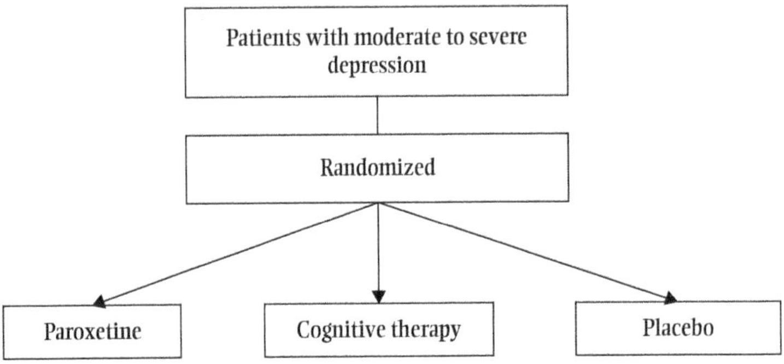

Figure 28.1 Summary of Study Design

Study Intervention: Patients were randomly assigned to receive paroxetine, pill placebo, or CT.

Patients in the paroxetine group received initial doses of 10 to 20 mg of paroxetine, which was increased in 10 to 20 mg increments up to a maximum of 50 mg daily based on response and side effects. Those who did not achieve a satisfactory response (HDRS $\leq$12) were given lithium or desipramine as augmentation, which was not blinded to the patient or prescriber.

Patients in the CT group received psychotherapy from trained psychologists in 50-minute sessions delivered twice weekly for four weeks, once or twice weekly for the next eight weeks, and weekly for the final four weeks. Most of the therapists were PhD psychologists, and many had training from the Beck Institute, a main center for cognitive psychotherapy.

Patients assigned to the placebo group received placebo therapy mimicking the active therapy protocol in the paroxetine group.

Follow-Up: Eight weeks, at which point the patients were followed for an additional eight weeks open label

Endpoints: A modified 17-item HDRS used to define "response" and "remission" rates. At eight weeks, response was defined as HDRS ≤12. Response at 16 weeks was defined as either of the following:

- HDRS ≤12 at 16 weeks and ≤14 at 14 weeks or ≤12 at 10 or 12 weeks
- HDRS ≤12 at 12, 14, and 18 weeks

Remission was defined using similar criteria as the "response" criteria except that patients were required to have an HDRS ≤7.

RESULTS

- At eight weeks, both paroxetine and CT were significantly superior with respect to response rate relative to the placebo group (Table 28.1).

Table 28.1 Summary of the Study's Key Findings

Outcome	Paroxetine	P value[a]	Cognitive therapy	P value[b]	P value[c]	Placebo
8-week response rate (95% CI)	50% (41%–59%)	0.001	43% (31%–56%)	0.04	0.40	25% (16%–38%)
16-week response rate (95% CI)	58% (48%–66%)	N/A	58% (45%–70%)	N/A	0.92	N/A
16-week remission rate (95% CI)	46% (37%–55%)	N/A	40% (28%–53%)	N/A	0.37, 0.05[c]	N/A

[a]Compared to placebo.
[b]Comparing paroxetine to cognitive therapy.
[c]There was a treatment X site interaction, so P values were calculated by site, for University of Pennsylvania and Vanderbilt, respectively.

- Effect sizes were 0.60 for paroxetine and 0.44 for CT compared to placebo, indicating a "medium" effect of these treatments.

Criticisms and Limitations: The generalizability of the findings of this study may be limited because CT may vary in how it is performed by individual practitioners. The therapists in this study were highly trained from major CT academic institutions. In addition, therapy was delivered multiple times per week, which may not be available in most parts of the country. Also, only one class of antidepressant medication, a selective serotonin reuptake inhibitor, was used. Moreover, patients with common comorbidities including substance abuse and personality disorders were excluded, further limiting the generalizability. The fact that there was a significant site X treatment interaction (i.e., different outcomes at different treatment sites) highlights these concerns related to generalizability.

Finally, the study became open-label after eight weeks, and the placebo arm was stopped.

Other Relevant Studies and Information:

- The NIMH Treatment of Depression Collaborative Research Program study found that while there were no differences between psychotherapy and antidepressant medications for depression overall, those with moderate to severe depression had more benefit with medications compared to psychotherapy.[2]
- The most recent American Psychiatric Association (APA) guidelines recommend psychotherapy or antidepressants alone for mild to moderate depression depending on patient and clinician preference and resource availability. For patients with severe depression; however, either pharmacotherapy or combination pharmacotherapy and psychotherapy are recommended.[3]

Summary and Implications: This study compared paroxetine, cognitive therapy, and pill placebo for patients with moderate to severe depression. It found that paroxetine and cognitive therapy both lead to a significant improvement in depression compared to placebo with medium effect size. However, cognitive therapy in this study was performed at a high frequency by exceptionally well-trained psychologists, which may not be widely available, and as a result these findings may not be broadly generalizable.

CLINICAL CASE: A PATIENT WITH MODERATE TO SEVERE DEPRESSION

Case History

A 29-year-old man presents to an outpatient psychiatry clinic with complaints of low appetite, insomnia, anhedonia, and feelings of depression for the past three months leading to him missing work and having marital problems. He has no other medical, substance use, or psychiatric problems. The patient was found to have a 17-item HDRS score of 18. He asks what the next course of treatment would be and is particularly worried about starting an antidepressant medication based on previous experience and side effects. As the treating psychiatrist, based on the results of this study, how should this patient be treated?

Suggested Answer

This study found that cognitive psychotherapy can be used alone in the treatment of those with moderate to severe depression. Subsequent studies have shown that while this decision may appear simple, the clinical situation is complex and includes considerations of level of CT expertise (in the mental health provider) and of economy.[4] A course of antidepressant is much more inexpensive and standardizable than a course of CT that focuses on psychosocial aspects of depression, but it is unclear which will help in individual patients across the board.

The patient in the vignette has been diagnosed with moderate depression leading to problems in his daily functioning. While APA guidelines would recommend the use of psychotherapy and/or antidepressant medication for this patient, the psychiatrist should ultimately respect patient preference in this situation, especially considering this study's finding that psychotherapy alone was equally effective in 16 weeks of follow-up. Furthermore, the physician should note that, according to this study, there is no evidence that placebo alone would not lead to spontaneous remission. Given the debilitating effect of depression, it would seem prudent to recommend that the patient avail himself of both treatments if an expert CT is available and if economic considerations allow.

References

1. DeRubeis R. J., Hollon S. D., Amsterdam J. D., Shelton R. C., Young P. R., Salomon R. M., . . . Gallup, R. (2005). Cognitive therapy vs medications in the treatment of moderate to severe depression. *Archives of General Psychiatry, 62*(4), 409–416.
2. Elkin, I., Shea, M. T., Watkins, J. T., Imber, S. D., Sotsky, S. M., Collins, J. F., . . . Parloff, M. B. (1989). National Institute of Mental Health Treatment of Depression Collaborative Research Program: General effectiveness of treatments. *Archives of General Psychiatry, 46*(11), 971–982.
3. Gelenberg, A. J. Freeman, M. P., Markowitz, J. C., Rosenbaum, J. F., Thase, M. E., Trivedi, M. H., & Van Rhoads, R. S. (2010). *APA Practice guideline for the treatment of patients with major depressive disorder* (3rd ed.). Washington, DC: American Psychiatric Association.
4. Forand, N. R., DeRubeis, R. J., & Amsterdam, J. D. (2013). Combining medication and psychotherapy in the treatment of major mental disorders. In M. J. Lambert (Ed.), *Bergin and Garfield's Handbook of Psychotherapy and Behavior Change* (pp. 735–774). New York: Wiley.

SECTION 8

Obsessive-Compulsive Disorder

29

Exposure and Ritual Prevention, Clomipramine, or Their Combination for Obsessive-Compulsive Disorder

BRANDON M. KITAY AND MICHAEL H. BLOCH

> Intensive exposure and ritual prevention may be superior to clomipramine and, by implication, to monotherapy with the other [serotonin reuptake inhibitors].
>
> —FOA ET AL.[1]

Research Question: Is the combination of exposure and ritual prevention (a cognitive behavior therapy-based intervention) along with clomipramine more efficacious than monotherapy with either treatment for adults with obsessive-compulsive disorder (OCD)?

Funding: National Institute of Mental Health (NIMH)

Year Study Began: 1990

Year Study Published: 2005

Study Location: University of Pennsylvania (Philadelphia), New York State Psychiatric Institute, and St. Boniface General Hospital (Winnipeg, Manitoba, Canada).

Who Was Studied: Adults 18 to 70 years old with clinically significant DSM-III-R or DSM-IV OCD (Yale–Brown Obsessive Compulsive Scale[2] [Y-BOCS], score ≥16) and stable (≥1-year illness duration).

Who Was Excluded: Individuals currently in a major depressive episode, suicidal ideation, alcohol or substance dependence within six months of recruitment, schizotypal or borderline personality disorder, significant abnormalities in electrocardiogram, past treatment with clomipramine (≥150mg/day for more than four weeks), or exposure and response prevention (EX/RP; more than three visits/week for more than two weeks). Qualified participants on psychotropic medications during screening underwent a wash-out prior to pretreatment assessment.

How Many Participants: 149

Study Overview: See Figure 29.1 for a summary of the study design.

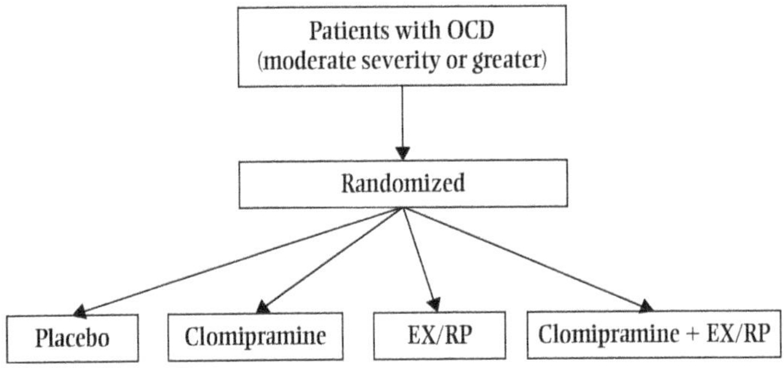

Figure 29.1 Summary of Study Design
NOTES: OCD = obsessive-compulsive disorder. EX/RP = exposure and response prevention.

Study Intervention: Subjects randomized to EX/RP underwent a manualized procedure consisting of two information gathering sessions of the OCD symptoms, each lasting 2 hours. At these sessions, clinicians also presented the rationale for EX/RP treatment and outlined the treatment plan. Subsequently, patients received 15 exposure sessions, each lasting two hours over a three-week period, with daily exposure and ritual prevention homework. In vivo exposure exercises were used in each treatment session and imaginal exposure were used as needed, depending on the nature of the OCD symptoms. Homework consisted of self-monitoring and further stimuli exposure as designed by the therapist. Ritual prevention entailed instructions to abstain from behaviors throughout the three-week period, with two home visits by the therapist in week 4 to conduct context relevant exposures with patients in their living environment. The remaining eight weeks consisted of weekly, 45-minute sessions to promote maintenance without conducting in-session exposures.

Those receiving placebo or clomipramine were seen weekly for 30 minutes by their psychiatrist for medication adjustment with a fixed dosage schedule: starting at 25 mg/day of clomipramine (or placebo) increasing to 200 mg/day as tolerated for the first five weeks with an optional increase to 250 mg/day if indicated. Participants were encouraged to expose themselves to situations evoking obsessions while refraining from rituals without systematic exposure instructions or homework.

Psychiatrists titrating medications were blind to patients' medication assignment and therapy status. Therapists providing EX/RP were blind to patients' medication.

Follow-Up: 12 weeks

Endpoints: Primary outcome: OCD symptom severity on the Y-BOCS. Secondary outcomes: Clinical Global Impression (CGI) scales for severity, the NIMH Global Obsessive-Compulsive Scale,[3] and "response," defined as scoring at least "much improved" on the CGI Improvement scale.

RESULTS

- By week 12, all active treatments outperformed placebo with respect to all key outcomes (Table 29.1).

Table 29.1 SUMMARY OF THE OCD TREATMENT STUDY'S KEY FINDINGS

Outcome at 12 weeks	Clomipramine	P value[a]	EX/RP	P value[b]	EX/RP + Clomipramine	P value[b]	Placebo
Y-BOCS	18.2	.04	11.0	≤0.01	10.5	<0.01	22.2
CGI	4.1	.04	2.7	≤0.01	2.9	<0.01	4.7
NIMH-GOCS	7.1	.04	4.3	≤0.01	4.7	<0.01	8.8

[a]Clomipramine monotherapy compared to placebo.
[b]Compared to clomipramine monotherapy.
NOTES: OCD = obsessive-compulsive disorder. Y-BOCS = Yale–Brown Obsessive Compulsive Scale. CGI = Clinical Global Impression scale. NIMH-GOCS = National Institute of Mental Health Global Obsessive-Compulsive Scale.

- By week 12, EX/RP and EX/RP plus clomipramine was superior to clomipramine alone on all measures.
- No significant difference was detected between EX/RP plus clomipramine and EX/RP plus placebo on any measure at week 12 ($p > 0.20$).

Criticisms and Limitations: Although patients were randomized and the study ratings performed by blinded raters, the research subjects were not blind to whether or not they received EX/RP therapy. The lack of blinding of subjects to the therapy condition could lead to a reporting bias that might influence the findings.

The study excluded patients with concurrent major depressive disorder, which is common in among patients with OCD, thus limiting generalizability of the study.

Finally, the trial employed clomipramine, a tricyclic antidepressant, rather than selective serotonin reuptake inhibitors (which are now the first-line treatment in OCD).

Other Relevant Studies and Information:

- The pediatric OCD treatment study (POTS; see Chapter 12) also found superiority of the combination of cognitive therapy and SSRIs as compared to either treatment alone. In contrast, POTS did not find a significant difference between cognitive therapy alone and SSRIs alone.[4]
- There is some evidence to support the use of antipsychotic medications in patients who do not respond adequately to psychotherapy and SSRIs.[5]
- Based on this and other studies,[6] American Psychiatric Association (APA) guidelines recommend psychotherapy such as EX/RP and/or SSRIs in the treatment of OCD, depending on case-by-case factors.[7]

Summary and Implications: This randomized, placebo-controlled trial evaluated the efficacy of clomipramine, exposure and ritual prevention therapy, and combined treatment for patients with OCD. All three active treatments proved superior to placebo after 12 weeks; however, EX/RP monotherapy and EX/RP plus clomipramine were superior to clomipramine monotherapy. Practice guidelines from the APA recommend EX/RP, SSRI's, or their combination for the treatment of OCD.

CLINICAL CASE: TREATMENT OF OCD

Case History

A 23-year-old man presents to an outpatient psychiatrist after he was fired from his job as a clerical worker. He describes himself as a perfectionist and explains that he was fired because he spent too much time arranging files in the perfect order. He explains that he also spends two to three hours per day washing his hands and checks to make sure that his door is locked up to 50 times daily before leaving the house. These behaviors help alleviate some anxiety, and although he feels some relief after performing them, he overall is quite anxious. The patient is diagnosed with OCD.

Based on this study, what treatment might the psychiatrist consider?

Suggested Answer

This randomized placebo-controlled trial supports the use of EX/RP either with or without clomipramine in the treatment of OCD. Now, based on an improved side-effect profile, SSRIs are recommended over clomipramine as an initial medication for OCD.

Based on the patient's reported history, symptoms have risen to the point of functional decline since he recently lost a job as a result of symptoms of OCD. Given his current level of functioning, it would be reasonable to offer a trial of an SSRI in addition to EX/RP. The psychiatrist should consider side effects of the SSRI and practical feasibility of EX/RP when contemplating treatment options and, of course, consider the patient's preference as well.

References

1. Foa, E. B., Liebowitz, M. R., Kozak, M. J., Davies, S., Campeas, R., Franklin, M.E., . . . Tu, X. (2005). Randomized, placebo-controlled trial of exposure and ritual prevention, clomipramine, and their combination in the treatment of obsessive-compulsive disorder. *American Journal of Psychiatry, 162*(1), 151–161.
2. Goodman, W. K., Price, L. H. (1992). Assessment of severity and change in obsessive compulsive disorder. *Psychiatric Clinics of North America, 15*(4), 861–869.
3. Storch, E., Benito, K., & Goodman, W. (2011). Assessment scales for obsessive-compulsive disorder. *Neuropsychiatry, 1*(3), 243–250.
4. Pediatric, O. C. D. (2004). Cognitive-behavior therapy, sertraline, and their combination for children and adolescents with obsessive-compulsive disorder: The Pediatric OCD Treatment Study (POTS) randomized controlled trial. *JAMA, 292*(16), 1969–1976.
5. Bloch, M., Landeros-Weisenberger, A., Kelmendi, B., Coric, V., Bracken, M. B., & Leckman, J. F. (2006). A systematic review: Antipsychotic augmentation with treatment refractory obsessive-compulsive disorder. *Molecular Psychiatry, 11*(7), 622–632.
6. Abramowitz, J. S., Whiteside, S. P., & Deacon, B. J. (2005). The effectiveness of treatment for pediatric obsessive-compulsive disorder: A meta-analysis. *Behavior Therapy, 36*(1), 55–63.
7. Koran, L. M., Hanna, G. L., Hollander, E., Nestadt, G., & Simpson, H. B. (2007). Practice guideline for the treatment of patients with obsessive-compulsive disorder. *American Journal of Psychiatry, 164*(Suppl 7), 5–53.

30

Meta-Analysis of the Dose–Response Relationship of SSRIs in Adult Patients with Obsessive-Compulsive Disorder

EUNICE YUEN AND MICHAEL H. BLOCH

> The results of this meta-analysis support expert opinion that higher doses of SSRI are more effective in the treatment of adults with OCD. This greater treatment efficacy is somewhat counterbalanced by the greater sider-effect burden with higher doses of SSRIs.
>
> —BLOCH ET AL.[1]

Research Question: Are there any differences in efficacy and tolerability among different doses of selective serotonin reuptake inhibitors (SSRIs) in the treatment of obsessive compulsive disorder (OCD)?

Funding: The National Institute of Mental Health, the National Institutes of Health Loan Repayment Program, the Doris Duke Charitable Foundation and the Tourette's syndrome Association

Year Study Began: Studies between 1992 and 2006

Year Study Published: Nine studies performed from 1993 to 2007

Study Location: Multicenter, multicountry, multiple treatment settings

Who Was Studied: Patients 18 to 65 years old with OCD for at least one year diagnosed using DSM-III-R, DSM-IV-TR, or DSM-IV (depending on the year of the study).

Who Was Excluded: Based on the three major studies included in this meta-analysis, patients were excluded if they had axis I diagnoses other than OCD or significant medical illnesses, such as diabetes, neurological disorders, renal or liver complications.[2,3,4]

How Many Participants: 2,268

Study Overview: PubMed was searched for relevant randomized clinical trials. Only placebo controlled trials that compared doses of SSRIs and used the Yale–Brown Obsessive Compulsive Scale (Y-BOCS) were included in the study (Figure 30.1). Nine studies were included in the meta-analysis.

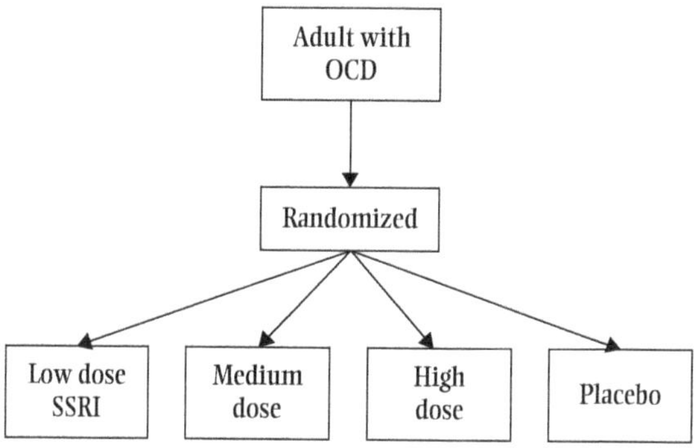

Figure 30.1 Example of a Typical Study Included in the Meta-Analysis
NOTES: OCD = obsessive-compulsive disorder. SSRI = selective serotonin reuptake inhibitor.

Study Intervention: This meta-analysis included nine previous trials that were randomized and double-blinded, which compared multiple fixed doses of SSRIs to placebo. Of these studies, three included fluoxetine, two included sertraline, and one study examined each fluvoxamine, citalopram, escitalopram, and paroxetine. To make comparison among different SSRIs, low, medium, and high dose of SSRIs were defined using calculation based on fluoxetine equivalents of SSRIs used in previous meta-analysis and from the American Psychiatric Association (APA) guideline for treating patients with OCD.[5,6,7] Low, medium, and high dose of fluoxetine were defined as 20 to 30 mg, 40 to 50 mg, and 60 to 90 mg, respectively.

Follow-Up: 8 to 13 weeks

Endpoints: Primary: the average change in Y-BOCS to detect changes before and after SSRI treatment. Secondary: proportion of treatment responders (either decrease in Y-BOCS by 25% or Clinical Global Impression <3), total dropouts, and dropouts due to side effects.

RESULTS

- Compared to placebo, low, medium, and high doses of SSRIs showed significantly greater improvement in symptom severity measured by Y-BOCS scores and the proportion of responders.
- High doses of SSRIs were superior to medium and low doses of SSRIs. Medium dose was not significantly better than low dose SSRIs.
- High doses of SSRIs had a greater proportion of dropouts due to side effects than low doses of SSRIs, but not significantly different from medium doses of SSRIs (Tables 30.1 and 30.2).

Table 30.1 Dose–Response versus Placebo

Outcome	**Low dose**	**Medium dose**	**High dose**	**P value**
Improvement in Y-BOCS – weighted mean difference	2.5	2.6	3.9	<0.001
Proportion improved – Absolute risk difference	0.16	0.16	0.22	<0.001

NOTE: Y-BOCS = Yale–Brown Obsessive Compulsive Scale.

Table 30.2 Dose–Response versus Each Other

Outcome	**High vs. Low dose (P value)**	**High vs. Medium dose (P value)**	**Medium vs. Low dose (P value)**
Improvement in Y-BOCS – Weighted mean difference	2.1 (<0.001)	1.8 (0.001)	0.4 (0.4)
Proportion improved– Absolute risk difference	0.07 (<0.05)	0.08 (0.02)	0.01 (0.86)
Dropout due to side effects – Absolute risk difference	0.05 (0.03)	0.01 (0.60)	0.04 (0.11)

NOTE: Y-BOCS = Yale–Brown Obsessive Compulsive Scale.

Criticisms and Limitations: This meta-analysis integrates nine studies using different SSRIs with distinct pharmacological profiles, which may generate heterogeneity among studies. The dose–response differences among individual SSRIs was not addressed in this study. All nine studies also had different treatment duration from 8 to 13 weeks, which may influence the measurement of efficacy.

This meta-analysis has limited data to address whether higher dose of SSRIs may produce similar beneficial effect in pediatric population. Several studies share similar conclusions that children with OCD often show partial response to SSRI, and augmentation by cognitive behavioral therapy or antipsychotic (such as risperidone), have been shown to provide great therapeutic effect in OCD symptoms.[8,9]

Other Relevant Studies and Information: Significant symptom improvement is seen with higher dose of sertraline (up to 400 mg per day) in OCD patients who are nonresponding to the standard recommended treatment of sertraline 200 mg per day. Both dosages have a similar side-effect profile.[10]

Other smaller randomized trials using high doses of SSRI in patients with OCD have come to similar conclusions with this meta-analysis.[11]

This study supports American Psychiatric Association guidelines that recommend the use of high dose SSRIs as a treatment for OCD in adults.[5]

Summary and Implications: This meta-analysis demonstrates the superiority of high doses of SSRIs relative to low doses of SSRIs in the management of OCD in adults. High doses are associated with higher rates of side effects, however. This study supports practice guidelines offered by the APA that recommend setting a high target dose of SSRIs to treat OCD.

CLINICAL CASE: META-ANALYSIS OF THE DOSE–RESPONSE RELATIONSHIP OF SSRIS IN ADULT PATIENTS WITH OCD

Case History

A 23-year-old graduate student with a history of OCD presents to an outpatient clinic. She compulsively counts the number of vowels in her textbook in an effort to prevent her family member from being murdered. Her symptoms are interfering with her performance at school. She denies any mood symptoms other than feeling anxious when she fails to count the vowels as described. She also denies other perceptual disturbance and a history of drug use. The patient was titrated to fluoxetine 50 mg daily with partial improvement of OCD symptoms and does not have any major side effects.

Based on the results from this meta-analysis, how should this patient be treated?

Suggested Answer

The meta-analysis by Bloch et al.[1] and APA guidelines suggest that higher doses of SSRIs are more effective than low and medium doses of SSRIs in the treatment of adults with OCD. Higher doses of SSRIs also correlate with a greater side effect profile.

The patient in this vignette is typical of patients from studies included in this meta-analysis. Given that this patient is a young and healthy individual without other medical and psychiatric comorbidities, she could be titrated to a higher dose of fluoxetine to target the OCD symptoms. Patients should be advised that higher doses of SSRIs are associated with greater side effects and should make an informed decision with their doctor.

References

1. Bloch, M. H., McGuire, J., Landeros-Weisenberger, A., Leckman, J. F., & Pittenger, C. (2010). Meta-analysis of the dose–response relationship of SSRI in obsessive-compulsive disorder. *Molecular Psychiatry, 15*(8), 850–855.
2. Tollefson, G. D., Rampey, A. H., Jr., Potvin, J. H., Jenike, M. A., Rush, A. J., Kominguez, R. A., Koran, L. M., . . . Genduso, L. A. (1994). A multicenter investigation of fixed-dose fluoxetine in the treatment of obsessive-compulsive disorder. *Archives of General Psychiatry, 51*, 559–567.
3. Montgomery, S. A., Kasper, S., Stein, D. J., Bang Hedegaard, K., & Lemming, O. M. (2001). Citalopram 20 mg, 40 mg and 60 mg are all effective and well tolerated compared with placebo in obsessive-compulsive disorder. *International Clinical Psychopharmacology, 16*(2), 75–86.
4. Hollander, E., Allen, A., Steiner, M., Wheadon, D. E., Oakes, R., & Burnham, D. B. (2003). Acute and long-term treatment and prevention of relapse of obsessive-compulsive disorder with paroxetine. *Journal of Clinical Psychiatry, 64*, 1113–1121.
5. Koran, L. M., Hanna, G. L., Hollander, E., Nestadt, G., & Simpson, H. B. (2007). *Practice guideline for the treatment of patients with obsessive-compulsive disorder.* Washington, DC: American Psychiatric Association.
6. Gelenberg, A. J. Freeman, M. P., Markowitz, J. C., Rosenbaum, J. F., Thase, M. E., Trivedi, M. H., & Van Rhoads, R. S. (2010). *APA Practice guideline for the treatment of patients with major depressive disorder* (3rd ed.). Washington, DC: American Psychiatric Association.
7. Bollini, P. Pampallona, S., Tibaldi, G., Kupelnick, B., & Munizza, C. (1999). Effectiveness of antidepressants: Meta-analysis of dose-effect relationships in randomised clinical trials. *British Journal of Psychiatry, 174*, 297–303.

8. Romanelli, R. J., Wu, F. M., Gamba, R., Mojtabai, R., & Segal, J. B. (2014). Behavioral therapy and serotonin reuptake inhibitor pharmacotherapy in the treatment of obsessive-compulsive disorder: A systematic review and meta-analysis of head-to-head randomized controlled trials. *Depression and Anxiety, 31*, 641–652.
9. Wheaton, M. G. Rosenfield, D., Foa, E. B., & Simpson, H. B. (2015). Augmenting serotonin reuptake inhibitors in obsessive-compulsive disorder: What moderates improvement? *Journal of Consulting and Clinical Psychology, 83*(5), 926–937.
10. Ninan, P. T., Koran, L. M., Kiev, A., Davidson, J. R., Rasmussen, S. A., Zajecka, J. M., . . . Austin, C. (2006). High-dose sertraline strategy for nonresponders to acute treatment for obsessive-compulsive disorder: a multicenter double-blind trial. *Journal of Clinical Psychiatry, 67*(1), 15–22.
11. Dougherty, D. D., Jameson, M., Deckersbach, T., Loh, R., Thompson-Hollands, J., Jenike, M., & Keuthen, N. J. (2009). Open-label study of high (30 mg) and moderate (20 mg) dose escitalopram for the treatment of obsessive-compulsive disorder. *International Clinical Psychopharmacology, 24*(6), 306–311.

SECTION 9

Personality Disorders

31

Psychotherapy for Borderline Personality Disorder

A Multiwave Study

DAVID GRUNWALD, ERICA ROBINSON, AND SARAH FINEBERG

> The general equivalence of outcome across the three [psychotherapy] treatments suggests that there may be different routes to symptom change in patients with Borderline Personality Disorder.
>
> —Clarkin et al.[1]

Research Question: How does transference-focused psychotherapy (TFP), supportive therapy, and dialectical behavioral therapy (DBT) compare in the treatment of borderline personality disorder (BPD)?

Funding: The Borderline Personality Disorder Research Foundation

Year Study Began: 1998

Year Study Published: 2007

Study Location: Three academic sites in the New York area

Who Was Studied: Patients 18 to 50 years old meeting DSM-IV criteria for BPD.

Who Was Excluded: Patients with psychotic disorders, bipolar I disorder, delusional disorder, delirium, dementia, and/or amnestic or other cognitive disorders were excluded. People with comorbid active substance dependence were also excluded.

How Many Participants: 90

Study Overview: See Figure 31.1 for a summary of the study design.

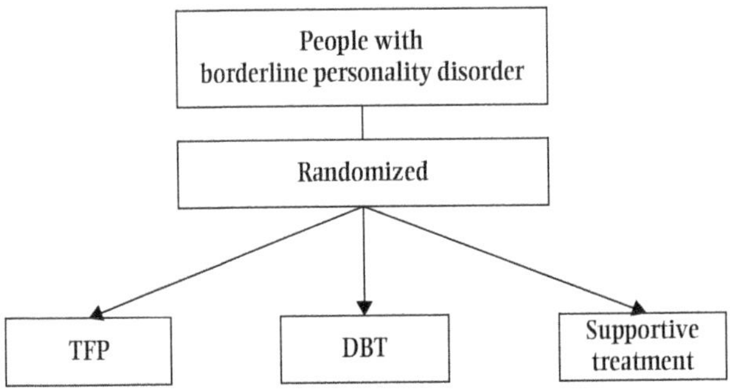

Figure 31.1 Summary of Study Design
NOTES: TFP = transference-focused psychotherapy. DBT = dialectical behavioral therapy.

Study Intervention: Patients with BPD were randomly assigned to TFP, DBT, or supportive treatment.

TFP is a psychodynamic-informed therapy that focuses on "borderline" psychological organization. Treatment examines patterns in outside life through the lens of situations occurring between patient and therapist. Individual TFP sessions were offered twice weekly.

DBT is a behavioral therapy that treats symptoms as maladaptive behaviors arising when a sensitive person is in an invalidating environment. Treatment teaches skills to regulate emotions; the therapist is highly supportive. Weekly individual and group sessions and as-needed telephone consultation were provided.

Supportive therapy provides emotional support and the therapist offers advice on practical problems. Supportive treatment involved 1 weekly session plus additional sessions as needed.

In all study arms, subjects were evaluated before study onset and medicated as needed by separate blinded study psychiatrists. At baseline and at 4-month intervals, raters assessed suicidal behavior, aggression, impulsivity, anxiety, depression, and social adjustment.

Follow-Up: 4, 8, and 12 months

Endpoints: Primary outcomes (measure used listed in parentheses): suicidality (Overt Aggression Scale–Modified), aggression (Anger, Irritability, and Assault Questionnaire), and impulsivity (Barratt Impulsiveness Scale II). Secondary outcomes: anxiety (Brief Symptom Inventory), depression (Beck Depression Inventory), and social adjustment (Global Assessment of Functioning Scale and Social Adjustment Scale).

RESULTS

- All three treatments significantly improved depression, anxiety, global functioning, and social adjustment.
- TFP showed significant improvement across 10 of 12 domains versus 6 of 12 domains in the supportive treatment, and 5 of 12 in the DBT groups.
- Suicidality significantly decreased with both TFP and DBT.
- Anger significantly decreased with TFP and supportive treatment.
- Only TFP significantly decreased motor impulsivity, irritability, verbal assault, and direct assault.[2]
- Only supportive therapy significantly improved self-control.[2]
- None of the groups significantly improved on attention-based impulsivity.[2]
- 62 of 90 enrolled subjects continued 9+ months. Intent to treat analysis suggested that attrition did not substantially alter the findings (Table 31.1).

Table 31.1 Summary of BPD Multiwave Study's Key Findings

Outcome	TFP	P value	DBT	P value	Supportive treatment	P Value
Suicidality	0.33	0.01	0.44	0.01	0.18	>0.05
Anger	0.44	0.001	0.25	>0.05	0.28	0.05
Irritability	0.33	>0.05	0.11	>0.05	0.16	>0.05
Verbal assault	0.43	0.001	0.21	>0.05	0.19	>0.05
Impulsivity	0.36	0.005	0.05	>0.05	0.31	>0.02
Anxiety	0.37	0.004	0.50	0.001	0.48	0.001
Depression	0.50	0.001	0.38	0.003	0.49	0.001
Social adjustment	0.28	0.03	0.44	0.001	0.59	0.001

Notes: The data presented here represents the effect size regarding improvement relative to baseline. A higher value represents a larger effect. P values represents the outcome measure post-treatment and at baseline. BPD = borderline personality disorder. TFP = transference-focused psychotherapy. DBT = dialectical behavior therapy.

Criticisms and Limitations: The study had limited statistical power for assessing differences between the treatment groups, so it is not possible to know whether the study interventions are significantly better than no intervention. Also, the study population (92% female) differed from epidemiologic data on BPD[3] (50% female). These factors limit the ability to generalize the findings.

Also, ethical constraints prevented the authors from including a control group that did not receive any intervention, so it is not possible to know whether the study interventions are significantly better than no intervention. Although the supportive treatment arm was intended to approximate usual care, study therapists likely had more support than many typical community clinicians.

Treatment dose also differed among the groups: the TFP group had two visits per week, the DBT group had three visits per week, and the supportive treatment group had one visit per week. Therefore, therapy dose rather than content may have driven study outcomes.

Though there are no FDA-approved medications for BPD, many subjects in this study received pharmacologic therapy. Rates of pharmacotherapy also differed among groups, and information about specific medications, classes, and numbers of medications is not reported. Subgroup analysis suggested that medicated subjects had similar outcomes to the full study cohort.

Other Relevant Studies and Information:

- A 2012 Cochrane Systemic Review found that both comprehensive (defined as therapy that includes one-to-one treatment) as well as noncomprehensive psychotherapeutics for BPD show beneficial effects on core pathology and associated general psychopathology.[3] DBT has been studied most extensively, followed by mentalization-based treatment (MBT), TFP, schema-focused therapy and systems training for emotional predictability and problem-solving for BPD (STEPS).
- Polypharmacy is common in BPD despite evidence only for mood stabilizers, second generation antipsychotics, and symptom-focused use of selective serotonin reuptake inhibitors.[4] There are no FDA-approved medications for BPD, and no evidence for using benzodiazepines.
- American Psychiatric Association (APA) guidelines for BPD promote psychodynamic or DBT approaches and treating co-occurring psychiatric diagnoses with therapy and/or medications.[4] A 2017 meta-analysis supports this approach, finding significant but modest and unstable benefits of the main evidence-based psychotherapies for BPD.[5]

Summary and Implications: This study was the first randomized controlled trial that examined and compared three manualized psychotherapeutic treatments for BPD. Each of the three therapies led to significant improvement in multiple symptoms over one year of outpatient treatment relative to baseline. Notably, patients treated with TFP improved in more domains than did those assigned to other treatment groups.

CLINICAL CASE: PSYCHOTHERAPIES FOR BPD

Case History

A 43-year-old man with BPD including mood instability, irritability, and chronic passive suicidality was sent to a local emergency department after describing increasing suicidal urges to his therapist. The patient was discharged from the ED, and at a follow-up therapy session two days later, asked for a referral to a new clinician. The patient now presents to a new outpatient psychiatrist for treatment.

Based on the results of this study, what modality of psychotherapy should the psychiatrist choose?

Suggested Answer

This and other studies contributed to APA guidelines supporting DBT or psychodynamic psychotherapy (e.g. TFP, MBT, etc.) to treat BPD.

The patient in this vignette is typical of patients in this study, and thus any of the three psychotherapies may be appropriate. Considering the patient's suicidality and irritability, a trial of TFP should be strongly considered if logistically feasible. In this study, TFP was the only treatment with significant improvement in both suicidality and irritability. However, psychoeducation about the format and content of various treatment options (such as the 3 modalities described in this chapter) will be important to help connect the patient to an appropriate care setting where he is likely to follow through.

References

1. Clarkin, J. F., Levy, K. N., Lenzenweger, M. F., & Kernberg, O. T. (2007). Evaluating three treatments for borderline personality disorder: A multiwave study. *American Journal of Psychiatry, 164*(6), 922–928.
2. Stoffers, J. M., Völlm, B. A., Rücker, G., Timmer, A., Huband, N., & Lieb, K. (2012). Psychological therapies for people with borderline personality disorder. *Cochrane Database of Systematic Reviews, 8*, CD005652.
3. Grant, B. F., Chou, S. P., Goldstein, R. B., Huang, B., Stinson, F. S., Saha, T. D., . . . Ruan, W. J. (2008). Prevalence, correlates, disability, and comorbidity of DSM-IV

borderline personality disorder: Results from the Wave 2 National Epidemiologic Survey on Alcohol and Related Conditions. *Journal of Clinical Psychiatry, 69*(4), 533–545.
4. Oldham, J. M., Gabbard, G. O., Goin, M. K., Gunderson, J., Soloff, P., Spiegel, D., . . . Phillips, K. A. (2001). Treatment of patients with borderline personality disorder. American Psychiatric Association Practice Guidelines. *American Journal of Psychiatry, 158*(10 Suppl), 1–52.
5. Cristea, I. A., Gentili, C., Cotet, C. D., Palomba, D., Barbui, C., & Cuijpers, P. (2017). Efficacy of psychotherapies for borderline personality Disorder: A systematic review and meta-analysis. *JAMA psychiatry, 74*(4), 319–328.

32

Dialectical Behavior Therapy versus Community Treatment by Experts for Reducing Suicidal Behaviors among Patients with Borderline Personality Disorder

DAVID SAUNDERS, ERICA ROBINSON, AND SARAH FINEBERG

> This is not a "horse race" study pitting one complex active treatment against another. Rather, it is a dismantling study designed to begin answering questions as to the unique effects of DBT.... Dialectical behavior therapy appears to be uniquely effective in reducing suicide attempts.
>
> —LINEHAN ET AL.[1]

Research Question: Is dialectical behavior therapy (DBT) more effective than treatment offered by nonbehavioral psychotherapy experts in reducing suicidal behaviors and treating borderline personality disorder (BPD)?

Funding: National Institutes of Mental Health

Year Study Began: Not indicated

Year Study Published: 2006

Study Location: University of Washington

Who Was Studied: Women aged 18 to 45 with BPD and "at least 2 suicide attempts or self-injuries in the past 5 years with at least 1 in the past 8 weeks."

Who Was Excluded: Individuals with a history of a serious mental illness, "a seizure disorder requiring medication, a mandate to treatment, or the need for primary treatment for another debilitating condition."

How Many Participants: 101

Study Overview: See Figure 32.1 for a summary of the study design.

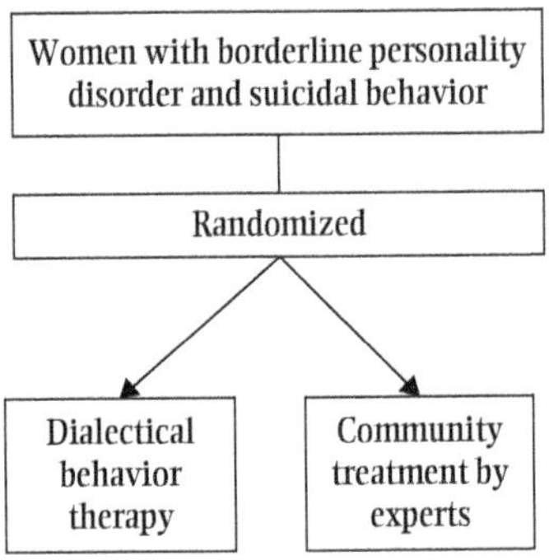

Figure 32.1 Summary of Study Design

Study Intervention: DBT targets suicidal behavior and behaviors that interfere with treatment or are otherwise dangerous, severe, or destabilizing. In this study, treatment included weekly one-hour individual psychotherapy and weekly 2.5-hour group skills training with licensed DBT psychotherapists, telephone consultations, and weekly therapy supervision for approximately one year. The group sessions consisted of a short mindfulness meditation exercise, a discussion of personal experiences implementing the previous week's skill, and teaching on the new skill. Individual psychotherapy targets motivation and the application of skills, tailored to each unique patient. Assessments of suicidal behaviors, emergency services usage and general psychological functioning were performed every 12 weeks.

The control group was community treatment by experts (CTBE), with therapists randomized by age, sex, level of education, and years clinical experience. The content of CTBE was not prescribed by researchers, though they were instructed to provide "the type and dose of therapy that they believed was most suited, with a minimum of 1 scheduled individual session per week" for one year. Controls were also monitored every 12 weeks.

Follow-Up: 24 months

Endpoints: Scores on the Suicide Attempt Self-Injury Interview, which measures the severity of suicide attempts and self-injury; scores on the Suicide Behaviors Questionnaire, which measures suicidal ideation; and scores on the Reasons for Living Inventory. Emergency service use and depression severity as measured by the Hamilton Rating Scale for Depression–17 item were also assessed.

RESULTS

- DBT is more effective than CTBE in reducing suicide attempts.
- Both DBT and CTBE were effective in reducing nonsuicidal self-injuries, and there was no difference between the two groups.
- Among subjects with a suicide attempt or intentional self-injury during the treatment year, the medical consequences resulting from suicide attempts and self-injurious acts were significantly less severe for the DBT group than for CTBE.
- Patients in both treatment groups experienced significant reductions in suicidal ideation and improvements in reasons for living relative to the beginning of the study period.
- The DBT group used crisis services significantly less than the control group (Table 32.1).

Table 32.1 SUMMARY OF KEY FINDINGS FOR THE DBT VERSUS CTBE FOR BPD STUDY

Outcome	DBT	CTBE	NNT	P value
Suicide Attempts	23.1%	46%	4.24 (2.4–18.07)	0.005
Hospitalizations for SI	14.9%	18.4%	3.88 (2.26–13.71)	0.004
Psychiatric hospitalizations	23.4%	23.7%	9.09 (3.30–12.04)	0.007
Psychiatric ER visits for SI	19.6%	18.4%	4.42 (2.49–19.76)	0.02
Psychiatric ER visits	23.4%	28.9%	4.46 (2.53–19.17)	0.04

NOTES: DBT = dialectical behavior therapy. CTBE = community treatment by experts. BPD = borderline personality disorder. NNT = number needed to treat. SI = suicide ideation. ER = emergency room.

Criticisms and Limitations: A major limitation is that subjects dropped out of the control condition more often than DBT, though statistical analysis showed that this factor did not explain the differences in outcomes. Results may also be limited by the heterogeneity of the control treatments offered in the CTBE. While the DBT was strictly supervised and regimented, the CTBE group was not as critically supervised, and each individual therapist had considerable flexibility in implementing their treatment plan.

Other Relevant Studies and Information:

- There have been several smaller randomized controlled trials to evaluate the efficacy of various treatments for BPD[2,3,4] including partial [3]hospitalization[5] and DBT.[6,7] These studies have suggested beneficial effects of several different manualized treatments, including transference-focused psychodynamic (TFP) therapy and mentalization-based treatment, Systems Training for Emotional Predictability and Problem Solving.
- Clarkin et al.[3] compared DBT, TFP, and supportive therapy finding that DBT and TFP were similarly effective in decreasing suicidal ideation in BPD patients and that all three groups led to symptom improvement across multiple symptom groups (see Chapter 31).
- The American Psychiatric Association (APA) recommends DBT for the treatment of BPD owing to its demonstrated efficacy in randomized-controlled trials such as this one.
- While the number of DBT providers is growing, access to care is still a significant limitation for BPD patients. Finding ways to train more nonexpert providers in the basics of treatment of BPD patients is one way to provide more access to patients. One example of this is Good Psychiatric Management, a manual of BPD-tailored treatment guidance for nonexpert providers.

Summary and Implications: This study found that, for patients with BPD and a history of suicide attempts, DBT reduced the rate of suicide attempts and the use of emergency services relative to a rigorous control condition of treatment by experts. Because of this large study and others, the APA has recommended DBT in the treatment of BPD.

CLINICAL CASE: DBT VERSUS CTBE IN SUICIDAL BORDERLINE PERSONALITY DISORDER PATIENTS

Case History

After being fired from her job last week and breaking up with her boyfriend, a 21-year-old woman attempted suicide by overdosing on 45 acetaminophen pills and was admitted to the medical intensive care unit. She has a history of two prior suicide attempts, self-injurious behavior and unstable interpersonal relationships. She carries the diagnosis of BPD and requires more intensive outpatient treatment for her suicidal behaviors. What are the options for alternative treatments?

Suggested Answer

According to clinical studies including this one on the treatment of BPD patients with suicidal behaviors, DBT is a very effective treatment at reducing suicidality in patients. This paper also reports that DBT patients utilized emergency resources and psychotropic medications less that did those in non-DBT community treatment by experts. However, DBT providers are limited in quantity, and many patients have difficulty gaining access. As such patients could also be referred for TFP, or supportive therapy, as it tends to be more readily available. Both providers and patients should also be aware of studies such as Gunderson et al.[9] (see Chapter 33) that show that patients with BPD tend to have high levels of remission with low relapse rates but continued severe impairments in social functioning.

This troubled young woman is typical of one included in this study considering her demographics and suicide attempts. Based on the results of this study, BPD-focused psychotherapy will help. The data suggest that DBT may provide some additional benefits over nonmanualized supportive therapy by a BPD expert, but in low-resource areas, BPD-informed supportive therapy can also help patients to improve.

References

1. Linehan, M. M., Comtois, K. A, Murray, A. M., Brown, M. Z., Gallop, R. J., . . . Lindenboim, N. (2006). Two-year randomized controlled trial and follow-up of dialectical behavior therapy vs therapy by experts for suicidal behaviors and borderline personality disorder. *Archives of General Psychiatry, 63*(7), 757–766.
2. Meares, R. & Stevenson, J. (1992). An outcome study of psychotherapy for patients with borderline personality disorder. *American Journal of Psychiatry, 149*(3), 358–362.
3. Clarkin, J. F., Levy, K. N., Lenzenweger, M. F., & Kernberg, O. F. (2007). Evaluating three treatments for borderline personality disorder: A multiwave study. *American Journal of Psychiatry, 164*(6), 922–928.
4. Doering, D., Hörz, S., Rentrop, M., Fischer-Kern, M., Schuster, P., Benecke, C., . . . Buchheim, P. (2010). Transference-focused psychotherapy v. treatment by community psychotherapists for borderline personality disorder: Randomised controlled trial. *British Journal of Psychiatry, 196*(5), 389–395.
5. Bateman, A., & Fonagy, P. (1999). Effectiveness of partial hospitalization in the treatment of borderline personality disorder: A randomized controlled trial. *American Journal of Psychiatry, 156*(1), 1563–1569.

6. Koons, C. R., Robins, C. J., Tweed, J. L., Lynch, T. R., Gonzalez, A. M., Morse, J. Q., . . . Bastian, L. A. (2001). Efficacy of dialectical behavior therapy in women veterans with borderline personality disorder. *Behavior Therapy*, *32*(2), 371–390.
7. Verheul, R., van den Bosch, L. M., Koeter, M. W., De Ridder, M. A., Stijnen, T., & Van Den Brink, W. (2003). Dialectical behaviour therapy for women with borderline personality disorder. *British Journal of Psychiatry*, *182*(2), 135–140.
8. Gunderson, J. G., & Links, P. S. (2014). *Handbook of good psychiatric management for borderline personality disorder*. Washington, DC: American Psychiatric Association.

33

Ten-Year Course of Borderline Personality Disorder

The Collaborative Longitudinal Personality Disorders Study

KEVIN JOHNSON, ERICA ROBINSON, AND SARAH FINEBERG

> What is evident appears clinically counterintuitive: patients with BPD improve symptomatically more often, more quickly, and more dramatically than expected, and once better, maintain improvements more enduring than for many other major psychiatric disorders.
>
> —The Collaborative Longitudinal Personality Disorders Study Investigators[1]

Research Question: What is the long-term prognosis of those with borderline personality disorder?

Funding: The National Institute of Mental Health.

Year Study Began: 1985

Year Study Published: 2011

Study Location: 19 clinical sites affiliated with one of four academic medical centers

Who Was Studied: Adults aged 18 to 45 who met DSM-IV criteria for one of three personality disorders: borderline personality disorder (BPD; 5+ DSM criteria), avoidant personality disorder (AVPD; 4+ DSM criteria), or obsessive-compulsive personality disorder (OCPD; 4+ DSM criteria). The study also recruited participants with major depressive disorder (MDD; 5+ DSM criteria) with no concurrent personality disorder.

Who Was Excluded: Those with schizotypal personality disorder, or MDD with comorbid personality disorder.

How Many Participants: 582

Study Overview: See Figure 33.1 for an overview of the study.

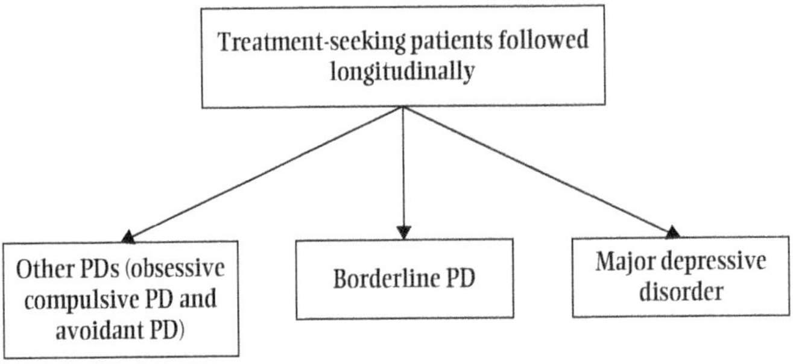

Figure 33.1 Overview of Study
NOTE: PD = personality disorder.

This was an observational study with no interventions. Participants were assessed at fixed periods over 10 years: at baseline, 6 months, 12 months, and 2, 4, 6, 8, and 10 years. At each assessment, personality disorder criteria were reassessed via the Diagnostic Interview for DSM-IV Personality Disorders, a Global Assessment of Functioning (GAF) score, the Global Social Adjustment (GSA) scale, and the Longitudinal Interval Follow-Up Evaluation (LIFE).

Ongoing psychiatric treatment was not required, and the study does not indicate how many participants were engaged in active psychiatric treatment during the course of the 10-year study.

Follow-Up: 10 years

Endpoints: Primary outcome: (a) Remission of symptoms (defined by meeting two or more diagnostic criteria); (b) Relapse of symptoms (among those who achieved remission). Secondary outcomes: (a) functional remission (defined by achieving a GAF score >70 for at least two months); (b) rate of remission of each BPD symptom (affective instability, unstable relationships, self-injurious behavior, etc.).

RESULTS

- At the 10-year mark, 91% of patients had achieved remission for at least two months. 85% of the patients remitted for a full 12 months. These rates were comparable to those of either MDD or cluster C personality disorders.
- BPD patients take longer to achieve remission relative to MDD or cluster C personality disorders (PDs).
- BPD patient were less likely to relapse once remitted relative to those with MDD or cluster C PDs (21% BPD; 67% MDD; 36% cluster C PDs).
- Over 10 years of follow-up all nine DSM-IV criteria for BPD decreased in rate and level similarly.
- Functional remission (getting back to life roles) was less frequent in BPD than psychiatric controls (21% in BPD vs. approximately 50%; Table 33.1).

Table 33.1 Summary of the CLPS Key Findings

Outcome	BPD	Other PDs	P value Other PDs vs BPD	MDD	P value MDD vs. BPD
% achieving 2 month remission	91% [86%, 96%]	NR	NR	NR	NR
% achieving 12 month remission	85% [78%, 91%]	NR	NR	NR	NR
10-year relapse rate	11% [4%, 17%]	25% [18%, 31%]	0.008	21% [13%, 29%]	0.001
% achieving functional remission at 10 years	21%	48%		61%	

NOTES: CLPS = Collaborative Longitudinal Personality Disorders Study.
PDs = personality disorders BPD = borderline personality disorder. MDD = major depressive disorder. NR = not reported.

Criticisms and Limitations: The study did not report patients' involvement (if any) with treatment and did not analyze factors that may predict remission or recovery.

Study patients lived in predominately urban areas on the East Coast. Access to mental health care, especially for people with personality disorders, may be far less outside academic and urban centers, and thus these findings may not be generalizable to other regions of the country.

Only 66% of patients completed the full 10-year follow-up period. Survivorship bias may artificially inflate remission rates if lower-functioning BPD patients were disproportionately likely to drop out.

The results also rely on self-report—raising the question of recall bias. However, recent data on personality-disordered patients showed that self-report was highly concordant with information reported (collateral) behavior.[2]

Other Relevant Studies and Information:

- The only other 10+ year longitudinal study of people with BPD is the McLean Study of Adult Development (MSAD).[3] These authors also report significant functional impairment over time though many more people did recover in their sample (60% in 16 years). Predictors of social recovery in the MSAD included no past psychiatric hospitalizations, higher baseline IQ, recent work, absence of an anxious cluster personality disorder, high extroversion, and high agreeableness.[4]
- Evidence is accumulating to demonstrate the biologic basis and heritability of BPD. BPD is at least as prevalent and heritable as schizophrenia.[5]
- Others have found that the clinical course for BPD is impacted by strong affect and stigma from families and providers.[6] The Collaborative Longitudinal Personality Disorders Study results can help instill hope and decrease stigma.

Summary and Implications: Though stigma persist among patients and health-care providers, and many may still believe borderline personality disorder to be nearly untreatable, the Collaborative Longitudinal Personality Disorder Study found long-term remission of symptoms to be very common for BPD patients. In fact, long-term remission rate in BPD was comparable to that for other personality disorders and MDD. Nevertheless, almost 80% of patients remained socially/functionally impaired at the end of the 10-year study period, highlighting the importance of assessing social functioning and psychosocial supports among patients with BPD.

CLINICAL CASE: BORDERLINE PERSONALITY DISORDER AND TREATMENT

Case History

A 31-year-old chronically unemployed woman with past psychiatric diagnoses of bipolar disorder, self-injurious behavior, and alcohol use disorder is admitted to the hospital after a suicide attempt in the setting of an argument with her partner. During her hospitalization, her treatment team initiated a discussion about the diagnosis of borderline personality disorder. They reviewed with the patient her life-long history of affect instability, anger outbursts, impulsive behavior, unstable interpersonal relationships, feelings of chronic emptiness, and history of self-injurious behavior and provided psychoeducation about BPD symptoms and prognosis.

Based on the results of this study, what is her likely long-term prognosis? What sort of outpatient treatment options should be discussed with the patient?

Suggested Answer

According to this 10-year longitudinal study, it is highly likely that this woman will improve psychiatrically and show fewer BPD symptoms. However, she may have prolonged deficits in social functioning compared to those with other psychiatric illnesses. She may benefit from therapies that target her ability to form stable relationships and her ability to sustain stable employment or other occupational roles. As discussed in the Clarkin et al.[7] study on the effectiveness of therapy modalities for BPD patients (see Chapter 31), dialectical behavioral therapy and transference-focused psychodynamic therapy are both effective in treating suicidality in people with BPD. Importantly, the accessibility of these treatments must also be considered. That same study also showed that supportive therapy was associated with a significant positive effect on multiple symptom domains of BPD, and it tends to be a more readily accessible form of therapy across the country. John Gunderson and Paul Links have recently codified the principles of effective supportive therapy for BPD in their Good Psychiatric Management manual.[8] This approach aims to be more accessible to generalist providers than the specialized manualized treatments. While the information gained from this study should be provided to both BPD patients and families, providers must also expect that this information may be difficult for patients to accept. Most BPD patients are experiencing a great deal of distress and may have difficulty believing that their prognosis is not worse. Data about the very high likelihood of remission from studies such as this one can be provided to instill hope.

References

1. Gunderson, J. G., Stout, R. L., McGlashan, T. H., Shea, M. T., Morey, L. C., Grilo, C. M., . . . Skodol, A. E. (2011). Ten-year course of borderline personality disorder: Psychopathology and function from the Collaborative Longitudinal Personality Disorders Study. *Archives in General Psychiatry, 68*(8), 827–837.
2. Ready, R. E., Watson, D., & Clark, L. A. (2002). Psychiatric patient–and informant-reported personality: Predicting concurrent and future behavior. *Assessment, 9*(4), 361–372.
3. Zanarini, M. C., Frankenburg, F. R., Reich, D. B., & Fitzmaurice, G. (2010). Time to attainment of recovery from borderline personality disorder and stability of recovery: A 10-year prospective follow-up study. *American Journal of Psychiatry, 167*(6), 663–667.
4. Zanarini, M. C., Frankenburg, F. R., Reich, D. B., Wedig, M. M., Conkey, L. C., & Fitzmaurice, G. M. (2014). Prediction of time-to-attainment of recovery for borderline patients followed prospectively for 16 years. *Acta Psychiatrica Scandinavica, 130*(3), 205–213.
5. Schmahl, C., Herpertz, S. C., Bertsch, K., Ende, G., Flor, H., Kirsch, P., . . . Spanagel, R. (2014). Mechanisms of disturbed emotion processing and social interaction in borderline personality disorder: State of knowledge and research agenda of the German Clinical Research Unit. *Borderline Personality Disorder and Emotion Dysregulation, 1*(1), art. 12.
6. Bodner, E., Cohen-Fridel, S., Mashiah, M., Segal, M., Grinshpoon, A., Fischel, T., & Iancu, I. (2015). The attitudes of psychiatric hospital staff toward hospitalization and treatment of patients with borderline personality disorder. *BMC Psychiatry, 15*(1), art. 2.
7. Clarkin, J. F., Levy, K. N., Lenzenweger, M. F., & Kernberg, O. T. (2007). Evaluating three treatments for borderline personality disorder: A multiwave study. *American Journal of Psychiatry, 164*(6), 922–928.
8. Gunderson, J. G., & Links, P. S. (2014). *Handbook of good psychiatric management for borderline personality disorder*. Washington, DC: American Psychiatric Association.

SECTION 10

Psychiatry in Primary Care

34

Depressive Symptoms and Health-Related Quality of Life

The Heart and Soul Study

AMALIA LONDONO TOBON AND CATHERINE CHILES

> Among patients with coronary disease, we found that depressive symptoms were strongly associated with health status outcomes, including symptom burden, physical limitation, quality of life, and overall health. . . . Efforts to improve health status [in patients with coronary artery disease] should include assessment and treatment of depressive symptoms.
>
> —The Heart and Soul Study Investigators[1]

Research Question: What are the effects of depressive symptoms and cardiac function on health-related quality of life in patients with coronary artery disease?

Funding: The Department of Veterans Affairs, the Robert Wood Johnson Foundation, the American Federation for Aging Research, the Ischemia Research and Education Foundation, and the University of California, San Francisco

Year Study Began: 2000

Year Study Published: 2003

Study Location: 12 outpatient clinics in the San Francisco Bay Area

Who Was Studied: Adults with stable coronary heart disease defined by one or more of the following: a history of myocardial infarction, angiographic evidence of at least 50% stenosis in one or more coronary vessels, prior evidence of exercise-induced ischemia by treadmill or nuclear testing, a history of coronary revascularization, or a diagnosis of coronary artery disease by an internist or cardiologist.[2]

Who Was Excluded: Patients who could not be reached by telephone, had a history of myocardial infarction in the past six months, reported an inability to walk one block, or planned to move out of the area within three years

How Many Participants: 1,024

Study Overview: See Figure 34.1 for a summary of the study design.

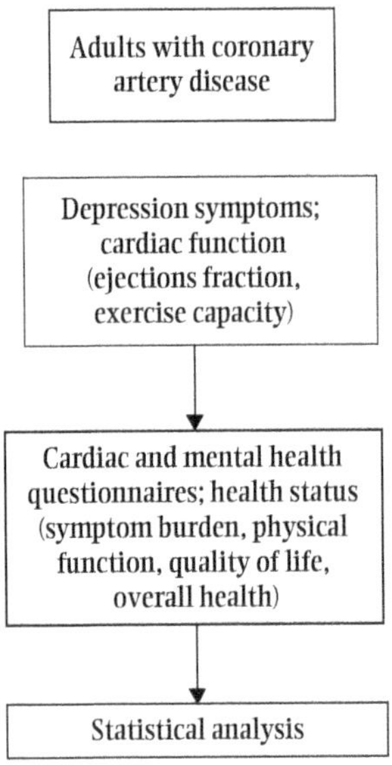

Figure 34.1 Summary of Study Design

This is a cross-sectional study in which participants were screened for inclusion in the study and asked to complete cardiac and mental health questionnaires, a physical examination, and cardiac testing. Depressive symptoms were assessed with the nine-item Patient Health Questionnaire (PHQ). Cardiac evaluation included measurements of ejection fraction by resting echocardiography, exercise capacity by an exercise treadmill test, and ischemia by stress echocardiography. Patients also completed the Seattle Angina Questionnaire to measure disease-specific health status, including symptom burden (two-item angina frequency scale), functional status (nine-item physical limitation scale), and disease-specific quality of life (three-item disease perception scale). To evaluate overall health status, participants were asked "Compared with other people your age, how would you rate your overall health?" A statistical analysis was performed to identify independent predictors of health status outcomes.

Follow-Up: This is a cross-sectional study.

Endpoints: Primary outcome: the contributions of depressive symptoms and cardiac function to patient-reported health status. Secondary outcomes: the association between independent variables (depression and cardiac function) and outcome variables (symptom burden, functional status, quality of life, and overall health).

RESULTS

- 20% of study participants had depressive symptoms.
- Compared to participants without depressive symptoms, those with depressive symptoms (PHQ score ≥10) were more likely to report cardiac symptom burden, physical limitation, diminished quality of life, and fair or poor overall health.
- These findings persisted after adjustment for objective measures of cardiac function and other patient characteristics.
- Depressive symptoms were not associated with objective measures of cardiac function.
- In adjusted models, decreased exercise capacity by treadmill testing was associated with greater symptom burden, greater physical limitation, worse quality of life, and worse overall health, but ejection fraction and ischemia were not (Table 34.1).

Table 34.1 SUMMARY OF HEART AND SOUL KEY FINDINGS

Outcome	Non-depressed group	Depressed group	P value
Mild cardiac symptoms burden or greater symptoms	33%	60%	<0.001
Mild physical limitation or greater limitation	40%	73%	<0.001
Mildly diminished quality of life or worse quality of life	31%	67%	<0.001
Fair or poor overall health	30%	66%	<0.001
Greater symptom burden	–	OR 1.8 (1.3–2.7)	0.002
Greater physical limitation	–	OR 3.1 (2.1–4.6)	<0.001
Worse quality of life	–	OR 3.1 (2.2–4.6)	<0.001
Worse overall health	–	OR 2.0 (1.3–2.9)	<0.001

Criticisms and Limitations: The study's cross-sectional design limits its ability to detect causality or directionality of effect (e.g., if depressive symptoms worsen quality of life or diminished quality of life worsens depressive symptoms). The study had a low response rate overall of 16.2%. The study population consisted mainly of older men, so generalizability of these results is limited. Furthermore, depression was diagnosed by scores on the PHQ-9, which has limitations including that it is a self-reported questionnaire and does not account for duration or recurrence of depressive symptoms.

Other Relevant Studies and Information:

- The Heart and Soul Study cohort was followed up for about 4.8 years. Longitudinal results of this cohort demonstrated that "after adjustment for comorbid conditions and disease severity, depressive symptoms were associated with a 31% higher rate of cardiovascular events."[2]
- Previous studies have found similar associations between depressive symptoms and health outcomes in patients with coronary disease and other medical illnesses.[3]
- Previous studies have also reported improvements in physical health status in patients with treated depression.[4,5] Furthermore, studies have demonstrated that improved self-reported health status has been associated with better health outcomes.[6]
- The American Heart Association recommends to screen for and treat depression in patients with coronary artery disease.[7]

Summary and Implications: The Heart and Soul study found that even after controlling for indicators of worsening cardiac status, patients with comorbid depressive symptoms reported greater symptom burden, worse quality of life, decreased physical functioning, and worse overall health. More recent studies have found that treating depressive symptoms in patients with coronary artery disease may lead to improved general health status.

CLINICAL CASE: ASSESSING DEPRESSION

Case History

A 60-year-old man with coronary artery disease presents to an integrated care clinic with increased difficulty walking due to chest discomfort. The symptoms are severely affecting his quality of life. An echocardiogram measures an unchanged ejection fraction. He demonstrates diminished capacity on an exercise treadmill test, yet no increase in ischemia by stress echocardiography.

Based on the Heart and Soul study, what else should you consider and how should this patient be treated?

Suggested Answer

The Heart and Soul study showed that patients with coronary artery disease who also had depressive symptoms tended to report increased coronary disease symptom burden, physical limitation, and decreased quality of life even after controlling for worsening cardiac disease.

The patient described has the characteristics of participants in the Heart and Soul Study. Even though the clinical indicators of cardiac disease are static, the patient is still experiencing a decline in health quality. Therefore, an informed cardiologist or consulting psychiatrist would screen for and treat depression to address the patient's worsening quality of life and cardiac symptom burden.

References

1. Ruo, B., Rumsfeld, J. S., Hlatky, M. A., Liu, H., Browner, W. S., & Whooley, M. A. (2003). Depressive symptoms and health-related quality of life: The Heart and Soul Study. *JAMA, 290*(2), 215–221.
2. Whooley, M. A., de Jonge, P., Vittinghoff, E., Otte, C., Moos, R., Carney, R. M., . . . Schiller, N. B. (2008). Depressive symptoms, health behaviors, and risk of cardiovascular events in patients with coronary heart disease. *JAMA, 300*(20), 2379–2388.
3. Sullivan, M. D., LaCroix, A. Z., Russo, J. E., & Walker, E. A. (2001). Depression and self-reported physical health in patients with coronary disease: Mediating and moderating factors. *Psychosomatic Medicine, 63*(2), 248–256.
4. Cossette, S., Frasure-Smith, N., & Lesperance, F. (2001). Clinical implications of a reduction in psychological distress on cardiac prognosis in patients participating in a psychosocial intervention program. *Psychosomatic Medicine, 63*(2), 257–266.
5. Glassman, A. H., O'Connor, C. M., Califf, R. M., Swedberg, K., Schwartz, P., Bigger, J. T., Jr., . . . Landau, C. (2002). Sertraline treatment of major depression in patients with acute MI or unstable angina. *JAMA, 288*(6), 701–709.
6. Spertus, J. A., Jones, P., McDonell, M., Fan, V., & Fihn, S. D. (2002). Health status predicts long-term outcome in outpatients with coronary disease. *Circulation, 106*(1), 43–49.
7. Lichtman, J. H., Bigger, J. T., Jr., Blumenthal, J. A., Frasure-Smith, N., Kaufmann, P. G., Lespérance, F., . . . Froelicher, E. S. (2008). Depression and coronary heart disease: Recommendations for screening, referral, and treatment: A science advisory from the American Heart Association Prevention Committee of the Council on Cardiovascular Nursing, Council on Clinical Cardiology, Council on Epidemiology and Prevention, and Interdisciplinary Council on Quality of Care and Outcomes Research: Endorsed by the American Psychiatric Association. *Circulation, 118*(17), 1768–1775.

35

The Canadian Cardiac Randomized Evaluation of Antidepressant and Psychotherapy Efficacy (CREATE) Trial

NIKHIL GUPTA AND CATHERINE CHILES

> Citalopram or sertraline plus clinical management should be considered as a first-step treatment for patients with CAD and major depression.
>
> —The CREATE Investigators[1]

Research Question: In the treatment of patients with major depression and coronary artery disease (CAD), what is the short-term efficacy of a selective serotonin reuptake inhibitor (SSRI; citalopram) and/or interpersonal therapy (IPT)?

Funding: Canadian Institutes of Health Research Clinical Trials Program grant and the foundations of the University of Montreal Hospital Research Center and the Montreal Heart Institute.

Year Study Began: 2002

Year Study Published: 2007

Study Location: Nine academic centers in Canada

Who Was Studied: Patients 18 years or older with stable CAD meeting DSM-IV criteria for major depression for four weeks or longer and a baseline score of 20 or higher on the 24-item Hamilton Depression Rating Scale (HAM-D).

Who Was Excluded: Patients with depression caused by a medical condition, bipolar disorder, depression with psychotic features, at high risk for suicide, substance abuse during the previous 12 months, cognitive impairment (Mini Mental State Examination score <24), current use of psychotherapy or medications for a mood disorder, and previous unsuccessful treatment response to citalopram or IPT. Patients with coronary artery bypass graft surgery planned in the next 4 months, or CAD with severe physical activity limitations were also excluded.

How Many Participants: 284

Study Overview: See Figure 35.1 for a summary of the study design.

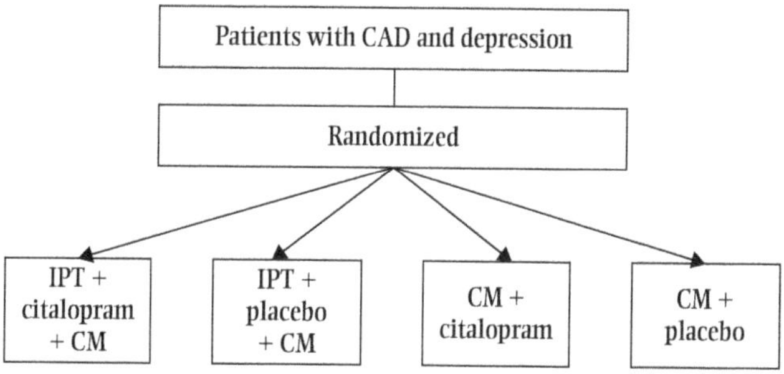

Figure 35.1 Summary of Study Design
NOTES: CAD = coronary artery disease. IPT = interpersonal psychotherapy. CM = clinical management.

Study Intervention: Participants randomized to citalopram received 10 mg/day of the drug for one week and then 20 mg/d. The dose was increased to 40 mg/d if there was inadequate response in six weeks. The other half of study participants received a placebo.

Participants randomized to IPT received 12 weekly therapy sessions from a certified therapist, immediately following weekly clinical management (CM) sessions. Therapists were at least masters-level clinicians with 4 or more years of experience. IPT is a short-term, semi-structured evidence based psychotherapy dealing with life transitions, grief, loss, and social isolation. IPT has been found superior to cognitive behavior therapy (CBT) in treating depression in patients with comorbid physical and mental health conditions. CM served as the psychotherapy control condition, consisting of information about depression and medication use, reassurance and encouragement to adhere to study protocol, evaluation of study medication side effects, serious adverse events, and depressive symptoms. CM was provided by the same therapists who delivered the IPT to other participants. Patients were blind to their therapy randomization group.

Follow-Up: 12 weeks

Endpoints: Primary outcome: centralized, telephone rated 24-item HAM-D. Secondary endpoints: self-report Beck Depression Inventory II (BDI-II).

RESULTS

- Citalopram was superior to placebo in reducing depressive symptoms in all efficacy measures, with an effect size of 0.33 between the citalopram and placebo groups in the changes in HAM-D scores between baseline and at 12 weeks (primary outcome). It demonstrated similar effect sizes for the secondary outcomes. The benefits were greater in patients with recurrent episodes of major depression than in patients with a first episode.
- There was no benefit for IPT over CM alone in any of the outcome measures (Table 35.1).

Table 35.1 SUMMARY OF CREATE'S KEY FINDINGS

Outcome	Citalopram vs Placebo	P value	IPT vs. Clinical management only	P value
12-week decrease in HAM-D	3.33	0.005	−2.26	0.06
12-week decrease in BDI-II scores	3.61	0.005	1.13	0.37

NOTES: CREATE = Canadian Cardiac Randomized Evaluation of Antidepressant and Psychotherapy Efficacy Trial. IPT = interpersonal therapy. HAM-D = Hamilton Depression Rating Scale. BDI-II = Beck Depression Inventory II.

Criticisms and Limitations: Participants were recruited through advertisements, and there were extensive exclusion criteria limiting the generalizability of the results. Most of the study population was moderately to severely depressed (HAM-D score >24), and the severity of illness, combined with an acute phase trial (12 weeks), may not have captured a treatment response. In patients with lower baseline social functioning, CBT may be a more effective therapeutic modality than IPT; however, in this trial all patients were provided with IPT irrespective of their level of functioning.

Other Relevant Studies and Information:

- The Sertraline Antidepressant Heart-Attack Randomized Trial (SADHART) found that sertraline is safe in patients with a recent MI or unstable angina. However, when compared to placebo,[2] sertraline did not demonstrate greater reduction in depression or improved cardiovascular status.
- The Enhancing Recovery in Coronary Heart Disease Patients (ENRICHD) study found that in patients with depression or perceived low social support after a myocardial infarction, the addition of a serotonin reuptake inhibitor did not decrease mortality risk. It did improve depression and social isolation, however.[3] A recent systematic review also noted that depression often spontaneously remits without treatment; in patients with persistent depression post-acute coronary syndrome, both antidepressants and psychotherapy may improve prognosis, although noradrenergic antidepressants should be prescribed cautiously.[4]
- The American Heart Association guidelines,[5] which were endorsed by the American Psychiatric Association, recommend to screen for and treat depression in patients post myocardial infarction with CBT and/or an SSRI depending on the severity and contraindications.

Summary and Implications: Patients with recent myocardial infarction or other cardiac disease are at an elevated risk of depression and mortality. This and other key studies demonstrate that SSRIs are safe in the treatment of depression in these patients. The CREATE study found that in patients with CAD, antidepressants such as citalopram are effective in reducing depressive symptoms in the acute-phase treatment of moderate to severe depression. In this group, interpersonal psychotherapy was not shown to be effective in the short term. The American Heart Association, with the endorsement of the American Psychiatric Association, supports the use of SSRIs and psychotherapy to treat depression in patients with cardiac comorbidities.

CLINICAL CASE: CITALOPRAM AND PSYCHOTHERAPY IN CAD AND DEPRESSION

Case History

A 55-year-old male realtor with an acute coronary event two months prior presents to an outpatient psychiatrist with depressed mood, anhedonia, poor sleep, decreased concentration, and low energy, affecting his work and personal life. The patient had been successfully treated for depression with citalopram years ago.

Based on the results of CREATE, how should this patient be treated?

Suggested Answer

According to the CREATE trial, after 12 weeks, citalopram in combination with weekly CM was found to be more effective than placebo and CM in reducing depressive symptoms, whereas IPT was not shown to have advantages in reducing depressive symptoms over CM alone.

This patient, in the post-acute coronary syndrome phase, meets criteria for a diagnosis of major depression and can be started on an SSRI after an adequate medical workup if there are no contraindications. Close monitoring is indicated as trial participants with a first episode of depression did not respond as well as those with recurrent episodes. IPT was not shown to be effective in this trial; however, he should be offered regular CM to improve compliance and develop and maintain coping strategies to help with the depression.

References

1. Lespérance, F., Frasure-Smith, N., Koszycki, D., Laliberté, M. A., van Zyl, L. T., Baker, B., . . . Guertin, M. C. (2007). Effects of citalopram and interpersonal psychotherapy on depression in patients with coronary artery disease: The Canadian Cardiac Randomized Evaluation of Antidepressant and Psychotherapy Efficacy (CREATE) trial. *JAMA, 297*(4), 367–379.
2. Glassman, A. H., O'Connor, C. M., Califf, R. M., Swedberg, K., Schwartz, P., Bigger, J. T., Jr., . . . Landau, C. (2002). Sertraline treatment of major depression in patients with acute MI or unstable angina. *JAMA, 288*(6), 701–709.
3. Berkman, L. F., Blumenthal, J., Burg, M., Carney, R. M., Catellier, D., Cowan, M. J., . . . Kaufmann, P. G. (2003). Effects of treating depression and low perceived social support on clinical events after myocardial infarction: The Enhancing Recovery in Coronary Heart Disease Patients (ENRICHD) Randomized Trial. *JAMA, 289*(23), 3106-3116.
4. Ramamurthy, G., Trejo, E., & Faraone, S. V. (2013). Depression treatment in patients with coronary artery disease: a systematic review. Primary Care Companion for CNS Disorders, 15(5).
5. Lichtman, J. H., Bigger, J. T., Blumenthal, J. A., Frasure-Smith, N., Kaufmann, P. G., Lespérance, F., . . . Froelicher, E. S. (2008). Depression and coronary heart disease. *Circulation, 118*(17), 1768–1775.

SECTION 11

Women's Mental Health

36

Buprenorphine versus Methadone During Pregnancy

The MOTHER Trial

RACHEL WURMSER AND KIRSTEN WILKINS

> Infants who had prenatal exposure to buprenorphine required significantly less morphine for the treatment of NAS [neonatal abstinence syndrome], a significantly shorter period of NAS treatment, and a significantly shorter hospital stay than did infants with prenatal exposure to methadone.
>
> —The MOTHER Investigators[1]

Research Question: Is buprenorphine an alternative treatment option associated with less severe neonatal abstinence syndrome (NAS) compared to methadone for pregnant women with opioid use disorders?

Funding: The National Institute on Drug Abuse

Year Study Began: 2005

Year Study Published: 2010

Study Location: Eight sites in the United States, Canada, and Austria (one site screened participants but did not complete randomization).

Who Was Studied: Pregnant women 18 to 41 years old with opioid dependence according to DSM-IV criteria between 6 and 30 weeks of gestation.

Who Was Excluded: Women with multigestation pregnancies, medical conditions, outstanding legal issues that could interfere with participation, disorders involving benzodiazepines or alcohol use, or who planned to give birth outside the hospital.

How Many Participants: 175

Study Overview: See Figure 36.1 for a summary of the study design.

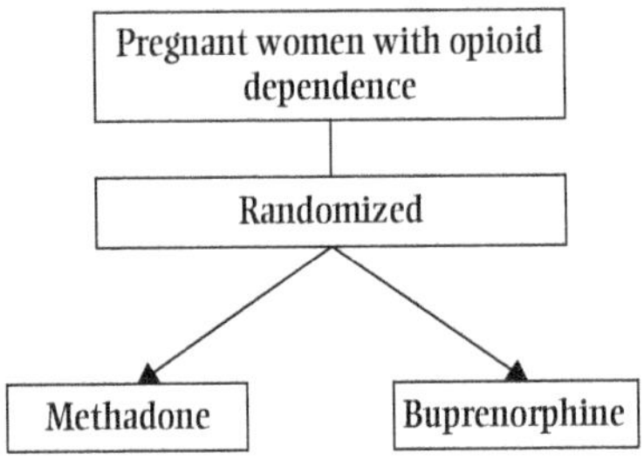

Figure 36.1 Summary of Study Design

Study Intervention: All participants received morphine sulfate prior to randomization to help with the transition to study medication. Participants were admitted to the hospital and randomized to receive buprenorphine (2 to 32 mg) or methadone (20 to 140 mg). The dosing schedule was blinded and individualized. Dose adjustments (buprenorphine 2 mg or methadone 5 or 10 mg) were double-blind and based on patient request, withdrawal or craving symptoms, adherence, and urine toxicology reports. A double dummy design was used for blinding purposes meaning patients received seven tablets of buprenorphine or indistinguishable placebo (three 8 mg tablets and four 2 mg tablets) and a fixed volume of liquid containing methadone or indistinguishable placebo. All participants were provided with "comprehensive care" including monetary vouchers in exchange for negative urine drug screens.

Follow-Up: Assessments were performed for a minimum of 10 days after birth and up to 36 months post-delivery.

Endpoints: Primary neonatal outcomes: the number of neonates requiring treatment for NAS, peak NAS score, amount of morphine needed for treatment of NAS, duration of hospital stay, and head circumference. Secondary neonatal outcomes: duration that medication was given for NAS, birth-related outcomes (e.g., birth weights, Apgar scores). Secondary maternal outcomes included (but not limited to) cesarean section, abnormal fetal presentation during delivery, anesthesia during delivery, medical complications at delivery, and number of prenatal obstetrical visits.

RESULTS

- Neonates exposed to buprenorphine spent less time in the hospital, required less morphine, and had a shorter duration of NAS treatment.
- There was no significant difference between groups with respect to neonates requiring NAS treatment, peak NAS score, or head circumference.
- The study did not detect a difference between the methadone and buprenorphine groups with respect to other secondary neonatal outcomes including birth weight and length, preterm birth, gestational age at delivery, and Apgar scores at one and five minutes.
- The study did not detect a difference between the groups for secondary maternal outcomes (e.g., cesarean section, weight gain, anesthesia during delivery, medical complications at delivery, and number of prenatal obstetrical visits).
- There were higher rates of nonserious maternal adverse events in the methadone group (e.g. blood-borne disorders, cardiovascular symptoms, gastrointestinal symptoms, genitourinary symptoms, dental problems, musculoskeletal symptoms, neuromuscular symptoms, postsurgical problems), but there were no differences between groups in terms of serious maternal or neonatal adverse events
- In total, 18% (16 of 89) of the methadone group and 33% (28 of 86) of the buprenorphine group discontinued treatment prior to delivery, though this was not statistically significant. Of these, 71% of buprenorphine noncompleters and 13% of the methadone noncompleters cited "dissatisfaction" with the medication as their reason for discontinuation. Again, no statistical significance was found. (Table 36.1).

Table 36.1 SUMMARY OF MOTHER's KEY FINDINGS

Outcome	**Methadone**	**Buprenorphine**	**P value**
% Treated for NAS	57	47	0.26
NAS peak score	12.8	11.0	0.04
Total amount of morphine for NAS (mg)	10.4	1.1	<0.009
Days of infant hospital stay	17.5	10.0	<0.009

NOTES: MOTHER = Maternal Opioid Treatment: Human Experimental Research. NAS = neonatal abstinence syndrome.

Criticisms and Limitations: Only 16% of women that were screened ended up getting randomized, raising questions about the generalizability of the results.

Other Relevant Studies and Information:

- The American College of Obstetrics and Gynecology (ACOG) recommends pharmacotherapy with either buprenorphine or methadone in pregnant patients with opioid use disorder.[2]
- A Cochrane Review of studies comparing methadone and buprenorphine in pregnant women did not find evidence that one was superior. However, the findings suggest that methadone has a lower attrition rate and buprenorphine appears to lead to less severe neonatal abstinence syndrome.[3]

Summary and Implications: The MOTHER study was a rigorous randomized controlled study demonstrating that neonates born to mothers with opioid dependence taking buprenorphine required less morphine for the treatment of NAS, experienced shorter periods of treatment for NAS, and had shorter hospital stays compared with neonates born to mothers treated with methadone. Based on the results of this study, either buprenorphine or methadone may be considered for the management of opioid use disorder in pregnancy.

CLINICAL CASE: BUPRENORPHINE VERSUS METHADONE FOR TREATMENT OF OPIOID DEPENDENCE IN PREGNANCY

Case History

A 28-year-old pregnant woman in her second trimester presents to an outpatient psychiatrist seeking treatment for opioid use disorder. She has no medical diagnoses and takes no other medications. She is open to taking opiate agonist treatment to reduce the risk of relapse during pregnancy. She is appropriately concerned about the effect of the medication on her baby.

Based on the results of this study, how should this patient be treated?

Suggested Answer

The MOTHER trial provided evidence that neonates with prenatal exposure to buprenorphine required less morphine for the treatment of NAS, shorter periods of treatment for NAS, and shorter hospital stays compared with neonates born to mothers treated with methadone. Based on this and other studies, ACOG recommends the use of buprenorphine or methadone for the treatment of opioid use disorders in pregnancy.

The patient in the vignette would likely meet inclusion criteria for this trial. A reasonable treatment strategy would be to offer a trial of an optimal dose of buprenorphine and assess satisfaction with treatment. If the patient is at risk of buprenorphine discontinuation and opioid relapse, the psychiatrist and patient could consider switching to methadone. It is also important to counsel the patient on the risks of taking other drugs of abuse during pregnancy and of combining alcohol and benzodiazepines with opiate agonist treatment. Other services such as counseling and case management are important components of treatment.

References

1. Jones, H. E., Kaltenbach, K., Heil, S. H., Stine, S. M., Coyle, M. G., Arria, A. M., . . . Fischer, G. (2010). Neonatal abstinence syndrome after methadone or buprenorphine exposure. *New England Journal of Medicine, 363*(24), 2320–2331.
2. Committee on Health Care for Underserved Women and the American Society of Addiction Medicine. (2012). Committee Opinion no. 524: Opioid abuse, dependence, and addiction in pregnancy. *Obstetrics & Gynecology, 119*(5), 1070–1076.
3. Minozzi, S,. Amato, L., Bellisario, C., Ferri, M., & Davoli, M. (2013). Maintenance agonist treatments for opiate-dependent pregnant women. *Cochrane Database of Systematic Reviews, 12,* CD006318.

SECTION 12

Schizophrenia

37

QTc-Interval Abnormalities and Psychotropic Drug Therapy in Psychiatric Patients

AMANDA SUN AND VINOD H. SRIHARI

> The confirmation of a link between QT-interval abnormalities and high-dose prescribing supports current guidelines for electrocardiographic screening, but our results suggest that monitoring is also needed in patients taking tricyclic antidepressants, droperidol, and thioridazine, particularly if other risk factors are present.
>
> —REILLY ET AL.[1]

Research Question: Is QTc prolongation associated with specific psychotropic medications, the dose, or other factors?

Funding: Northern Regional National Health Service and Medical Research Council

Year Study Began: 1994

Year Study Published: 2000

Study Location: Mental health facilities (inpatient, day hospital, outpatient) in six districts in northeast England

Who Was Studied: 18 to 74-year-old psychiatric patients, some of whom were on psychotropic medications, and healthy volunteers. Notably, subjects with pre-existing cardiac disease were included in the psychiatric patients group.

Who Was Excluded: Among the psychiatric patients, patients who failed to provide informed written consent, underwent a change in drug therapy within the last two weeks (or last three months for patients on depot medications), or had a history of atrial fibrillation or bundle branch block were excluded. Those with "overt cardiovascular disease" were excluded from the healthy reference group to minimize the impact of pre-existing cardiac disease on the measurement of normal QTc.

How Many Participants: 495 psychiatric patients, 101 healthy volunteers

Study Overview: See Figure 37.1 for a summary of the study design.

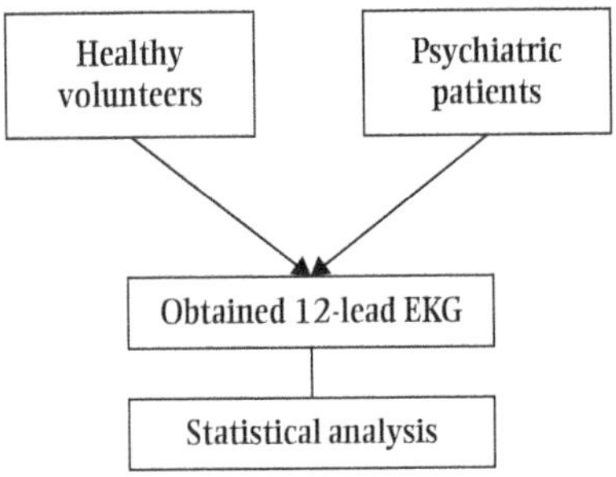

Figure 37.1 Summary of Study Design
NOTE: EKG = electrocardiography.

Study Implementation: The researchers performed 12-lead electrocardiograms (EKG) on the healthy volunteer group and psychiatric patients. The QTc values obtained from the healthy reference group were used to define abnormal QTc as greater than 456 ms, two standard deviations above the mean value in the group. The researchers then conducted logistic regression analyses to examine various predictive variables for QTc prolongation in the psychiatric patient group. They also examined the impact of QTc dispersion (defined as the difference between the minimum and maximum QTc on the 12-lead EKG) and T-wave abnormality (defined as the presence of inversion, flattening, or bifid T wave) as secondary outcomes, both of which are associated with increased cardiac events.

The investigators looked at the impact of demographic variables, psychiatric disorders and drug therapy such as antipsychotics, selective serotonin reuptake inhibitors, tricyclic antidepressants, monoamine oxidase inhibitors, benzodiazepines, and mood stabilizers on the presence of EKG changes. Pharmacotherapy use was defined as use for more than one week (for oral medications) and more than two months (for long-acting injectable medications). Antipsychotic dose category was determined by conversion into chlorpromazine equivalents (standard: 0–1,000 mg chlorpromazine equivalents per day; high: 1,001–2,000 mg chlorpromazine equivalents per day; very high: >2,000 mg chlorpromazine equivalents per day).

Follow-Up: This study was a cross-sectional study, and patients were not followed longitudinally.

Endpoints: Rate-corrected QT interval (QTc), unadjusted QTc dispersion, and T wave abnormalities (inversion, flattening, or bifid) on electrocardiogram

RESULTS

- Age over 65 years, use of tricyclic antidepressants, and use of droperidol or thioridazine were found to be significantly associated with QTc prolongation, based on logistic regression analyses and confirmed by backwards stepwise regression.
- Increased antipsychotic dose was associated with increased risk for QTc lengthening.
- QT dispersion and T-wave abnormalities were not significantly associated with antipsychotic treatment but were associated with lithium use (Tables 37.1 and 37.2).

Table 37.1 Summary of Study Key Findings: Significant Risk Factors for QTc Lengthening by Logistic Regression and Backwards Stepwise Regression

Risk factor	Adjusted odds ratio from full model	P value
Demographics		
Age >65	3.0	0.04
Drug Therapy		
Droperidol	6.7	0.004
Thioridazine	5.3	<0.001
Tricyclics	4.4	0.004

Table 37.2 Summary of Study Key Findings: Antipsychotic Dose and Risk of QTc Prolongation

Risk factor	Adjusted odds ratio from full model	P value
Antipsychotic		
Low dose	1.4	0.52
High dose	5.4	0.03
Very high dose	8.2	0.01

Criticisms and Limitations: The cross-sectional design with use of logistic regression can provide only weak evidence of causality, and these results should thus these findings should be interpreted with caution. The study excluded severely ill inpatients and those with atrial fibrillation and bundle branch block, which decreases generalizability. Additionally, the study evaluated over 30 different psychotropic drugs, and many patients were on more than one drug, which limited the study's ability to evaluate effects of individual drugs. Finally, the study used QTc as a surrogate risk factor for clinically significant cardiac events but did not report on frequency of arrhythmias or sudden death.

Other Relevant Studies and Information:

- For further information on QTc prolongation with antipsychotics (including more second-generation antipsychotics) and additional data on their comparative efficacy and tolerability, see the meta-analysis[2] on this topic.
- There have been other trials that studied the effects of psychotropic medications on QTc.[3,4]
- According to the Berkshire Healthcare National Health Service antipsychotic prescribing guidelines,[5] a baseline EKG should be obtained on initiation of an antipsychotic, and QTc should be followed at least annually. In the early stages of high-dose treatment and in patients with a cardiac history, the EKG should be repeated every few days during dose escalation and then every one to three months. Care should be taken especially with thioridazine, pimozide, droperidol, and haloperidol and the second-generation antipsychotic ziprasidone,[6] whereas lurasidone, clozapine, and arpiprazole may have lower risks of QTc prolongation.[7]
- According to the American Psychiatric Association, providers should reduce or discontinue the offending agent if the EKG shows an absolute

QTc interval of >500 msec or an increase of 60 msec from baseline.[8] Given the dose-dependent nature of QTc prolongation, prescribers should use the lowest dose of antipsychotic possible.

Summary and Implications: In patients on psychotropic medications, in particular tricyclic antidepressants, high-dose antipsychotics and droperidol or thioridazine, QTc interval should be closely monitored by routine electrocardiography. Caution should also be exercised among patients on these agents in combination with lithium. Findings from this and other studies have contributed to shifts in prescribing practices for antipsychotic agents, including a reduction in the use of droperidol and thioridazine and lower dosing of antipsychotics.

CLINICAL CASE: CHOICE OF PSYCHOTROPIC DRUG IN PATIENTS WITH PSYCHIATRIC ILLNESS AND QTC PROLONGATION

Case History

A 67-year-old veteran with a history of coronary artery disease, hypertension, and schizoaffective disorder, depressive type, presents to the Veterans Affairs psychiatric emergency department and is admitted for worsening psychosis (despite good adherence to high-dose droperidol), severe depressed mood, and suicidal ideation. He endorses poor sleep and appetite, low self-worth, depressed mood, and thoughts of suicide by hanging. He demonstrates profound thought disorganization and paranoia about staff at his rest home wanting to hurt him. On routine admission EKG, patient is found to have an increased QTc of 514. According to the patient, and confirmed in the record, he benefited significantly during past and separate trials of nortriptyline and sertraline (that had been added to his antipsychotic treatment) to target depressive symptoms.

Based on the results of this study, what psychopharmacological approaches are safest?

Suggested Answer

This study raises concerns that tricyclic antidepressants and droperidol could each have contributed to QTc lengthening in this patient. He is typical of patients included in this study and, given his older age, is also more susceptible to QTc prolongation. If selecting an antidepressant, the team should counsel the patient to prefer sertraline over nortriptyline. They should also consider switching the patient's antipsychotic (since dose reduction would threaten symptom control) and consider clozapine as one option that could multiply target worsening psychosis and suicidality, with a likely lower risk of QTc prolongation.

References

1. Reilly, J. G., Ayis, S. A., Ferrier, I. N., Jones, S. J., & Thomas, S. H. (2000). QTc-interval abnormalities and psychotropic drug therapy in psychiatric patients. *Lancet, 355*(9209), 1048–1052.
2. Leucht, S., Cipriani, A., Spineli, L., Mavridis, D., Orey, D., Richter, F., . . . Davis, J. M. (2013). Comparative efficacy and tolerability of 15 antipsychotic drugs in schizophrenia: A multiple-treatments meta-analysis. *Lancet, 382*(9896), 951–962.
3. Wenzel-Seifert, K., Wittmann, M., & Haen, E. (2011). QTc prolongation by psychotropic drugs and the risk of Torsade de Pointes. *Deutsches Ärzteblatt International, 108*(41), 687–693.
4. van Noord, C., Straus, S. M., Sturkenboom, M. C., Hofman, A., Aarnoudse, A. J. L., Bagnardi, V., . . . Stricker, B. H. (2009). Psychotropic drugs associated with corrected QT interval prolongation. *Journal of Clinical Psychopharmacology, 29*(1), 9–15.
5. Sims, K., Hewitt, K., Raynes, A., Tahir, O., and Booth, D. (2011). *Antipsychotic guidelines: Treatment of schizophrenia and psychosis*. Bracknell, UK: Berkshire Healthcare NHS Foundation Trust.
6. Glassman, A. H., & Bigger, J. T. (2001). Antipsychotic drugs: Prolonged QTc interval, torsade de pointes, and sudden death. *American Journal of Psychiatry, 158*(11), 1774–1782.
7. Ries, R., & Sayadipour, A. (2014). Management of psychosis and agitation in medical-surgical patients who have or are at risk for prolonged QT interval. *Journal of Psychiatric Practice, 20*(5), 338–344.
8. Lieberman, J. A., Merrill, D., & Parameswaran, S. (2009). *APA guidance on the use of antipsychotic drugs and cardiac sudden death*. Washington, DC: APA Council on Research.

38

Tardive Dyskinesia with Atypical versus Conventional Antipsychotic Medications

EMMA LO AND CENK TEK

> Our findings suggest that the incidence rate of TD with atypical antipsychotics, while modestly reduced, remains substantial.
>
> —TD Incidence Study Investigators[1]

Research Question: How does the incidence of tardive dyskinesia (TD) compare among users of atypical and conventional antipsychotics?

Funding: National Institute of Mental Health

Year Study Began: 2000

Year Study Published: 2010

Study Location: The Connecticut Mental Health Center in New Haven, Connecticut

Who Was Studied: Psychiatric outpatients receiving conventional antipsychotics, atypical antipsychotics, or both for at least 3 months.

Who Was Excluded: Patients with primary neurological diseases who therefore could not reliably be examined for TD as well as those with baseline persistent TD.

How Many Participants: 352

Study Overview: See Figure 38.1 for a summary of the study design.

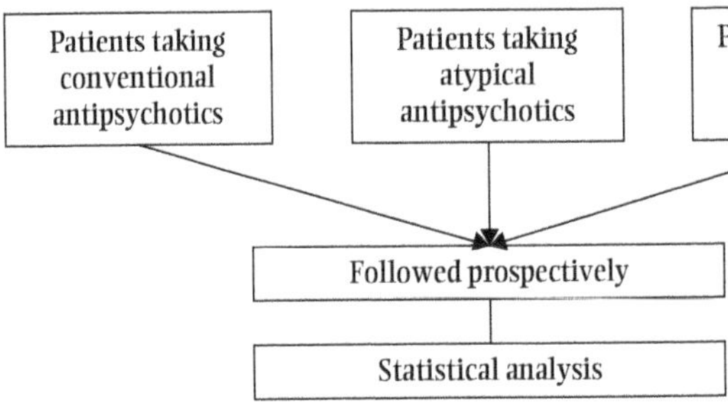

Figure 38.1 Summary of Study Design

Study Implementation: Using a prospective cohort study design, investigators followed patients without existing TD for up to 4 years, comparing the incidence of TD among those taking conventional antipsychotics, atypicals, or both. The comparisons were adjusted for medication dose, age, race, and length of exposure to antipsychotics.

Subjects were evaluated for TD using the Abnormal Involuntary Movement Scale (AIMS).[2]

Follow-Up: Every six months for up to four years

Endpoints: Incidence of TD as diagnosed using the AIMS.

RESULTS

- The relative risk of TD among patients exposed to atypical antipsychotics versus conventional antipsychotics was 0.68 (95% CI [0.29, 1.64]). In an analysis adjusting for the previously noted potential confounding factors , the risk ratio was 0.55 (95% CI [0.23, 1.36]).
- Incidence of TD in patients prescribed both atypical and conventional antipsychotics combined versus conventional antipsychotics alone yielded an adjusted rate ratio of 2.21 (95% CI [0.85, 5.8]).

- Surprisingly, patients treated with clozapine compared to conventional antipsychotics had an adjusted rate ratio of 2.27, suggesting much higher rate of TD among clozapine patients than in prior studies; however, the investigators note a small sample size of clozapine-exposed individuals, and the cumulative antipsychotic exposure may not have been fully accounted for in patients on clozapine, who are often refractory to initial therapy (Table 38.1).

Table 38.1 SUMMARY OF KEY FINDINGS—INCIDENCE RATES OF PERSISTENT TARDIVE DYSKINESIA

Outcome	Conventionals (CV) group	Atypicals (AT) group	AT (adjusted)	Combined CV and AT	Clozapine	P value[a]
Adjusted rate–ratio	1	0.55	0.68	2.21	2.27	0.004

[a]This is an overall p value for the comparisons.

Criticisms and Limitations: Of note, almost all study participants already had extensive histories of exposure to conventional antipsychotics prior to the initial examination, making it more difficult to attribute incident TD to current versus past medication exposure, and it is unclear whether prior exposure could affect future susceptibility to TD.

Even though the authors attempted to adjust for potential confounding factors, unmeasured confounders may have influenced the results.

About 45% of the initial cohort was lost to follow-up, but the dropout rates were adjusted for in the analysis and not felt to change the overall study results.

The dataset used for this sample had low use of ziprasidone and aripiprazole, two atypical antipsychotics with low D2 blockade. This may have falsely elevated the risk of TD in atypical compared to conventional antipsychotics.

Other Relevant Studies and Information:

- This study followed the methods of the Yale Tardive Dyskinesia Study, which was completed before the introduction of atypical antipsychotics, and found a similar incidence of TD among patients taking conventional antipsychotics.[3,4]

- A meta-analysis compiling results from nine prior studies demonstrated a relatively higher incidence rate of TD with conventional antipsychotics (0.085 annual incidence rate vs. 0.056 in this study), as well as a relatively lower rate of TD with atypical antipsychotics (0.31 annual incidence rate vs. 0.059 in this study). The relative risk of TD with atypical versus conventional antipsychotics was also lower than what was found in this study (0.24 vs. 0.68 in this study).[1]
- The findings of this study with respect to clozapine contrast with another study finding a rate one-tenth of the risk found here[5] but are consistent with several other small studies.[6,7]
- Contrary to the findings of this study, American Psychiatric Association guidelines suggest consideration of clozapine among patients with TD, pointing to studies in which severity of the dyskinetic movements improved after switching to clozapine, though these guidelines acknowledge there is little long-term evidence to support this claim.[8 9]
- Prior studies indicated a relative risk of 0.24,[10] suggesting less substantial protection from TD with atypical antipsychotics than had been previously thought.
- The overall prevalence of TD has remained relatively similar despite much increased use of atypical antipsychotics since the prior TD study was completed by this group in the 1980s.

Summary and Implications: This study demonstrated a lower incidence of TD with the use of atypical versus conventional antipsychotics, though the risk reduction was more modest than that reported in prior analyses. Patients on both atypical and conventional antipsychotics require close monitoring for this serious complication.

CLINICAL CASE: CONVENTIONAL VERSUS ATYPICAL ANTIPSYCHOTICS AND TD RISK

Case History

A 36-year-old obese woman with schizophrenia has been maintained on haloperidol for the past three years, which has allowed her to maintain relatively independent functioning with minimal symptoms. Recently, she was switched from haloperidol to risperidone due to concern for early signs of TD. Upon follow up in two months, the patient has gained 26 pounds and her psychotic symptoms are similar to how she appeared on the haloperidol. Her AIMS exam is also unchanged. Her sister, her primary caretaker, asks about whether it would be better to switch back to the haloperidol but is worried about "her tongue movements."

Based on the results of the study, how should this patient be treated?

Suggested Answer

The study by Woods et al.[1] reexaming the risk of TD among patients on conventional versus atypical antipsychotics suggests that the risk of TD associated with atypicals is about two thirds the risk compared with conventional antipsychotics. When considering the risks and benefits of various medications, it is important to weigh both efficacy and side-effect profiles. Both medications appear to have similar effects upon her psychotic symptoms, but she has unfortunately gained significant weight on risperidone, which is more commonly seen among atypical antipsychotics. Her early signs of TD are concerning, and based on the results of this study, the risk of TD for the patient is somewhat improved by switching to an atypical antipsychotic. To avoid worsening her metabolic syndrome, and considering that her risk of TD is reduced by about one third using an atypical, it would be reasonable to switch to a more weight-neutral atypical antipsychotic such as aripiprazole (assuming similar efficacy), but keeping in mind that the protection against TD conferred by an atypical agent is modest.

References

1. Woods, S. W., Morgenstern, H., Saksa, J. R., Walsh, B. C., Sullivan, M. C., Money, R., . . . Glazer, W. M. (2010). Incidence of tardive dyskinesia with atypical and conventional antipsychotic medications: Prospective cohort study. *Journal of Clinical Psychiatry, 71*(4), 463–474.
2. Guy, W. (1976). ECDEU assessment manual for psychopharmacology—Revised (DHEW Publication no. ADM 76–338). Rockville, MD: US Department of Health, Education, and Welfare.
3. Morgenstern, H., & Glazer, W. M. (1993). Identifying risk factors for tardive dyskinesia among long-term outpatients maintained with neuroleptic medications. Results of the Yale Tardive Dyskinesia Study. *Archives of General Psychiatry, 50*(9), 723–733.
4. Kane, J. M., Woerner, M., & Lieberman, J. (1988). Tardive dyskinesia: Prevalence, incidence, and risk factors. *Journal of Clinical Psychopharmacology, 8*(4 Suppl), 52S–56S.
5. Kane, J. M., Woerner, M. G., Pollack, S., Safferman, A. Z., & Lieberman, J. A. (1993). Does clozapine cause tardive dyskinesia? *Journal of Clinical Psychiatry, 54*(9), 327–330.

6. Chakos, M. H., Alvir, J. M., Woerner, M. G., Koreen, A., Geisler, S., Mayerhoff, D., . . . Lieberman, J. A. (1996). Incidence and correlates of tardive dyskinesia in first episode of schizophrenia. *Archives of General Psychiatry, 53*(4), 313–319.
7. Bunker, M. T., Sommi, R. W., Stoner, S. C., & Switzer, J. L. (1996). Longitudinal analysis of abnormal involuntary movements in long- term clozapine-treated patients. *Psychopharmacology Bulletin, 32*(4), 699–703.
8. Lehman, A. F., Lieberman, J. A., Dixon, L. B., McGlashan, T. H., Miller, A. L., Perkins, D. O., & Kreyenbuhl, J. (2004). Practice guideline for the treatment of patients with schizophrenia, second edition. *American Journal of Psychiatry, 161*(2 Suppl), 1–56.
9. Lieberman, J. A., Saltz, B. L., Johns, C. A., Pollack, S., Borenstein, M., & Kane, J. (1991). The effects of clozapine on tardive dyskinesia. *British Journal of Psychiatry, 158*, 503–510
10. Tenback, D. E., van Harten, P. N., Slooff, C. J., Belger, M. A., & van Os, J. (2005). Effects of antipsychotic treatment on tardive dyskinesia: A 6-month evaluation of patients from the Eur Schizophrneia Outpatient Health Outcomes (SOHO) study. *Journal of Clinical Psychiatry, 66*(9), 1130–1133.

39

Effectiveness of Antipsychotics in the Treatment of Schizophrenia

CATIE Phase 1

CHADRICK LANE AND MOHINI RANGANATHAN

> This outcome indicates that antipsychotic drugs, though effective, have substantial limitations in their effectiveness in patients with chronic schizophrenia.
>
> —CATIE AUTHORS[1]

Research Question: Are there measurable differences in effectiveness between antipsychotics (risperidone vs. olanzapine vs. ziprasidone vs. quetiapine vs. perphenazine) in the treatment of patients with schizophrenia?

Funding: National Institute of Mental Health and the Foundation of Hope of Raleigh, North Carolina

Year Study Began: 2001

Year Study Published: 2005

Study Location: 57 outpatient clinical sites across the United States

Who Was Studied: Adults between the ages of 18 to 65 who met DSM-IV criteria for a diagnosis of schizophrenia. The diagnosis was confirmed using the Structured Clinical Interview prior to randomization.

Who Was Excluded: Patients with prior diagnoses of intellectual disability, schizoaffective disorder, cognitive disorder, known intolerance to study medications, unstable medical conditions, pregnancy or active breastfeeding, a history of only one psychotic episode, or having met criteria for treatment resistance (continued severe symptoms even after a previous adequate trial of another antipsychotic in this study or clozapine).

How Many Participants: 1,432

Study Overview: See Figure 39.1 for a summary of the study design.

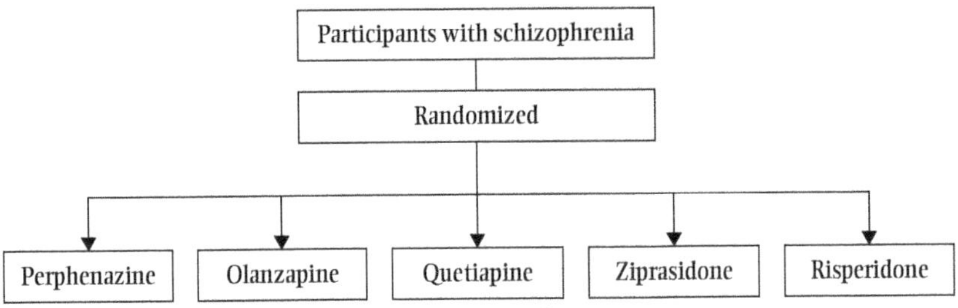

Figure 39.1 Summary of Study Design

Study Intervention: This double-blinded study randomized participants to one of five possible medications (mean daily dose): perphenazine (20.8 mg), which was the only first-generation drug tested; olanzapine (20.1 mg); quetiapine (543.4 mg); ziprasidone (112.8 mg); or risperidone (3.9 mg). An intention-to-treat analysis was used.

Participants with a diagnosis of tardive dyskinesia were not randomized to the perphenazine arm of the study. Of note, ziprasidone received FDA approval and was added approximately midway through the study. The study authors selected perphenazine for the first-generation agent due to its lower propensity for intolerable side effects contrasted with higher-potency medications like haloperidol.

Follow-Up: 18 months

Endpoints: The primary endpoint was all-cause discontinuation. The researchers selected this outcome measure in an effort to incorporate both participant and clinician considerations in determining efficacy and tolerability in treatment. Secondary outcomes included scores on the Positive and Negative Syndrome Scale (PANSS) and "successful treatment time," which was defined as the time in months the patient had a Clinical Global Impressions (CGI) score indicating mild or moderate illness with ≥2 points improvement from baseline, in addition to discerning reasons behind discontinuation.

RESULTS

- 74% of participants discontinued treatment with the medication they were randomized to prior to the end of this first phase of the Clinical Antipsychotic Trials of Intervention Effectiveness (CATIE) study.
- Time to discontinuation for any reason was longest for those treated with olanzapine (i.e., participants randomized to olanzapine remained on this medication for a longer period of time relative to the other agents). The difference was not significant for olanzapine when compared to perphenazine or ziprasidone when controlled for multiple comparisons.
- Time to discontinuation due to lack of efficacy was longest for olanzapine.
- There was no difference between medications in time to discontinuation due to side effects, though rates of discontinuation due to side effects were highest for olanzapine and lowest for risperidone.
- The amount of time categorized as "successful treatment" (as previously defined) was longest for the olanzapine group.
- The olanzapine group experienced the most improvement in PANSS and CGI scores early in treatment, though this effect lessened with time.
- Participants treated with olanzapine were less likely to be hospitalized for a worsening of psychotic symptoms.
- Olanzapine was associated with more weight gain, insulin resistance, and dyslipidemia that the other medications.
- No significant differences in extrapyramidal side effects (EPS) were noted between groups, though those treated with perphenazine were more likely to discontinue due to EPS (Table 39.1).

Table 39.1 SUMMARY OF CATIE PHASE 1 KEY OUTCOMES

Outcome	Olanzapine	P value	Quetiapine	P value	Risperidone	P value	Ziprasidone	P value	Perphenazine	P value
All-cause discontinuation (hazard ratio vs. olanzapine)	N/A	N/A	0.63	<0.001*	0.75	0.002*	0.76	0.028	0.78	0.021
Discontinuation secondary to lack of efficacy (hazard ratio vs. olanzapine)	N/A	N/A	0.41	<0.001*	0.45	<0.001*	0.59	0.026*	.47	<0.001
Discontinuation secondary to intolerable side effects (hazard ratio vs. risperidone)	0.62	0.27	0.65	<0.051	N/A	N/A	0.79	0.41	0.60	0.043
Duration of successful treatment (hazard ratio vs. olanzapine)	N/A	N/A	0.53	<0.001*	0.69	0.002*	0.75	0.017	0.73	0.013*

NOTE: CATIE = Clinical Antipsychotic Trials of Intervention Effectiveness.
*Statistically significant.

Criticisms and Limitations: Many participants were not treated with maximum doses of medications during the study, which could may be a limitation or a strength of this naturalistic design. Additionally, those with evidence of tardive dyskinesia were not allowed to enter the perphenazine treatment arm, which could have selected for participants with a lower propensity for EPS, thus increasing perceived safety.

Other Relevant Studies and Information:

- The Cost Utility of the Latest Antipsychotic Drugs in Schizophrenia Study (CUtLASS),[2] conducted in England, largely replicated the findings of CATIE. Though the primary outcome in CUtLASS measured quality of life rather than all-cause discontinuation, it supported the conclusion that there are no major differences in effectiveness between first- and second-generation antipsychotics.
- A meta-analysis by Leucht and colleagues[3] comparing the different antipsychotic agents found that olanzapine was the most likely to result in weight gain of the drugs included in their study. This analysis also demonstrated other modest differences in safety and efficacy among the agents.
- In those with first episode psychosis, the Schizophrenia Patients Outcome Research Team[4] recommends first-line treatment with antipsychotic medication. Due to a worse side-effect profile, these guidelines recommend against using clozapine or olanzapine as first-line agents.

Summary and Implications: The CATIE trial found that nearly three fourths of patients with schizophrenia stopped or changed their antipsychotic medications within 18 months of initiation. Participants remained on olanzapine for a longer duration of time compared to risperidone, quetiapine, ziprasidone, and perphenazine, but the comparisons with perphenazine and ziprasidone were not significant when adjusted for multiple comparisons. CATIE also suggested that perphenazine, a first-generation antipsychotic, was comparable on multiple measures relative to second-generation agents. While olanzapine appeared to have some advantages over the other medications, it had higher rates of discontinuation due to intolerability, with significant effects on weight gain, insulin resistance, and impaired lipid metabolism.

CLINICAL CASE: ANTIPSYCHOTIC EFFECTIVENESS

Case History

A 34-year-old homeless, obese man with a history of schizophrenia is admitted to an inpatient psychiatric ward after exhibiting erratic behavior and paranoia. He has intermittently been in outpatient care with two previous attempts at treatment with risperidone. He never received more than two weeks of medications prior to leaving follow-up care. On exam, his gait is stable, and there is no evidence of tremor, abnormal movements, or rigidity.

Based on the Phase 1 findings of the CATIE study, what medication should the psychiatrist consider?

Suggested Answer

The choice of antipsychotic medication in the treatment of schizophrenia should consider patient preference, potential adverse effects, past medication trials, and comorbidity. Phase 1 of CATIE would suggest that the vast majority of patients will discontinue their antipsychotic within a relatively short period of time, making the process of shared decision-making all the more important to promote medication adherence. While there is modest evidence that patients will remain on olanzapine for slightly longer periods of time and that improvement in symptoms may be greater for olanzapine, the decision to use this medication must be weighed with its high propensity for metabolic side effects. This particular patient is already obese, and the use of olanzapine may lead to additional weight gain and increased risk for diabetes and dyslipidemia. The use of perphenazine or a second-generation agent with less metabolic side effects may be better options for the patient. The American Diabetes Association along with the American Psychiatric Association and others released a consensus recommendation[5] to check baseline glucose and lipid levels with interval follow-up.

References

1. Lieberman, J. A., Stroup, T. S., McEvoy, J. P., Swartz, M. S., Rosenheck, R. A., Perkins, D. O., . . . Hsiao, J. K. (2005). Effectiveness of antipsychotic drugs in patients with chronic schizophrenia. *New England Journal of Medicine*, 353, 1209–1223.
2. Jones, P. B., Barnes, T. R., Davies, L., Dunn, G., Lloyd, H., Hayhurst, K. P. . . . Lewis, S. W. (2006). Randomized controlled trial of the effect on quality of life of second- vs first- generation antipsychotic drugs in schizophrenia. *Archives of General Psychiatry*, 63(10), 1079–1087.

3. Leucht, S., Cipriani, A., Spineli, L., Mavridis, D., Orey, D., Richter, F., . . . Davis, J. M. (2013). Comparative efficacy and tolerability of 15 antipsychotic drugs in schizophrenia: A multiple-treatments meta-analysis. *Lancet, 382*(9896), 951–962.
4. Kreyenbuhl, J., Buchanan, R. W., Dickerson, F. B., & Dixon, L. B. (2010). The Schizophrenia Patient Outcomes Research Team (PORT): Updated treatment recommendations 2009. *Schizophrenia Bulletin, 36*(1), 94–103.
5. American Diabetes Association, American Psychiatric Association, American Association of Clinical Endocrinologists, & North American Association for the Study of Obesity. (2004). Consensus Development Conference on Antipsychotic Drugs and Obesity and Diabetes. *Diabetes Care, 27*(2), 596–601.

40

Clozapine for Treatment-Resistant Schizophrenia

CHADRICK LANE AND VINOD H. SRIHARI

> For individuals suffering from treatment-resistant schizophrenia, the availability of clozapine, a potentially helpful treatment, is, in our view, a useful therapeutic advance.
>
> —KANE ET AL.[1]

Research Question: Is clozapine effective for patients with treatment-resistant schizophrenia who have not responded to past trials of first-generation antipsychotics?

Funding: Sandoz Research Institute and the Public Health Service

Year Study Published: 1988

Study Location: 16 inpatient psychiatric sites in the United States

Who Was Studied: Adults 20 to 59 years old with schizophrenia diagnosed using DSM-III and meeting criteria for treatment resistance, characterized as no response to at least three first-generation antipsychotics from two classes for at least six weeks (1,000 mg per day of a chlorpromazine equivalent dose). In addition, participants had poor functional status for the 5 years preceding the study. Patients were also required to have a score of ≥45 on the Brief Psychiatric Rating Scale (BPRS)[2] and a Clinical Global Impression (CGI) Scale[3] score of ≥4.

Who Was Excluded: There were no significant exclusion criteria.

How Many Participants: 319

Study Overview: See Figure 40.1 for a summary of the study design.

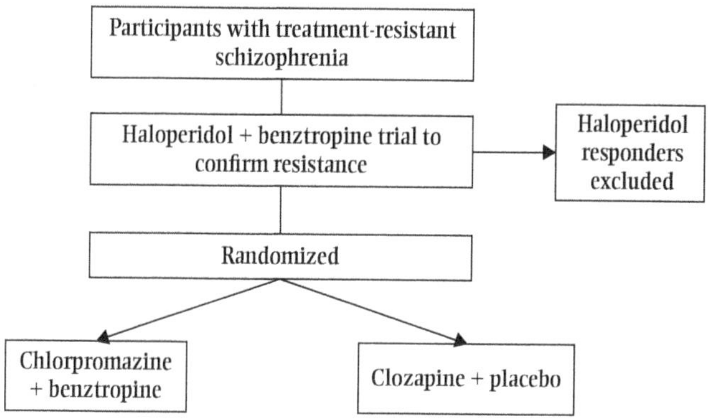

Figure 40.1 Summary of Study Design

Study Intervention: Participants meeting inclusion criteria were treated for a period of six weeks with haloperidol (up to 60 mg/day or more) and benztropine (up to 6 mg/day) to confirm treatment-resistance to other neuroleptics. Less than two percent responded to haloperidol (response criteria defined in the following discussion), and these responders were excluded from the next phase of the trial.

Participants were then randomized in a double-blind fashion to either chlorpromazine plus benztropine or to clozapine plus placebo. Researchers titrated the dose of chlorpromazine and benztropine based on treatment response, to a maximum 1,800mg/day and 6 mg/day, respectively. Clozapine was titrated to 500 mg/day up to a maximum of 900 mg/day based on response.

Follow-Up: Six weeks

Endpoints: The primary outcome was an "improvement" in symptoms, defined a priori as a post-treatment 20% decrease in total BPRS score from baseline plus either a CGI score of mild illness or a total BPRS score ≤35. Secondary measures included changes in scores on the Nurses' Observation Scale for Inpatient Evaluation (NOSIE-30),[4] the Simpson-Angus Scale for Extrapyramidal Side Effects,[5] and the Abnormal Involuntary Movements Scale (AIMS).[6]

RESULTS

- By week 1, patients receiving clozapine were already showing improvement relative to those receiving chlorpromazine and benztropine with respect to both BPRS total score and CGI Scale score; by week 6, patients in the clozapine group had three times as much improvement over the chlorpromazine group.
- Specific positive symptom and negative symptom BPRS items were significantly improved in favor of clozapine.
- Blinded nursing assessment via the NOSIE-30 scale significantly favored clozapine.
- 30% of participants receiving clozapine met the definition for "improvement" versus 4% of participants receiving chlorpromazine and benztropine.
- There were no cases of granulocytopenia in either group. The chlorpromazine + benztropine group was more likely to experience dry mouth and hypotension, while the clozapine group was more likely to experience increased salivation, benign hyperthermia, and tachycardia.
- Extrapyramidal symptoms ratings improved significantly in those treated with clozapine compared to those receiving chlorpromazine + benztropine (Table 40.1).

Table 40.1 Summary of Key Outcomes

Outcome	Chlorpromazine	Clozapine	P value
"Improvement" in symptoms (%)	4	30	<0.001
Mean BPRS score at 6 weeks	61 ± 11	45 ± 13	<0.001
Mean CGI score at 6 weeks	5.3 ± 0.8	4.4 ± 1.1	<0.001

NOTES: BPRS = Brief Psychiatric Rating Scale. CGI = Clinical Global Impression.

Criticisms and Limitations: In the initial phases of the study, participants were placed on what would now be considered extremely large doses of haloperidol, with an average dose of 61 mg/day. Participants randomized to chlorpromazine were also on relatively high doses, with peak average dose at 1,200 mg/day. It is possible the results would be different or current standard doses of haloperidol and chlorpromazine were used.

An additional limitation is the small percentage of female participants, only 20% at the start of the study, limiting the generalizability of the findings.

Other Relevant Studies and Information:

- Multiple studies[7,8,9,10] have corroborated the evidence for the superiority of clozapine to both first- and other second-generation antipsychotics in the management of treatment-resistant schizophrenia.
- Wider use of clozapine since the publication of this study has led to useful clinical wisdom on management of side effects and dose optimization.[11]
- While benefits on clozapine can gradually accumulate over 6 months to a year, inadequate response over the period of this study (6 weeks) should lead to measurement of serum levels and adjusting the dose to achieve a clozapine level above 350 µg/L.[12]
- The American Psychiatric Association (APA) guidelines[13] recommend considering a trial of clozapine for patients who have had a suboptimal response to two antipsychotics, with at least one being a second-generation agent.

Summary and Implications: This study demonstrated the efficacy of clozapine for treatment-resistant schizophrenia, both with respect to positive and negative symptoms. These findings culminated in the FDA's approval of clozapine for patients with treatment-resistant schizophrenia, and APA guidelines now recommend clozapine for such patients.

CLINICAL CASE: CLOZAPINE FOR TREATMENT-RESISTANT SCHIZOPHRENIA

Case History

A 42-year-old man, currently admitted to the inpatient psychiatric unit, has been titrated to 36 mg per day of perphenazine for the last 7 weeks with minimal benefit. He continues to endorse disparaging voices and persecutory delusions, notably of the nursing staff plotting to poison him through his morning coffee. He has been in and out of hospitals since the age of 28, having been treated with maximum doses of haloperidol, risperidone, and aripiprazole with no sustained period of clinical stability.

Based on the study conducted by Kane and colleagues,[1] how should this patient be treated?

Suggested Answer

In a landmark study, Kane et al.[1] illustrated the superiority of clozapine over chlorpromazine + benztropine combination in the management of treatment-resistant schizophrenia. This and other studies has led to APA guidelines that recommend the use of clozapine with close follow-up in patients with schizophrenia who have not responded to other antipsychotics.

The patient in the vignette would have met criteria for treatment-resistance and would have been included in the study. Given the history of more than three adequate trials of antipsychotic agents, continued symptoms of delusions and hallucinations, and the absence of a prolonged period of good functioning within the community, the CATIE study would support the use of clozapine. The likelihood of significant clinical improvement with clozapine is 30%, as contrasted with 4% in those treated with a first-generation agent (i.e., chlorpromazine). Given the need to monitor for leukopenia and granulocytopenia, a weekly complete blood count would be checked for the first six months, followed by every two weeks for an additional six months and then monthly as long as the patient is maintained on clozapine. The psychiatrist should present to this patient and salient caregivers the potentially significant benefits and the management of risks and engage in shared decision-making around a possible trial of clozapine.

References

1. Kane, J., Honigfeld, G., Singer, J., & Meltzer, H. (1988). Clozapine for the treatment-resistant schizophrenic: A double-blind comparison with chlorpromazine. *Archives of General Psychiatry, 45*(9), 789–796.
2. Overall, J. E. & Gorham, D. R. (1962). The brief psychiatric rating scale. *Psychological Reports, 10*(3), 799–812.
3. Guy, W. (1976). Clinical Global Impressions. In idem, *ECDEU assessment manual for psychopharmacology—Revised* (DHEW Publ No ADM 76–338; pp. 217–222). Rockville, MD: US Department of Health, Education, and Welfare.
4. Honigfeld, G., & Klett, C. J. (1965). The nurses' observation scale for inpatient evaluation: A new scale for measuring improvement in chronic schizophrenia. *Journal of Clinical Psychology, 21*(1), 65–71.
5. Simpson, G. M., & Angus, J. W. S. (1970). A rating scale for extrapyramidal side effects. *Acta Psychiatrica Scandinavica, 45*(Suppl 212), 11–19.

6. Guy, W. (1976). Abnormal involuntary movement scale (AIMS). In idem, *ECDEU assessment manual for psychopharmacology—Revised* (DHEW Publ No ADM 76-338; pp. 534–537). Rockville, MD: US Department of Health, Education, and Welfare.
7. Claghorn, J., Honigfeld, G., Abuzzahab, F. S., Sr., Wang, R., Steinbook, R., Tuason, V., & Klerman, G. (1987). The risks and benefits of clozapine versus chlorpromazine. *Journal of Clinical Psychopharmacology, 7*(6), 377–384.
8. Fischer-Cornelssen, K. A., & Ferner, U. J. (1976). An example of European multicenter trials: Multispectral analysis of clozapine. *Psychopharmacology Bulletin, 12*(2), 34–39.
9. McEvoy, J. P., Lieberman, J. A., Stroup, T. S., Davis, S. M., Meltzer, H. Y., Rosenheck, R. A., . . . Hsiao, J. K. (2006). Effectiveness of clozapine versus olanzapine, quetiapine, and risperidone in patients with chronic schizophrenia who did not respond to prior atypical antipsychotic treatment. *American Journal of Psychiatry, 163*(4), 611–622.
10. Wahlbeck, K., Cheine, M., Essali, A., & Adams, C. (1999). Evidence of clozapine's effectiveness in schizophrenia: a systematic review and meta-analysis of randomized trials. *American Journal of Psychiatry, 156*(7), 990–999.
11. Taylor, D., Paton, C., & Kapur, S. (2015). *The Maudsley prescribing guidelines* (12th ed.). London: Wiley Blackwell.
12. Schulte, P. (2003). What is an adequate trial with clozapine? Therapeutic drug monitoring and time to response in treatment-refractory schizophrenia. *Clinical Pharmacokinectics, 42*(7), 607–618.
13. Lehman, A. F., Lieberman, J. A., Dixon, L. B., McGlashan, T. H., Miller, A. L., Perkins, D. O., & Kreyenbuhl, J. (2004). Practice guideline for the treatment of patients with schizophrenia, second edition. *American Journal of Psychiatry, 161*(2 Suppl), 1–56.

41

Effectiveness of Clozapine versus Other Atypical Antipsychotics

Clinical Antipsychotic Trials for Interventions Effectiveness (CATIE)

EUNICE YUEN AND CENK TEK

> For these patients with schizophrenia who prospectively failed to improve with an atypical antipsychotic, clozapine was more effective than switching to another newer atypical antipsychotic. Safety monitoring is necessary to detect and manage clozapine's serious side effects.
>
> —The CATIE Investigators[1]

Research Question: What is the role of clozapine among patients with chronic schizophrenia who fail to respond to atypical antipsychotics?

Funding: The National Institute of Mental Health

Year Study Began: 2001

Year Study Published: 2006

Study Location: 57 sites in the United States in inpatient and outpatient settings at universities, state facilities, Virginia hospitals, private agencies, private practice, and mixed system sites.[2]

Who Was Studied: Adults 18 to 65 years old with a DSM-IV diagnosis of schizophrenia who could take oral antipsychotic medication. A broad spectrum of patients with schizophrenia were enrolled, including outpatients who remained symptomatic or continued to suffer from medication side effects, as well as inpatients who had acute exacerbation.[3]

Who Was Excluded: Patients that presented with first-episode psychosis and prior history of treatment resistance to antipsychotics. Also excluded were those who were pregnant or breast-feeding during the time of treatment, as well as those who were medically unstable.

How Many Participants: 1,493 in CATIE; 99 in this particular study.

Study Overview: See Figure 41.1 for a summary of the study design.

Study Intervention: First, patients were randomized to receive treatment with either an atypical antipsychotic (olanzapine, quetiapine, risperidone, or ziprasidone) or a typical antipsychotic (perphenazine). Those randomized to receive perphenazine whose treatment was discontinued for any reason were then randomized to receive olanzapine, quetiapine, or risperidone. The subjects were randomized further to various antipsychotics as indicated in Figure 41.1.

In the clozapine group, titration and maintenance dosing schedules were determined by physicians based on closely monitoring on patient's agranulocytosis and myocardial inflammation. Standard weekly white cell count, sedimentation rate, and creatine phosphokinase levels were performed. Moreover, electrocardiograms were performed prior to and at week 1, 2, and 4 weeks after treatment.

For subjects assigned to the newer atypical antipsychotics, dosing was initiated at one capsule a day of olanzapine (7.5 mg), quetiapine (200 mg), or risperidone (1.5 mg). Titration dosing schedules were adjusted by clinicians up to four capsules per day.

Decisions of treatment discontinuation were based on therapeutic effect, side effects, and patient preference.

Follow-Up: 18 months

Endpoints: The primary outcome measure was the time until treatment discontinuation due to tolerability and efficacy. Secondary outcome measures included the reasons for treatment discontinuation, including side effects, inefficacy, or patient preference. The Positive and Negative Syndrome Scale (PANSS) was used to measure clinical symptoms and the Clinical Global Impression (CGI) was used to assess illness severity.

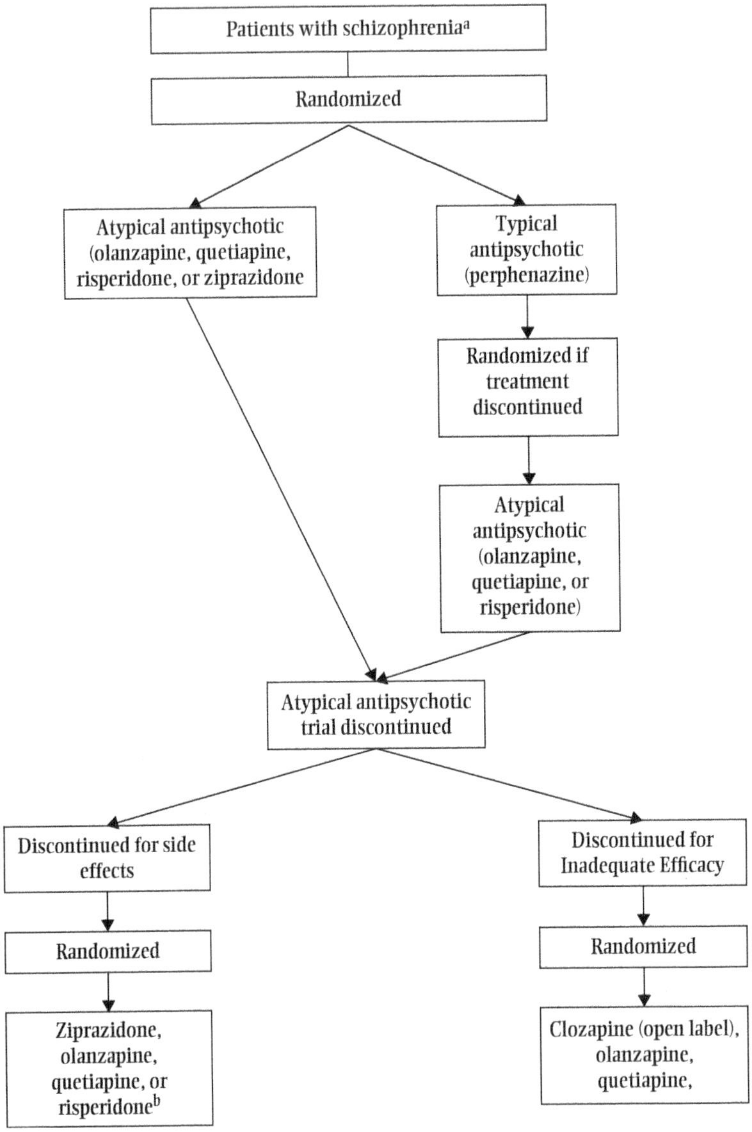

Figure 41.1 Summary of Study Design

[a]Patients with tardive dyskinesia at baseline were excluded from random assignment of perphenazine in phase 1.

[b]Subjects were not randomized to medications they had previously been given in the study.[3]

RESULTS

- Patients treated with clozapine had a significantly longer time before treatment discontinuation compared to those treated with quetiapine or risperidone. There was also a nonsignificant trend toward longer time before treatment discontinuation among patients treated with clozapine versus olanzapine.
- Clinical symptoms measured by PANSS were significantly improved among patients receiving clozapine compared to those receiving quetiapine or risperidone, though there was no difference relative to those receiving olanzapine. Clozapine-treated patients also had significant improvement in CGI severity at three months compared to the groups treated with olanzapine and quetiapine, though not risperidone.
- Clozapine had a distinct side effect profile compared to the other atypical antipsychotics. Clozapine was less associated with insomnia, elevated prolactin, and anti-cholinergic symptoms (dry mouth, urinary hesitancy, and constipation). Out of the 49 patients treated with clozapine, one developed agranulocytosis and another developed eosinophilia (Table 41.1).

Criticisms and Limitations: Unlike other antipsychotics given as blinded treatment, clozapine was administered in an open-label manner. Many clinicians view clozapine as the last resort medication. This perception could have influenced the study results.

While the entire CATIE trial had almost 1,500 patients, this study only utilized 99 patients. This relatively small sample size may not offer adequate power for reasonable comparisons across different atypical antipsychotics.

Other Relevant Studies and Information:

- A number of other studies comparing clozapine to alternative psychotics typically used in treating schizophrenia have come to similar conclusions as CATIE.[4,5,6]
- A follow-up study to CATIE found that risperidone and olanzapine are more effective than quetiapine and ziprasidone as reflected by longer time until discontinuation.[7]
- Another study suggests that in patients with treatment resistance to olanzapine, 41% of this population shows significant respond to clozapine.[8]

Table 41.1 SUMMARY OF CATIE: CLOZAPINE VERSUS OTHER ATYPICAL ANTIPSYCHOTICS KEY FINDINGS

Outcome	Clozapine	Olanzapine	P Value	Quetiapine	P Value	Risperidone	P value
Median time to treatment discontinuation in months (95% CI)	10.5 (7.3–16.1)	2.7 (1.9–11.9)		3.3 (1.0–4.9)		2.8 (1.1–4.0)	
Hazard ratio compared to clozapine for treatment discontinuation	N/A	0.57	0.12	0.39	0.01	0.42	<0.02
Hazard ratio compared to clozapine due to lack of efficacy	N/A	0.24	0.02	0.16	0.004	0.16	<0.003

NOTE: CATIE = Clinical Antipsychotic Trials for Interventions Effectiveness.

- Another recent study utilizing patients from the CATIE trial suggests that clozapine demonstrates superior antidepressant effects to quetiapine and comparable effects to olanzapine and risperidone in chronic schizophrenia.[9]
- International Suicide Prevention Trial (InterSePT) suggests that clozapine is significantly more effective in suicidal prevention than olanzapine for patients with schizophrenia and schizoaffective disorder.[10]
- Longitudinal cohort study suggests that patients taking clozapine have the lowest morality rate among second generation antipsychotics.[11]
- American Psychiatric Association (APA) treatment guidelines recommend the use of clozapine when there is an inadequate response to other antipsychotic medications or when a patient has persistent suicidal ideation.[12] Clozapine is considered a second-line agent due to its unfavorable side effect profile.

Summary and Implications: The CATIE trial investigated strategies to treat patients with chronic schizophrenia unresponsive to initial therapy with antipsychotics. The study found that switching to clozapine as compared to other atypical antipsychotics was significantly more effective. However, because clozapine may cause several side effects that warrant close monitoring, including agranulocytosis, myocarditis, seizure, diabetes, and other metabolic abnormalities, guidelines from the APA recommend that clozapine should be considered only among patients with an inadequate response to antipsychotic medications or those with persistent suicidal ideation.[12]

CLINICAL CASE: EFFECTIVENESS OF CLOZAPHINE VERSUS OTHER ATYPICAL ANTIPSYCHOTICS IN PATIENTS WITH CHRONIC SCHIZOPHRENIA

Case History

A 40-year-old man with a history of schizophrenia is admitted to the inpatient psychiatric ward for worsening bizarre behavior. On the unit, he is observed screaming at the microwave and told staff that he was worried that the machine could read his thoughts. He denies any mood symptoms and history of drug use. He does not have other active medical problems. Despite the patient's compliance with taking quetiapine (400 mg) twice per day for the past 6 months, he has not shown significant improvement. The patient recently decided to self-discontinue the medication for lack of efficacy. He has not noticed any significant side effects from quetiapine.

Based on the results of CATIE, how should this patient be treated?

Suggested Answer

CATIE found that for patients who do not respond to atypical antipsychotics, clozapine is superior to another atypical antipsychotics in terms of prolonging the time to stay on treatment and improving positive and negative symptomatology. Clozapine has been associated with significant side effects, so it is important to carefully weigh the risks and benefits of starting clozapine in any patient.

The patient in this vignette is typical of patients included in CATIE trial. Thus, he and the doctor should consider switching to clozapine. Fortunately, the patient does not have any significant side effects from quetiapine. If clozapine is started, the patient would need weekly blood draws for the first 6 months, biweekly thereafter, and be seen in clinic frequently to monitor for any side effects.

References

1. McEvoy, J. P. Lieberman, J. A., Stroup, T. S., Davis, S. M., Meltzer, H. Y., Rosenheck, R. A., . . . Hsiao, J. K. (2006). Effectiveness of clozapine versus olanzapine, quetiapine, and risperidone in patients with chronic schizophrenia who did not respond to prior atypical antipsychotic treatment. *American Journal of Psychiatry, 163*(4), 600–610.
2. Lieberman, J. A., Stroup, T. S., McEvoy, J. P., Swartz, M. S., Rosenheck, R. A., Perkins, D. O., . . . Hsiao, J. K. (2005). Effectiveness of antipsychotic drugs in patients with chronic schizophrenia. *New England Journal of Medicine, 353*, 1209–1223.
3. Stroup, T. S., McEvoy, J. P., Swartz, M. S., Byerly, M. J., Glick, I. D., Canive, J. M., . . . Lieberman, J. A. (2003). The National Institute of Mental Health Clinical Antipsychotic Trials of Intervention Effectiveness (CATIE) project: schizophrenia trial design and protocol development. *Schizophrenia Bulletin, 29*(1), 15–31.
4. Essock, S. M., Hargreaves, W. A., Covell, N. H., & Goethe, J. (1996). Clozapine's effectiveness for patients in state hospitals: Results from a randomized trial. *Psychopharmacology Bulletin, 32*(4), 683–697.
5. Rosenheck, R., Cramer, J., Xu, W., Thomas, J., Henderson, W., Frisman, L., . . . Charney, D. (1997). A comparison of clozapine and haloperidol in hospitalized patients with refractory schizophrenia: Department of Veterans Affairs Cooperative Study Group on Clozapine in Refractory Schizophrenia. *New England Journal of Medicine, 337*(12), 809–815.
6. Kane, J., Honigfeld, G., Singer, J., & Meltzer, H. (1988). Clozapine for the treatment-resistant schizophrenic: A double-blind comparison with chlorpromazine. *Archives of General Psychiatry, 45*(9), 789–796.

7. Stroup, T. S., Lieberman, J. A., McEvoy, J. P., Swartz, M. S., Davis, S. M., Rosenheck, R. A., . . . Hsiao, J. K. (2006). Effectiveness of olanzapine, quetiapine, risperidone, and ziprasidone in patients with chronic schizophrenia following discontinuation of a previous atypical antipsychotic. *American Journal of Psychiatry, 163*(4), 611–622.
8. Conley, R. R., Tamminga, C. A., Kelly, D. L., & Richardson, C. M. (1999). Treatment-resistant schizophrenic patients respond to clozapine after olanzapine non-response. *Biological Psychiatry, 46*(1), 73–77.
9. Nakajima, S., Takeuchi, H., Fervaha, G., Plitman, E., Chung, J. K., Caravaggio, F., . . . Graff-Guerrero, A. (2015). Comparative efficacy between clozapine and other atypical antipsychotics on depressive symptoms in patients with schizophrenia: Analysis of the CATIE phase 2E data. Schizophrenia Research, 161(2–3), 429–433.
10. Meltzer, H. Y. Alphs, L., Green, A. I., Altamura, A. C., Anand, R., Bertoldi, A., . . . Potkin, S. (2003). Clozapine treatment for suicidality in schizophrenia: International Suicide Prevention Trial (InterSePT). *Archives of General Psychiatry, 60*(1), 82–91.
11. Tiihonen, J., Lönnqvist, J., Wahlbeck, K., Klaukka, T., Niskanen, L., Tanskanen, A., & Haukka, J. (2009). 11-year follow-up of mortality in patients with schizophrenia: A population-based cohort study (FIN11 study). *Lancet, 374*(9690), 620–627.
12. American Psychiatric Association. (2007). *Practice guideline for the treatment of patients with obsessive-compulsive disorder*. Washington, DC: Author.

42

Atypical Antipsychotic Drugs and the Risk of Sudden Cardiac Death

HAMILTON GAIANI AND CENK TEK

> Current users of typical and atypical antipsychotic drugs had a similar, dose-related increased risk of sudden cardiac death.
>
> —The Antipsychotic Risk of Sudden Cardiac Death Investigators[1]

Research Question: Are atypical antipsychotic drugs associated with a lower risk of sudden cardiac death (SCD) versus typical antipsychotics?

Funding: National Heart, Lung, and Blood Institute and the Agency for Healthcare Quality and Research Centers for Education and Research on Therapeutics

Year Study Began: 1990

Year Study Published: 2005

Study Location: Nashville, Tennessee

Who Was Studied: Tennessee Medicaid patients between the ages of 30 and 74 years who were enrolled for at least 730 days and received at least one antipsychotic prescription.

Who Was Excluded: Patients at high risk of death from noncardiac causes

How Many Participants: 279,900

Study Overview: See Figure 42.1 for a summary of the study design.

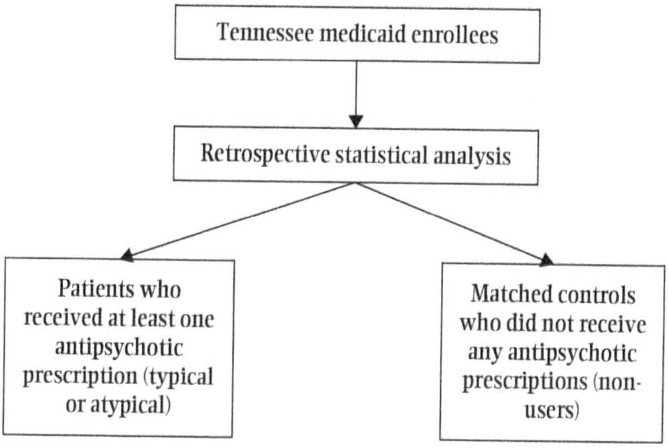

Figure 42.1 Summary of Study Design

Study Implementation: Electronic records of all 30 to 74-year-old Medicaid utilizers between January 1, 1990 and December 31, 2005 were evaluated. The cohort of antipsychotic medication users included all enrollees with at least one person-day of antipsychotic use during the analysis period. Death certificates were searched to identify community occurring SCD. These were defined as acute pulseless conditions consistent with tachy-arrhythmias. Deaths occurring in the hospital were excluded.

Each antipsychotic user was matched to two control patients who were not receiving antipsychotics. Matching was based on age, sex, and first day of follow-up. An additional analysis was performed on a secondary cohort of all antipsychotic users without a primary psychotic disorder. This group was matched in a 1:2 ratio to controls based on a calculated probability that the person would be prescribed antipsychotic medications.

Antipsychotic doses were classified as low, moderate, or high in each cohort based on chlorpromazine equivalents. Low dose was <100 mg, moderate dose was between 100 mg and 299 mg and high dose was considered more than 300 mg daily.

Follow-Up: Cohorts were monitored retrospectively over a 16-year period.

Endpoints: Primary endpoints: SCD in the community among users of typical and antipsychotics and matched controls who did not use antipsychotics. Secondary endpoints: SCD among users of specific medications (haloperidol, thioridazine, clozapine, olanzapine, quetiapine, risperidone.)

RESULTS

- The risk of SCD among antipsychotic users increased significantly in a dose-dependent manner for both the typical antipsychotic and atypical antipsychotic cohorts.
- The risk of SCD was not statistically different for typical versus atypical users.
- Former antipsychotic users did not have an increased risk of cardiac death versus current users.
- Of the individually analyzed medications, thioridazine and clozapine were associated with the highest risk for SCD (Table 42.1).

Table 42.1 SUMMARY OF KEY FINDINGS: INCIDENCE RATE RATIOS FOR SUDDEN CARDIAC DEATH

	Atypical IRR vs. non-users (95% CI)	**P value**	**Typical IRR vs. non-users (95% CI)**	**P value**	**Atypical IRR vs. typical (95% CI)**
Any dose	2.26 (1.88–2.72)	<0.001	1.99 (1.68-2.34)	<0.001	1.14 (0.93–1.39)
Low-dose	1.59 (1.03–2.46)	<0.001*	1.31 (0.97–1.77)	0.01*	–
Moderate-dose	2.13 (1.70–2.65)	<0.001*	2.01 (1.62–2.50)	0.01*	–
High-dose	2.86 (2.25–3.65)	<0.001*	2.42 (1.91–3.06)	0.01*	–
Cohort on atypical antipsychotics without a schizophrenia diagnosis	1.99 (1.61–2.46)	<0.001	1.84 (1.50–2.26)	<0.001	–

NOTE: IRR = incidence rate ratio.
*P values testing for a dose–response relationship.

Criticisms and Limitations: The study was an observational study, and while efforts were made to control for potential confounding factors it is possible that unmeasured confounders influenced the findings.

In-hospital deaths were excluded from this analysis; however, it is possible that use of antipsychotics among hospitalized patients is a risk factor for SCD.

Other Relevant Studies and Information:

- A meta-analysis of related studies also found similarly increased risk of SCD with use of atypical or typical antipsychotics.[2]
- American Psychiatric Association guidelines do not indicate whether typical versus atypical antipsychotics are associated with lower risk for SCD, though the guidelines do suggest that for patients with cardiovascular risk factors, clinicians should closely monitor potassium levels and use the lowest dose possible when using antipsychotics, particularly thioridazine, mesoridazine, pimozide, or ziprasidone. The guidelines do not recommend serial electrocardiograms (ECGs) for patients receiving any antipsychotic, as a prolonged QTc is not necessarily specific to predict risk of fatal arrhythmias.[3]

Summary and Implications: Prior to this analysis, it was widely assumed that atypical antipsychotics were associated with a lower risk of SCD versus typical antipsychotics. However, this study found that both atypical and typical antipsychotics increase risk of SCD approximately twofold.

CLINICAL CASE: ATYPICAL ANTIPSYCHOTIC DRUGS AND THE RISK OF SUDDEN CARDIAC DEATH

Case History

An otherwise healthy 25-year-old with schizophrenia is brought to the psychiatric emergency department by police. Police report she was verbally threatening to family members. She is disheveled and slightly malodorous and noted to be repeatedly glancing at the security camera. She reports her sister is colluding with the emergency room staff and plans to have her killed.

Per family, in recent weeks, she has become more delusional, paranoid, and aggressive at home. They report she has been hiding knives around the house and talking to herself. They are concerned for their own safety.

The patient's family members dissuaded her from initiating antipsychotics in previous mental health visits. They reported concern about long-term consequences of these medications.

Based on the study results, how should this patient be treated?

Suggested Answer

Antipsychotic treatment is indicated for this patient. Once stabilized and long-term treatment is discussed, a risk–benefits discussion of long term antipsychotic use should occur with the patient and her family supports. The risk of untreated schizophrenia is likely significantly higher than no treatment for this patient. However, increased risk of SCD as well as other potential side effects should be discussed. A careful history should be obtained to identify cardiac risk factors. Guidelines do not suggest ECG monitoring for antipsychotics other than ziprasidone, thioridazine, mesoridazine, or pimozide. However, many clinicians prefer to obtain electrolytes and ECG for patients treated with any antipsychotic, particularly at higher doses. ECG may also be considered with significant dose changes or addition of QTc prolonging medications.

References

1. Ray, W. A., Chung, C. P., Murray, K. T., Hall, K., & Stein, M. C. (2009). Atypical antipsychotic drugs and the risk of sudden cardiac death. *New England Journal of Medicine, 360*, 225–235.
2. Salvo, F., Pariente, A., Shakir, S., Robinson, P., Arnaud, M., Thomas, S., . . . Sturkenboom, M. (2016). Sudden cardiac and sudden unexpected death related to antipsychotics: A meta-analysis of observational studies. *Clinical Pharmacology & Therapeutics, 99*(3), 306–314.
3. American Psychiatric Association. (2004). American Psychiatric Association practice guidelines for the treatment of psychiatric disorders: Compendium. Washington, DC: Author.

43

Switching Antipsychotics to Reduce Metabolic Risk

The CAMP Trial

ERIC LIN AND JOHN CAHILL

> Switching to aripiprazole led to improvement of non-HDL cholesterol levels and other metabolic parameters . . . but switching to aripiprazole was associated with a higher rate of treatment discontinuation.
>
> —The CAMP Investigators[1]

Research Question: Does switching to aripiprazole from olanzapine, quetiapine, or risperidone confer metabolic benefits, and did the switch to aripiprazole cause clinical destabilization?

Funding: National Institute of Mental Health and the Foundation for National Institutes of Health. Bristol-Myers Squibb provided aripiprazole but did not participate in the study.

Year Study Began: 2007

Year Study Published: 2011

Study Location: Multisite study at 27 clinical research centers affiliated with the Schizophrenia Trials Network across 18 US states

Who Was Studied: Adults with an average age of 41 years with schizophrenia or schizoaffective disorder who were stable on olanzapine, quetiapine, or risperidone. Participants were on one of these three medications for at least three months and no other antipsychotic at least one month prior. Subjects were required to have a body mass index ≥27 and a non-high-density lipoprotein (HDL) cholesterol ≥130 mg/dl (if non-HDL cholesterol was 130–139 mg/dL, then low-density lipoprotein [LDL] cholesterol was required to be ≥100 mg/dl).

Who Was Excluded: Patients with minimal metabolic issues or those with severe metabolic issues requiring immediate treatment. Individuals with diabetes or treatment with oral diabetes medications or insulin, with non-HDL cholesterol ≥300 mg/dL, with triglycerides ≥500 mg/dL, in the first episode of psychosis, or currently on weight-loss medications.[2]

How Many Participants: 215

Study Overview: See Figure 43.1 for a summary of the study design.

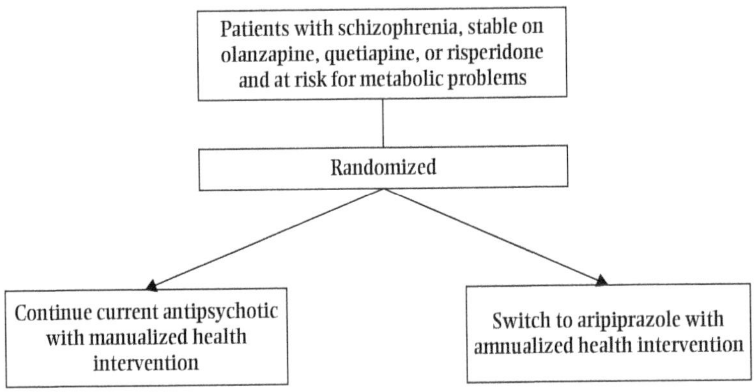

Figure 43.1 Summary of Study Design

Study Intervention: Patients in the switch group were cross-tapered to aripiprazole over four weeks according to a standard study protocol.

Patients assigned to continue their current antipsychotic continued taking the regimen they were already on; dosages were adjusted during the trial if clinically indicated.

For both groups, the addition of lithium, valproate, lipid-lowering agents, or drugs prescribed for weight loss were not allowed during the trial, but if subjects were already on such medications, the regimens were allowed to be continued.

Both groups also received a manualized behavioral intervention designed to improve exercise and diet habits with the goal of reducing cardiovascular disease risk. Patients came weekly to clinic for the first month and then followed up every four weeks after that. The behavioral intervention was provided in person at all study visits, and telephone calls to reinforce the behavioral treatment were provided between monthly visits.

Follow-Up: 24 weeks

Endpoints: Primary outcome: change in non-HDL cholesterol. Secondary outcome: "efficacy failure" defined as psychiatric hospitalization, 25% increase in the total Positive and Negative Syndrome Scale (PANSS) score, or ratings of "much worse" or "very much worse" on the Clinical Global Impressions (CGI) change subscale. Additional metabolic outcomes about weight change, total cholesterol, triglycerides, and fasting glucose were also measured.

RESULTS

- For the primary outcome, non-HDL cholesterol decreased more for the switch to aripiprazole group than stay group (–20.2 mg/dl compared to –10.8mg/dl) with difference of –9.4 mg/dl (95% CI [–2.2, –16.5], p = 0.010).
- For the secondary outcome, 20.6% of the switch group and 17% of the stay group experienced "efficacy failure." There was no detectable statistically significant difference in time to "efficacy failure," hazard ratio 95% CI [0.395, 1.413] (p = 0.370). No differences in psychopathology changes between the two groups on the PANSS score, change in CGI score, or the 12-Item Short-Form Health Survey mental health score.
- Improvements in non-HDL cholesterol and triglycerides were mostly realized after 4 weeks, but weight continued a downward trend over the 24 weeks.
- Overall, 47.7% of the switch group and 27.4% of the continue group went off the protocol treatments (discontinued assigned antipsychotic or beginning a prohibited medication) before the 24-week protocol was completed (Table 43.1).

Table 43.1 SUMMARY OF CAMP'S KEY FINDINGS

Outcome	Switch to aripiprazole group	Continue current antipsychotic group	P value
Change in non-HDL cholesterol (mg/dL)	−20.2	−10.8	0.0100
Change in weight (kg)	−3.6	−0.7	<0.0001
Change in total cholesterol (mg/dL)	−19.6	−10.8	0.0180
Change in triglycerides (mg/dL)	−25.7	7.0	0.0020
Change in fasting glucose (mg/dL)	0.5	4.0	0.0610
Antipsychotic "efficacy failure"	20.6%	17.0%	0.4782
PANSS total	−5.0	−3.9	0.5180
CGI severity subscale score	−0.2	−0.2	0.8560

NOTES: CAMP = Comparison of Antipsychotics for Metabolic Problems in Schizophrenia or Schizoaffective Disorder. HDL = high-density lipoprotein. PANSS = Positive and Negative Syndrome Scale. CGI = Clinical Global Impression.

Criticisms and Limitations: The study focused on non-HDL cholesterol as a marker for cardiovascular morbidity and mortality; however, this is a surrogate marker that may not actually reflect cardiovascular risk.

Since this was an open-label study, clinician bias may have influenced the results.

Other Relevant Studies and Information:

- One study suggested that a switch from olanzapine to aripiprazole improved weight and lipids and did not result in a significant worsening of psychiatric symptoms.[3]
- Another study found that switching to ziprasidone from risperidone or olanzapine led to improvements in metabolic measures.[4]
- A Cochrane review came to similar conclusions. Switching antipsychotics may yield benefits to weight and metabolic risks; however, switching is associated with increased risk of relapse and treatment dropout.[5]
- An experiment demonstrated that rosuvastatin significantly decreased triglycerides, total cholesterol, LDL, and non-HDL in schizophrenic

patients with severe dyslipidemia when compared against treatment as usual.[6]

- American Psychiatric Association guidelines for the treatment of schizophrenia recommend diet and exercise for antipsychotic-related weight gain and recommend considering an antipsychotic with lower weight gain risk.[7]

Summary and Implications: This study found that with careful cross-titration and close monitoring, switching from antipsychotics associated with significant metabolic effects to aripiprazole can lead to substantial improvements in non-HDL cholesterol levels, serum triglyceride levels, and weight loss. Switching from a stable antipsychotic regimen led to lower sustained medication adherence, however. The decision to switch patients to an antipsychotic agent like aripiprazole with a better metabolic profile must weigh the potential metabolic benefits against the potential risk of psychiatric destabilization.

CLINICAL CASE: METABOLIC SIDE EFFECTS FROM ATYPICAL ANTIPSYCHOTICS

Case History

A 45-year-old patient with schizophrenia who has been stable on olanzapine for many years wants to lose more weight than she has previously achieved with consistent diet and exercise. What risks and benefits should be considered before a switch to aripiprazole?

Suggested Answer

The CAMP trial provides hope, finding that triglycerides and non-HDL cholesterol may improve after a switch to aripiprazole (in the context of lifestyle modifications) without detecting a statistically significant loss of efficacy. There were, however, limitations to the study surround the open-label nature of the design, degree of generalizability, and risk of underemphasizing reduction in efficacy.

When counseling the patient in the vignette, the psychiatrist and patient should consider the benefit of improved metabolic measures against the risks of possible psychiatric destabilization amongst other potential effects of a switch. Risks can be mitigated by close monitoring and timely intervention. A structured diet and exercise program should be considered in parallel. Other options to consider may include the addition of medications such as metformin and/or statins in collaboration with a patient's primary care provider.

References

1. Stroup, T. S., McEvoy, J. P., Ring, K. D., Hamer, R. H., LaVange, L. M., Swartz, M. S., . . . Lieberman, J. A. (2011). A randomized trial examining the effectiveness of switching from olanzapine, quetiapine, or risperidone to aripiprazole to reduce metabolic risk: Comparison of Antipsychotics for Metabolic Problems (CAMP). *American Journal of Psychiatry, 168*(9), 947–956.
2. National Institute of Mental Health. (2007). *Comparison of Antipsychotics for Metabolic Problems in Schizophrenia or Schizoaffective Disorder (CAMP)*. Retrieved from https://clinicaltrials.gov/ct2/show/NCT00423878
3. Newcomer, J. W., Campos, J. A., Marcus, R. N., Breder, C., Berman, R. M., Kerselaers, W., . . . McQuade, R. D. (2008). A multicenter, randomized, double-blind study of the effects of aripiprazole in overweight subjects with schizophrenia or schizoaffective disorder switched from olanzapine. *Journal of Clinical Psychiatry, 69*(7), 1046–1056.
4. Weiden, P. J., Newcomer, J. W., Loebel, A. D., Yang, R., & Lebovitz, H. E. (2008). Long-term changes in weight and plasma lipids during maintenance treatment with ziprasidone. *Neuropsychopharmacology, 33*(5), 985–994.
5. Mukundan, A., Faulkner, G., Cohn, T., & Remington, G. (2010). Antipsychotic switching for people with schizophrenia who have neuroleptic-induced weight or metabolic problems. *The Cochrane Database of Systematic Reviews, 12*, CD006629.
6. De Hert, M., Kalnicka, D., van Winkel, R., Wampers, M., Hanssens, L., Van Eyck, D., . . . Peuskens, J. (2006). Treatment with rosuvastatin for severe dyslipidemia in patients with schizophrenia and schizoaffective disorder. *Journal of Clinical Psychiatry, 67*(12), 1889–1896.

44

Cost Utility of Atypical Antipsychotics

CUtLASS-1

NIKHIL GUPTA AND JOHN CAHILL

> In people with schizophrenia whose medication is changed for clinical reasons, there is no disadvantage . . . in using FGAs rather than nonclozapine SGAs.
>
> —The CUtLASS Investigators[1]

Research Question: Are second-generation antipsychotics (SGAs) better than first-generation antipsychotics (FGAs) for individuals with schizophrenia needing an antipsychotic change? Additionally, are there improvements in quality of life and savings in health service use to justify the additional costs of SGAs over FGAs?

Funding: United Kingdom National Health Service Health Technology Assessment Program

Year Study Began: 1999

Year Study Published: 2006

Study Location: 14 community psychiatric services in the English National Health Service.

Who Was Studied: 18 to 65-year-old patients with schizophrenia or a related disorder diagnosed by DSM-IV for more than one-month duration and needing a change in treatment due to inadequate clinical response or intolerance to the current antipsychotic.

Who Was Excluded: Individuals with a medical condition or substance use accounting for psychosis or with a history of neuroleptic malignant syndrome.

How Many Participants: 227

Study Overview: See Figure 44.1 for a summary of the study design.

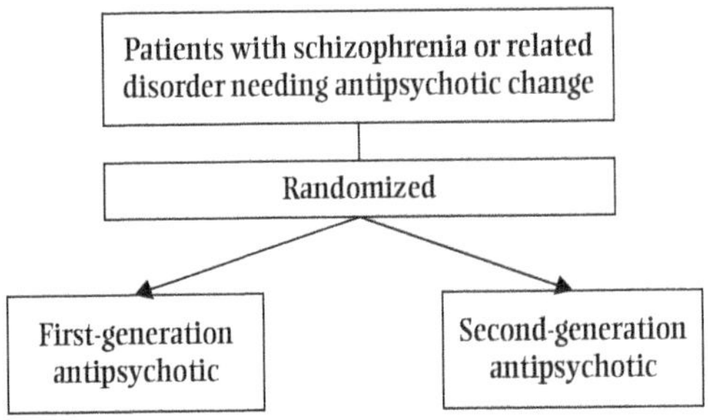

Figure 44.1 Summary of Study Design

Study Intervention: The psychiatrists who decided to switch antipsychotic treatment for their patients recruited participants into the trial. After a baseline assessment, participants were randomized to receive either an FGA or an SGA. The psychiatrist and the patient made the choice of which specific drug to use in that class and, hence, were not blinded to treatment. Clinicians tried to keep patients in the allotted treatment arm for 52 weeks, with a minimum of 12 weeks. They were encouraged to choose another antipsychotic from the same class if they wanted to change the antipsychotic that patients were started on after randomization, but there was significant crossover between the two groups (with an attrition rate of 46% in the FGA arm and 35% in the SGA arm at 52 weeks, $p = 0.1$). Antipsychotic polypharmacy was discouraged, but 11% to 14% of the patients in the two groups were on more than one antipsychotic agent at baseline.

Patients in the FGA arm were started on one of the following drugs: chlorpromazine, flupenthixol, fluphenazine, haloperidol, loxapine, methotrimeprazine, pipothiazine, sulpiride, trifluoperazine, or zuclopenthixol,

Patients in the SGA arm were started on one of the following drugs: risperidone, olanzapine, amisulpride, zotepine, or quetiapine.

Cost measures included inpatient and outpatient services, medical services, and medications.

Follow-Up: 12, 26, and 52 weeks

Endpoints: Primary outcome: total score on the Quality of Life Scale (QLS), with a five-point difference considered clinically meaningful. Secondary outcomes: positive and Negative Syndrome Scale, Calgary Depression Scale, participant adherence and satisfaction scales, global functioning, and adverse effects scales.

RESULTS

- The study did not detect a significant difference in QLS for patients randomized to FGAs versus SGAs, interpreted as excluding a clinically meaningful advantage for SGAs.
- The study did not detect a statistically significant difference between the two treatment arms in the costs of treatment (from a health systems perspective), or any of the secondary outcomes including symptom scores, adverse effect scales (e.g., extrapyramidal symptoms), or patient satisfaction (Table 44.1).

Table 44.1 Summary of CUtLASS-1 Key Findings

Outcome	**First generation antipsychotic**	**Second generation antipsychotic**	**P value**
QLS score at baseline, mean	43.3	43.5	not reported
QLS score at 12 weeks, mean	49.2	46.6	0.31
QLS score at 26 weeks, mean	49.2	50.4	not reported
QLS score at 52 weeks, mean	53.2	51.3	0.24

Notes: CUtLASS-1 = Cost Utility of Atypical Antipsychotics. QLS = Quality of Life Scale.

Criticisms and Limitations: This study focused on patients with an inadequate response to treatment and thus may not be generalizable to other populations of patients with schizophrenia. Additionally, the psychiatrists were not blinded to the treatment choice and, hence, may have been influenced by their perception of the medication's efficacy, which may have led to the high crossover rates between the two groups.

Cost information was based on the United Kingdom as part of the National Health Service, which may not be generalizable to health-care costs in the United States.

Metabolic side effects, a known complication of antipsychotic agents, were not systematically studied. Finally, dosing was based on the psychiatrist's clinical decision, which was not standardized.

Other Relevant Studies and Information:

- The CUtLASS 2 study randomized treatment refractory patients to receive either clozapine or another SGA. Results found a statistically significant advantage in those treated with clozapine.[2]
- CATIE was a randomized, double-blind trial that compared the FGA perphenazine to SGAs including olanzapine, quetiapine, risperidone, and ziprasidone. It found no significant difference in effectiveness between perphenazine and nonclozapine SGAs and found it to be the most cost-effective drug.[3]
- The American Psychiatric Association (APA) treatment guidelines for schizophrenia recommend the use of a FGA or SGA and recommend to consider side-effect profiles when deciding on antipsychotic choice.

Summary and Implications: This study failed to detect an advantage in terms of quality of life, symptoms, or associated costs of care for SGAs versus FGAs over a - year period among patients with schizophrenia requiring a medication change due to intolerance or inadequate response. The choice of antipsychotic agents among patients with schizophrenia should generally be based on the profile of adverse effects.

CLINICAL CASE: FIRST-GENERATION VERSUS SECOND-GENERATION ANTIPSYCHOTICS

Case History

A 23-year-old man presents to an outpatient psychiatrist experiencing ongoing derogatory auditory hallucinations, severe thought disturbance, social isolation, and inability to function properly at his work as a cook for the past two years. He has not been using any substances. He was diagnosed with schizophrenia one year ago, started on haloperidol, but has had inadequate response. The psychiatrist is considering switching the antipsychotic, and the patient's family is concerned about how this would affect the patients' quality of life.

According to the CUtLASS trial, which (class of) antipsychotic should the psychiatrist prescribe?

Suggested Answer

The CUtLASS 1 trial found no detectable difference between nonclozapine SGAs and FGAs in terms of a clinically meaningful difference in quality of life, positive or negative symptoms, adverse effects, or patient satisfaction at one year. APA guidelines also support the use of both FGA and SGA medications in individuals with schizophrenia.

Based on the questions raised by CUtLASS 1, the psychiatrist should consider the drug side-effect profiles, patient preferences, and economic considerations when choosing an individual agent from either generation of antipsychotics.

References

1. Jones, P. B., Barnes, T. R., Davies, L., Dunn, G., Lloyd, H., Hayhurst, K. P., . . . Lewis, S. W. (2006). Randomized controlled trial of the effect on quality of life of second- vs first-generation antipsychotic drugs in schizophrenia: Cost Utility of the Latest Antipsychotic Drugs in Schizophrenia Study (CUtLASS 1). *Archives of General Psychiatry, 63*(10), 1079–1087.
2. Lewis, S. W., Barnes, T. R. E., Davies, L., Murray, R. M., Dunn, G., Hayhurst, K. P., . . . Jones, P. B. (2006). Randomized controlled trial of effect of prescription of clozapine versus other second-generation antipsychotic drugs in resistant schizophrenia. *Schizophrenia Bulletin, 32*(4), 715–723.
3. Lieberman, J. A., Stroup, T. S., McEvoy, J. P., Swartz, M. S., Rosenheck, R. A., Perkins, D. O., . . . Severe, J. (2005). Effectiveness of antipsychotic drugs in patients with chronic schizophrenia. *New England Journal of Medicine, 353*(12), 1209–1223.

45

North American Prodrome Longitudinal Study

NIKHIL GUPTA AND VINOD H. SRIHARI

> Prospective ascertainment of individuals at risk for psychosis is feasible, with a level of predictive accuracy comparable to that in other areas of preventive medicine.
>
> —CANNON ET AL.[1]

Research Question: In patients identified clinically to be at high risk for psychosis, which variables (or their combinations) best predict conversion to schizophrenia or another psychotic disorder?

Funding: National Institute of Mental Health, Staglin Music Festival for Mental Health

Year Study Began: 1998

Year Study Published: 2008

Study Location: Eight research sites in North America

Who Was Studied: Referred subjects from 1998 to 2005 with prodromal psychotic symptoms. To be eligible for inclusion, patients were required to have symptoms in at least one of the five domains in the past 12 months on the Structured Interview for Prodromal Syndromes (SIPS) criteria[2]:

- Unusual thought content
- Suspicion/paranoia
- Perceptual anomalies
- Grandiosity
- Disorganized communication

Who Was Excluded: There were no exclusion criteria listed in the study.

How Many Participants: 291

Study Overview: See Figure 45.1 for a summary of the study design.

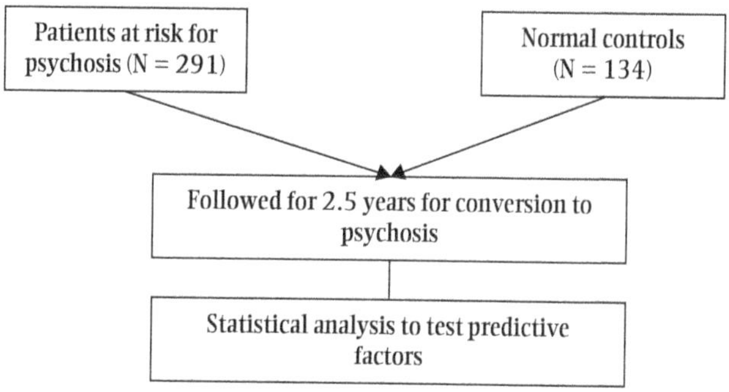

Figure 45.1 Summary of Study Design

Study Intervention: Patients with prodromal symptoms of psychosis were referred to the study sites by community clinicians. They were assessed at baseline for multiple variables possibly predictive for transition to schizophrenia. These results were compared to normal controls. This was a longitudinal, observational study with prospective follow-up.

Follow-Up: 6, 12, 18, 24, and 30 months.

Endpoints: Time from baseline evaluation to conversion to full blown psychosis according to SIPS criteria.

RESULTS

- 81 of 291 patients experienced conversion to psychosis with a mean time to conversion of 275.5 days from the baseline evaluation. This indicates that the SIPS criteria have a positive predictive power (PPP) of 35% during 2.5 years of follow-up. None of the 134 normal control subjects developed a psychotic disorder.
- There was a decelerating rate of conversion: 13% in the first 6 months, 9% from 7 to 12 months, 5% from 13 to 24 months, and 2.7% from 25 to 30 months.
- Of the 77 variables, 37 were associated with conversion to psychosis in univariate analysis but only 5 survived cross-domain multivariate analysis. These variables are listed in Table 45.1.

Table 45.1 Summary of the North American Prodrome Longitudinal Study Key Findings

Predictor	Base rate	Positive predictive power	Sensitivity	Specificity	P value
1. Genetic risk with functional decline	48	52	66	59	<0.001
2. Unusual thought content	43	48	56	62	0.002
3. Suspicion/paranoia	32	43	79	37	0.006
4. Social functioning	36	46	80	43	0.03
5. Any substance abuse	20	43	29	83	0.003
1 and 2	21	69	38	85	0.001
1, 2, and 4	16	81	30	90	<0.001
1, 2, 3, and 4	13	81	28	92	<0.001
1, 2, 3, 4, and 5	3	79	8	98	<0.001

- The adjunctive use of these predictor variables led to a marked increase in the positive predictive value (and specificity), but with a loss of sensitivity. For example, the combination of two variables (genetic risk with functional decline, and unusual thought content) has a PPP of 69, and adding a third variable (e.g., impaired social functioning) can increase the PPP up to 81.
- Treatment was not standardized across patients or sites; hence, details of antipsychotic treatment were not available for analysis in most cases, but presence or absence of treatment was not significantly associated with conversion to psychosis in the multivariate analysis.

Criticisms and Limitations: The predictive variables were derived empirically from this particular clinical sample and will need to be confirmed in an independent population. Also, the subjects had been referred to the clinical sites and already had some prodromal symptoms of psychosis. Thus, these are quantitative predictions of progression in an already ill, help-seeking population and cannot be extrapolated to screening of a general population. Finally, low base rates of certain variables (grandiosity, perceptual abnormalities, substance use) limited the researchers' ability to assess them as potential predictors of conversion to psychosis.

Other Relevant Studies and Information:

- A similar study was conducted as part of the European Prediction of Psychosis Study.[3] This study followed 245 individuals for 18 months and reported 19% conversion rates, with a similar group of predictors.
- Pharmacologic trials to prevent or delay the onset of psychosis among those showing prodromal symptoms have either shown unacceptable risks[4] or unclear results,[5] however this remains an active area of investigation.

Summary and Implications: The North American Prodromal Longitudinal Study (NAPLS) was an observational study to detect specific factors that may predict the conversion to psychosis among patients experiencing prodromal symptoms. The study found that a combination of genetic risk with deterioration in functioning, unusual thought content, paranoia, social impairment, and substance abuse were associated with an increased risk of conversion. This and subsequent studies offer insights regarding the detection of those at risk for chronic psychotic disorders and offer the possibility of studying the neurobiology of psychosis onset and developing approaches for delaying or preventing the progression of schizophrenia-spectrum illnesses.

CLINICAL CASE: PREDICTION OF PSYCHOSIS

Case History

A 17-year-old male is referred to a psychiatrist by a school counselor for endorsing bizarre ideas in the classroom and falling grades for the past year. His parents report increasing preoccupation for the past year with "aliens" accompanied by social withdrawal and a decline in academic performance. His aunt had schizophrenia. On initial interview, the young man is preoccupied with talk about spaceships and aliens and seems to believe that his internal experiences are linked in some way with cosmic events. There is no evidence of overt paranoia. He denies hearing voices and looks puzzled when asked about abnormal perceptual experiences. He denies overt mood fluctuations or thoughts of self-harm. He denies any drug use, and parents are confident he does not use drugs. The parents are concerned that he may be showing signs of a disease similar to his aunt.

Based on the results of this study, how should the clinician explain the prognosis?

Suggested Answer

According to NAPLS, he has two important signs associated with a chronic psychotic illness, namely, genetic risk with recent functional decline and unusual thought content. This profile in NAPLS is associated with a 69% probability of conversion to a diagnosable psychotic illness in the next 2.5 years. Hence, it would be prudent for the psychiatrist to educate the parents broadly about the varied manifestations of psychosis, explore environmental supports (e.g., school based academic assistance), offer psychotherapy to address social withdrawal related to prodromal symptoms, and to closely follow the patient to ensure early diagnosis and treatment.

References

1. Cannon, T. D., Cadenhead, K., Cornblatt, B., Woods, S. W., Addington, J., Walker, E., . . . Heinssen. R. (2008). Prediction of psychosis in youth at high clinical risk: A multisite longitudinal study in North America. *Archives of General Psychiatry*, *65*(1), 28–37.
2. Miller, T. J., McGlashan, T. H., Woods, S. W., Stein, K., Driesen, N., Corcoran, C. M., . . . Davidson, L., 1999. Symptom assessment in schizophrenic prodromal states. *Psychiatric Quarterly*, *70*(4), 273–287.
3. Ruhrmann, S., Schultze-Lutter, F., Salokangas, R. K., Heinimaa, M., Linszen, D., Dingemans, P., . . . Morrison, A. (2010). Prediction of psychosis in adolescents and young adults at high risk: results from the prospective European prediction of psychosis study. *Archives of General Psychiatry*, *67*(3), 241–251.
4. McGlashan, T. H., Zipursky, R. B., Perkins, D., Addington, J., Miller, T. J., Woods, S. W., & Breier, A. (2003). The PRIME North America randomized double-blind clinical trial of olanzapine versus placebo in patients at risk of being prodromally symptomatic for psychosis: I. Study rationale and design. *Schizophrenia Research*, *61*(1), 7–18.
5. McGorry, P. D., Nelson, B., Markulev, C., Yuen, H. P., Schäfer, M. R., Mossaheb, N., . . . Amminger, G. P. (2017). Effect of ω-3 polyunsaturated fatty acids in young people at ultrahigh risk for psychotic disorders: The NEURAPRO randomized clinical trial. *JAMA Psychiatry*, *74*(1), 19–27.

46

Clozapine for Suicidality in Schizophrenia

The International Suicide Prevention Trial (InterSePT)

DANIEL BARRON AND NOAH CAPURSO

> Clozapine therapy demonstrated superiority to olanzapine therapy in preventing suicide attempts in patients with schizophrenia and schizoaffective disorder.
>
> —THE INTERSEPT INVESTIGATORS[1]

Research Question: Does clozapine reduce suicidal events in patients with schizophrenia?

Funding: Novartis Pharmaceuticals Corp, William K Warren Research Foundation, and the Donald Test Foundation Trust and Lydia Bryant Test.

Year Study Began: 1998

Year Study Published: 2003

Study Location: 67 sites in 11 countries including the United States and Canada

Who Was Studied: Patients 18 to 65 years old diagnosed with schizophrenia or schizoaffective disorder by DSM-IV criteria at high risk for committing suicide, defined as having a history of previous suicide attempts or hospitalizations to prevent suicide attempt in the three years prior, depressive symptoms with current suicidal ideation, or command hallucinations for self-harm in the prior one week.

Who Was Excluded: Patients with a history of intolerance to clozapine or olanzapine.

How Many Participants: 980

Study Overview: See Figure 46.1 for a summary of the study design.

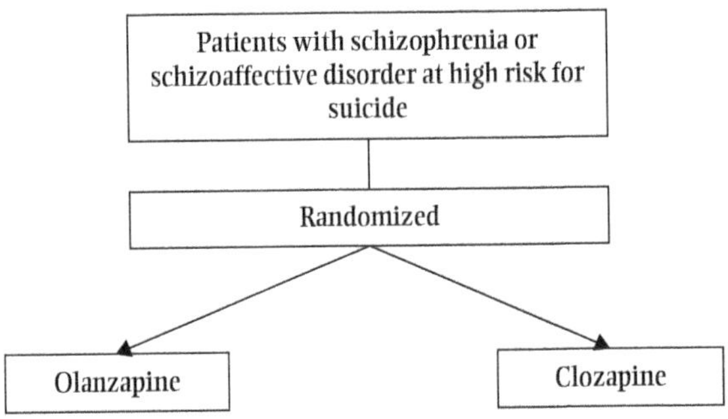

Figure 46.1 Summary of Study Design

Study Intervention: Patients were treated with open-label olanzapine or clozapine for two years. Patients were seen weekly for six months, then biweekly for 18 months. Blood monitoring was performed in the clozapine group as indicated, and those in the olanzapine group had their vitals taken. Clinicians were allowed to add other medications or make changes in doses to prevent suicide attempts. If research staff determined that the patient's risk for suicide had increased, the patient was referred to an independent psychiatrist for clinical management to ensure that the treating study psychiatrist remained blind to assignment.

A blinded, three-member suicide monitoring board evaluated whether a putative suicide event met the criteria for a suicide attempt or a hospitalization related to suicidality.

Follow-Up: Two years

Endpoints: Primary outcomes: "suicidal behavior," defined as completed suicide, serious suicide attempt, or psychiatric hospitalization to mitigate suicide risk as confirmed by the blinded suicide monitoring board. Secondary outcomes: ratings from a masked psychiatrist on the Clinical Global Impression–Suicide Severity (CGI-SS) of "much worse" or "very much worse" from baseline.

RESULTS

- The number needed to treat for a suicidal event in two years was 13, meaning that for every 13 high-risk patients treated, a suicidal event would occur in one fewer patient treated with clozapine versus olanzapine.
- Clozapine was associated with significantly less suicidal behavior than olanzapine (hazard ratio, 0.76; 95% CI, [0.58, 0.97], p = 0.03).
- There were five deaths by suicide in the clozapine group compared to three in the olanzapine group, though this did not differ statistically (p = 0.73).
- Those in the clozapine group received less rescue interventions (p = 0.01) and less adjunctive antidepressants (p = 0.01) or anxiolytics or soporifics (p = 0.03).
- Discontinuation and dropout rates were similar between groups (Table 46.1).

Table 46.1 Summary of InterSePT's Key Findings

Outcome	**Olanzapine**	**Clozapine**	**P value**
Patients with significant suicide attempts	11.2%	6.9%	0.03
Patients with psychiatric hospitalizations related to suicidality	21.8%	16.7%	0.05
CGI-SS of "much worse" or "very much" from baseline	32.9%	24.5%	0.005
Suicide deaths	0.6%	1.0%	0.73
Hazard ratio for suicide attempts or psychiatric hospitalizations related to suicidality		0.76[a]	0.03

[a]Compared to the olanzapine group.
Notes: InterSePT = International Suicide Prevention Trial. CGI-SS = Clinical Global Impression–Suicide Severity.

Criticisms and Limitations: Since this study was not fully blinded, clinicians may have been biased in favor of clozapine, which already had an established track record at the time of this study. Furthermore, inclusion of other comparators, particularly a first-generation antipsychotic, would have strengthened the study design.

Other Relevant Studies and Information:

- A retrospective study found decreased suicidal behavior and decreased serious suicidal behavior among patients with schizophrenia who were taking clozapine versus those who were not.[2]
- A meta-analysis of six studies representing 24,564 patients with schizophrenia or schizoaffective disorder showed decrease in suicidal risks with clozapine versus other treatments. The study concluded that patients with clozapine were three times less likely to attempt or complete suicide when treated with clozapine as compared with other medications.[3,4]
- The CATIE study and other have found that clozapine can be more effective than other antipsychotic medications for treatment of schizophrenia.[5]
- Clozapine is an effective treatment for bipolar disorder as well as psychotic disorders. Its ability to decrease suicidality in this population has been suggested, though not as thoroughly studied.[6]
- The FIN11 study found that that long-term treatment with clozapine is associated with lower mortality than other antipsychotics.[7]
- Based on this and other studies, American Psychiatric Association (APA) guidelines acknowledge the antisuicidal properties of many antipsychotic medications, however these guidelines suggest consideration of clozapine in patients found to be at particularly high risk for suicide.[8]

Summary and Implications: The InterSePT trial found that clozapine has considerable benefit in preventing suicidality in patients at high risk for suicide with schizophrenia or schizoaffective disorder vs. olanzapine. APA guidelines suggest consideration of clozapine in patients considered at high risk for suicide.

CLINICAL CASE: SUICIDALITY IN SCHIZOPHRENIA

Case History

A 35-year-old woman with schizophrenia is admitted to the inpatient psychiatric ward following a serious suicide attempt by hanging requiring a medical intensive care unit admission. She explained that prior to the attempt she was hearing voices telling her that a death by hanging would lead to salvation. She is currently being treated with olanzapine for schizophrenia and has previously been on haloperidol, which was discontinued due to inadequate efficacy. Based on the result of the InterSePT trial, how should this patient be treated?

Suggested Answer

The InterSePT trial randomized patients with schizophrenia or schizoaffective disorder and at high risk for suicide to receive clozapine or olanzapine. It found that clozapine was more effective in preventing suicidal behaviors compared to olanzapine.

The patient presented is typical of a patient included in InterSePT. Considering the recent serious suicide attempt, the psychiatrist should consider a trial of clozapine after discussing the risks and benefits of this medication with the patient and screening the patient for hematologic abnormalities.

References

1. Meltzer, H. Y., Alphs, L., Green, A. I., Altamura, A. C., Anand, R., Bertoldi, A., . . . Potkin, S. (2003). Clozapine treatment for suicidality in schizophrenia: International Suicide Prevention Trial (InterSePT). *Archives of General Psychiatry, 60*(1), 82–91.
2. Modestin, J., Dal Pian, D., & Agarwalla, P. (2005). Clozapine diminishes suicidal behavior: A retrospective evaluation of clinical records. *Journal of Clinical Psychiatry, 66*(4), 534–538.
3. Hennen, J., & Baldessarini, R. J. (2005). Suicidal risk during treatment with clozapine: a meta-analysis. Schizophrenia Research, 73(2–3), 139–145.
4. Kane, J., Honigfeld, G., Singer, J., & Meltzer, H. (1988). Clozapine for the treatment-resistant schizophrenic: A double-blind comparison with chlorpromazine. *Archives of General Psychiatry, 45*(9), 789–796.
5. McEvoy, J. P., Lieberman, J. A., Stroup, T. S., Davis, S. M., Meltzer, H. Y., Rosenheck, R. A., . . . Severe, J. (2006). Effectiveness of clozapine versus olanzapine, quetiapine, and risperidone in patients with chronic schizophrenia who did not respond to prior atypical antipsychotic treatment. *American Journal of Psychiatry, 163*(4), 600–610.
6. Li, X. B., Tang, Y. L., Wang, C. Y., & de Leon, J. (2015). Clozapine for treatment-resistant bipolar disorder: A systematic review. *Bipolar Disorders, 17*(3), 235–247.
7. Tiihonen, J., Lönnqvist, J., Wahlbeck, K., Klaukka, T., Niskanen, L., Tanskanen, A., & Haukka, J. (2009). 11-year follow-up of mortality in patients with schizophrenia: A population-based cohort study (FIN11 study). *Lancet, 374*(9690), 620–627.
8. Lehman, A. F., Lieberman, J. A., Dixon, L. B., McGlashan, T. H., Miller, A. L., Perkins, D. O., & Kreyenbuhl, J. (2004). Practice guideline for the treatment of patients with schizophrenia. *American Journal of Psychiatry, 161*(2 Suppl), 1–56.

47

A Cohort Study of Oral and Depot Antipsychotics after First Hospitalization for Schizophrenia

STEPHANIE NG AND CENK TEK

> In a pairwise comparison between depot injections and their equivalent oral formulations, the risk of rehospitalization for patients receiving depot medications was about one-third of that for patients receiving oral medications.
>
> —Tiihonen et al.[1]

Research Question: In patients hospitalized for the first time with a diagnosis of schizophrenia, what is the risk of rehospitalization, drug discontinuation, and total mortality? Also, which antipsychotics and routes of administration are most effective for maintenance after the first hospitalization for schizophrenia?

Funding: The Ministry of Health and Welfare of Finland and Janssen-Cilag

Year Study Began: 2000

Year Study Published: 2011

Study Location: Finland

Who Was Studied: 16- to 65-year-old patients hospitalized for the first time with a diagnosis of schizophrenia between 2000 and 2007

Who Was Excluded: Patients who used antipsychotics in outpatient care during the 6 months preceding the study period

How Many Participants: 2,588

Study Overview: See Figure 47.1 for a summary of the study design.

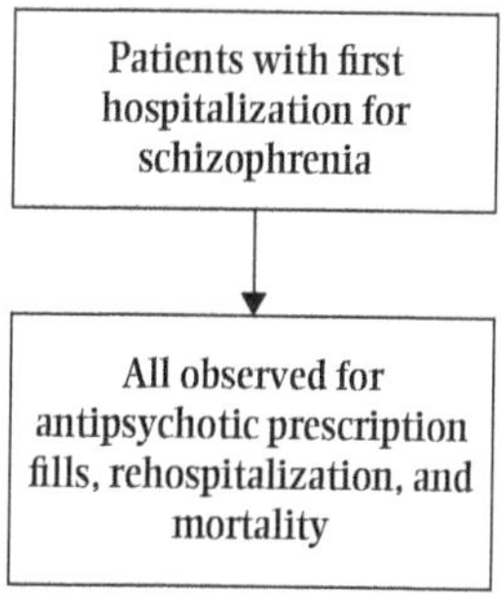

Figure 47.1 Summary of Study Design

Study Implementation: This was an observational cohort study. All patients were identified consecutively and diagnosed with schizophrenia.

Data regarding medication were obtained from the Finnish prescription database. Of note, the cost of outpatient antipsychotics is fully reimbursed by the government, and in Finland there is no involuntary outpatient treatment.

From the database, antipsychotic use was included based on predefined minimum daily doses (and from which data about duration of treatment was inferred). The daily doses were as follows: olanzapine (10 mg), risperidone oral (5 mg), clozapine (300 mg), quetiapine (400 mg), risperidone long-acting injection (2.7 mg), perphenazine long-acting injection (7 mg), perphenazine oral (30 mg), zuclopenthixol long-acting injection (15 mg), haloperidol long-acting injection (3.3 mg), haloperidol oral (8 mg), and zuclopenthixol oral (30 mg).

Risperidone, haloperidol, perphenazine, and zuclopenthixol are the most widely used antipsychotics in both oral and depot formulations.

Follow-Up: Seven years

Endpoints: Discontinuation of initial antipsychotic medication for any reason, the rate of rehospitalization for schizophrenia, and mortality.

RESULTS

- 58.2% of patients used an antipsychotic during the first 30 days after discharge; 45.7% continued the initial antipsychotic medication for ≥30 days.
- 57.8% of patients were rehospitalized because of relapse of schizophrenia symptoms.
- Use of any antipsychotic was associated with lower risk of mortality compared with no use of antipsychotic (adjusted hazard ratio was 0.45) (Table 47.1).

Criticisms and Limitations: The mean age of patients was 37.8 years, which is higher than the age at which people usually have their first episode of psychosis. Moreover, many patients likely had symptoms before their index hospitalization, and 21.1% of patients had temporary antipsychotic treatment earlier than 6 months before index hospitalization, so the stage of disease in which these patients were hospitalized may have varied.

There are inherent limits to all observational studies. For example, because patients collected a prescription (which is the collectible data), it is not clear that they were actually taking medications. Additionally, diagnoses were made through International Classification of Diseases codes rather than being verified by an independent set of clinicians. Whether the difference in relapse was due to oral versus depot antipsychotics is difficult to tell in a nonrandomized controlled trial in which confounders may not have been identified.

Finally, the generalizability of this study to the United States has limits, as this study was conducted in Finland, where medications are provided free of cost and the population is more homogenous than that of the United States.

Other Relevant Studies and Information:

- Compared with other studies including the Clinical Antipsychotics Trials of Intervention Effectiveness (CATIE)[2] and the European First Episode Schizophrenia (EUFEST),[3] all-cause discontinuation rate at 2 months in this study was much higher. This might be related to study design. This study was observational, while CATIE and EUFEST were both randomized controlled trials (RCTs). RCTs can have more intensive follow-up than observational studies.
- A meta-analysis of RCTs comparing long-acting injectable versus oral antipsychotics found that depot formulation generally did not reduce relapse compared with oral formulations in patients with schizophrenia

Table 47.1 SUMMARY OF KEY ADJUSTED HAZARD RATIOS

Outcome	Overall oral vs. equivalent depot	Depot haldol	Oral haldol	Clozapine	Olanzapine	Depot risperi-done	Quetia-pine
All-cause drug discontinuation pf depot compared to oral equivalent (P value)[a]	0.41 (<0.0001)	0.27 (0.03)	–	No depot	No depot	0.44 (<0.0001)	No depot
Rehospitalization (P value)[b]	0.36 (0.007)	0.21 (0.13)	1.79 (0.28)	0.48 (0.001)	0.54 (<0.0001)	0.57 (0.09)	1.11 (0.60)

[a]Adjusted hazard ratios vs. oral equivalent.
[b]Adjusted hazard ratios vs. oral risperidone.

(exception: first-generation depot in studies conducted before 1991). The authors speculate that this was related to cohort bias from RCTs, rather than reflecting a real-world phenomenon.

- The finding of clozapine and olanzapine being associated with lowest all-cause discontinuation and rehospitalization rates is similar to findings from CATIE[2] and EUFEST.[3]
- The American Psychiatric Association (APA) practice guidelines state that long-acting injectable antipsychotic medications should be considered for patients with recurrent relapses due to nonadherence, as well as patients who prefer this route of administration.[4] Similarly, the United Kingdom's National Institute for Health and Care Excellence (NICE) suggests that depot antipsychotic medications can be considered as an option for people with schizophrenia who "prefer such treatment after an acute episode" or when avoiding nonadherence is a clinical priority.[5]

Summary and Implications: This observational study using the Finnish national database found that only 58% of patients presenting with an initial hospitalization due to psychosis filled their antipsychotic prescription 30 days after discharge. It also found that, overall, depot injectable antipsychotics were associated with a 64% lower risk of rehospitalization compared to oral antipsychotics. Based on this and other studies, clinical guidelines from the APA and NICE recommend the use of depot injections among patients with recurrent relapses due to nonadherence or patient preference.

CLINICAL CASE: ANTIPSYCHOTIC CHOICE FOLLOWING FIRST HOSPITALIZATION

Case History

A 24-year-old man with no prior psychiatric history is brought to the hospital by worried family members. They have noticed him talking to himself when no one else is in the room, acting suspiciously toward them in fear that they may be reincarnations of the devil and stating that the police are going to jail him. The patient was found to meet criteria for schizophrenia and was hospitalized on an inpatient psychiatric ward. He was started on risperidone and titrated to a dose of 6 mg/day without side effects. After a 3-week hospitalization, what medication and formulations should be considered upon discharge?

Suggested Answer

The Finnish depot study found that patients with their first hospitalization for schizophrenia were not likely to continue with their medications after discharge. Long-acting injectable antipsychotics were associated with lower relapse rates than their oral counterparts. A long-acting injectable may thus be indicated.

The patient in this vignette is similar to patients included in the trial. Thus, after a discussion of the risks/benefits of different medications, a long-acting injectable formulation of risperidone may be indicated to promote adherence to antipsychotic use and thus decrease risk of relapse.

References

1. Tiihonen, J., Haukka, J., Taylor, M., Haddad, P. M., Patel, M. X., Korhonen, P. (2011). A nationwide cohort study of oral and depot antipsychotics after first hospitalization for schizophrenia. *American Journal of Psychiatry, 168*(6), 603–609.
2. Lieberman, J. A., Stroup, T. S., McEvoy, J. P., Swartz, M. S., Rosenheck, R. A., Perkins, D. O., . . . Severe, J. (2005). Effectiveness of antipsychotic drugs in patients with chronic schizophrenia. *New England Journal of Medicine, 353*(12), 1209–1223.
3. Kahn, R. S., Fleischhacker, W. W., Boter, H., Davidson, M., Vergouwe, Y., Keet, I. P., . . . Grobbee, D. E. (2008). Effectiveness of antipsychotic drugs in first-episode schizophrenia and schizophreniform disorder: An open randomised clinical trial. *Lancet, 371*(9618), 1085–1097.
4. Lehman, A. F., Lieberman, J. A., Dixon, L. B., McGlashan, T. H., Miller, A. L., Perkins, D. O., & Kreyenbuhl, J. (2004). Practice guideline for the treatment of patients with schizophrenia, second edition. *American Journal of Psychiatry, 161*(2 Suppl), 1–56.
5. National Institute for Health and Care Excellence. (2014). *Psychosis and schizophrenia in adults: Prevention and management.* Retrieved from https://www.nice.org.uk/guidance/cg178/chapter/1-recommendations?unlid=390905176201711613539

SECTION 13

Substance Use Disorders

48

Methadone Maintenance versus Detoxification and Psychosocial Treatment for Opioid Dependence

The M180 Study

HAMILTON GAIANI AND SRINIVAS MUVVALA

> Methadone maintenance therapy resulted in greater treatment retention . . . and lower heroin use rates than did detoxification [and psychosocial treatment].
>
> —METHADONE MAINTENANCE STUDY INVESTIGATORS[1]

Research Question: Should patients with opioid dependence be treated with methadone maintenance treatment or prolonged and psychosocially enriched methadone-assisted detoxification?

Funding: National Institute on Drug Abuse

Year Study Began: 1995

Year Study Published: 2000

Study Location: San Francisco, California

Who Was Studied: Patients 18 years or older with a DSM-III-R diagnosis of opioid dependence

Who Was Excluded: Those who were pregnant, those with psychiatric or medical conditions that would interfere with treatment, and those with recent substance abuse treatment

How Many Participants: 179

Study Overview: See Figure 48.1 for a summary of the study design.

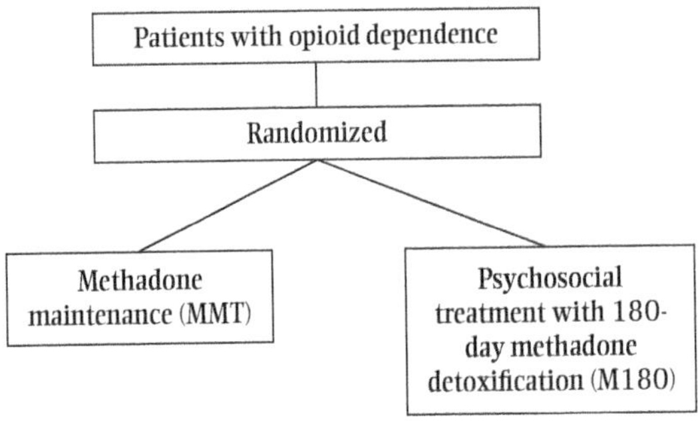

Figure 48.1 Summary of Study Design

Study Intervention: Opioid dependent study participants were treated with 30 mg/day of methadone, which was titrated to 80 mg/day in 3 weeks. The dose was further titrated based on illicit opioid use (assessed via urine screens) to as much as 100 mg/day.

Patients in the methadone maintenance treatment (MMT) arm received methadone therapy for 14 months. In the first 6 months, they received 4 to 5 hours of group therapy per month as well as 1 hour of monthly individual therapy.

Patients in the psychosocial treatment with detoxification (M180) arm received 120 days of methadone, which was tapered over the subsequent 60 days. In addition, they received more individual and group therapy than the MMT group. For the remaining months, patients were no longer on methadone but were eligible for aftercare services (weekly individual and group therapy, as well as medical, social, and legal services).

Follow-Up: 12 months

Endpoints: Primary outcome: frequency of heroin use, heroin abstinence, and treatment retention. Secondary outcomes: drug-use HIV risk behavior (Risk of

AIDS Behavior scale), Addiction Severity Index score, psychosocial functioning, alcohol use, and cocaine use.

RESULTS

- MMT resulted in significantly lower heroin use rates than the M180 group.
- MMT had significantly better treatment retention (439 vs. 174 days), lower HIV-risk drug use behavior, and less legal problems in the last 6 months of assessment.
- Many participants in both groups continued to use heroin throughout the study despite adequate doses. The proportion of those that used heroin was lower in the MMT group in the final 6 months of assessment, when the detox arm was no longer receiving methadone.
- There was no significant difference between groups in psychosocial functioning in several domains: employment, psychiatric, family, alcohol use, and high risk sexual behaviors (Table 48.1).

Table 48.1 Summary of Key Findings

Outcome	**MMT group**	**M180 (psychosocial treatment) group**	**P value**
Mean days of heroin use per month (months 7–12)	6.70[a]	13.95[b]	0.001[c]
Treatment retention – median days	438.5	174.0	<0.001
Injection risk score (ASI) at 6 months	4.07	3.07	not reported
Injection risk score at 12 months	3.73	2.17	not reported

[a]Mason et al.[5]
[b]Mattick et al.[3]
[c]Data originate from a later publication using original study data. Initial study presented these data in graphical format.
NOTES: MMT = methadone maintenance treatment. ASI = Addiction Severity Index.

Criticisms and Limitations: The psychosocial services provided in this study were not standardized, which may have biased the results as some patients may have received more intensive manualized treatment and/or vocational rehabilitational services than others. It is difficult to ascertain the impact of psychotherapy on the study participants as it was administered in both groups. Additionally, study participant's use of illicit heroin while undergoing treatment was quantified and discussed; however, it is unclear if other opioids were used illicitly. Finally, a longer follow-up period may have provided additional insight towards the treatment of chronic opioid dependence.

Other Relevant Studies and Information:

- A number trials have replicated the efficacy of buprenorphine[2] and methadone[3] treatment as compared to nonpharmacologic treatment for opioid abuse disorders.
- Substance Abuse and Mental Health Services Administration (SAMHSA) guidelines[4] recommend methadone maintenance therapy or suboxone therapy for patients with opioid use disorders.

Summary and Implications: The M180 study showed that MMT is more effective in decreasing heroin use and increasing treatment retention than prolonged, psychosocially enriched, methadone-assisted detoxification. Maintenance therapy also decreased high-risk injection behavior. There exists a growing body of evidence that MMT and buprenorphine maintenance are significantly more efficacious than detoxification or abstinence-based treatment at reducing frequency of use.

CLINICAL CASE: METHADONE MAINTENANCE VERSUS PSYCHOSOCIALLY ENRICHED DETOXIFICATION

Case History

A 25-year-old woman self-presents to the addiction treatment clinic asking for help for her intravenous heroin addiction. She has tried naltrexone in the past but continued to relapse. She has taken buprenorphine but did not like the medication. She has had extensive individual and group therapy exposure, which she found helpful. She reports two serious accidental overdoses in the past few years. She has made progress and developed a supportive network with the aid of 12-step meetings but continues to use on weekends. She has been sober for 24 hours and appears diaphoretic and pale. She recently started a new job and is motivated to continue improving her life. Her only medications are oral contraceptives. She has been told by some in her 12-step meetings that if she is on a medication she is "not really sober." She states "I just can't kick this, I am so tired of being sick." Recent labs were unremarkable.

Based on the results of this study, how should this patient be treated?

Suggested Answer

The M180 study showed that methadone maintenance reduces heroin use, strengthens treatment retention, and reduces high risk behaviors which could lead to Hepatitis C or HIV.

The patient in this vignette is typical of patients included in the study and is at especially high risk for overdose and medical complications secondary to intravenous drug use. Based on the results of this and other studies, SAMHSA has recommended the use of opioid agonist treatment (methadone or buprenorphine) in addition to psychosocial treatment for patients with opioid use disorders. It would likely help her to reduce heroin use and reduce behaviors that might lead to serious infections. As with all medications, the doctor and patient should discuss the risks and benefits before initiating treatment.

References

1. Sees, K. L., Delucchi, K. L., Masson, C., Rosen, A., Clark, H. W., Robillard, H., Hall, S. M. (2000). Methadone maintenance vs 180-day psychosocially enriched detoxification for treatment of opioid dependence: A randomized controlled trial. *JAMA, 283*(10), 1303–1310.
2. Mattick, R.P., Breen, C., Kimber, J., & Davoli, M. (2014). Buprenorphine maintenance versus placebo or methadone maintenance for opioid dependence. *Cochrane Database of Systematic Reviews*, 2, CD002207.
3. Mattick, R. P., Breen, C., Kimber, J., & Davoli, M. (2009). Methadone maintenance therapy versus no opioid replacement therapy for opioid dependence. *Cochrane Database of Systematic Reviews*, 3, CD002209.
4. Center for Substance Abuse Treatment. (2005). *Medication-assisted treatment for opioid addiction in opioid treatment programs*. Rockville, MD: Author.
5. Masson, C. L., Barnett, P. G., Sees, K. L., Delucchi, K. L., Rosen, A., Wong, W., & Hall, S. M. (2004). Cost and cost-effectiveness of standard methadone maintenance treatment compared to enriched 180-day methadone detoxification. *Addiction, 99*(6), 718–726.

49

Combined Pharmacotherapies and Behavioral Interventions for Alcohol Dependence

The COMBINE Study

KEVIN JOHNSON AND SRINIVAS MUVVALA

> [Regarding treating alcohol dependence] no combination [of treatments] produced better efficacy than naltrexone or [combined behavioral intervention] alone in the presence of medical management.
>
> —The COMBINE Study Research Group[1]

Research Question: What is the efficacy of medications, behavioral therapies, and their combinations in the treatment of alcohol dependence?

Funding: National Institute on Alcohol Abuse and Alcoholism. Lipha Pharmaceuticals donated medications and placebo.

Year Study Began: 2001

Year Study Published: 2006

Study Location: 11 academic sites across the United States

Who Was Studied: Treatment-seeking adults who met DSM-IV criteria for alcohol dependence with 4 to 21 days of abstinence. Participants were women and men who used at least 14 and 21 drinks per week, respectively, for at least a month within the previous 90 days with at least 2 days of heavy drinking, defined as >3 drinks per day for women and >4 drinks per day for men.

Who Was Excluded: Those who reported history of using other substances aside from nicotine or cannabis in the past 90 days, those who have another psychiatric disorder that requires medication, and those who are medically unstable (e.g., elevated liver enzyme levels).

How Many Participants: 1,383

Study Overview: See Figure 49.1 for a summary of the study design.

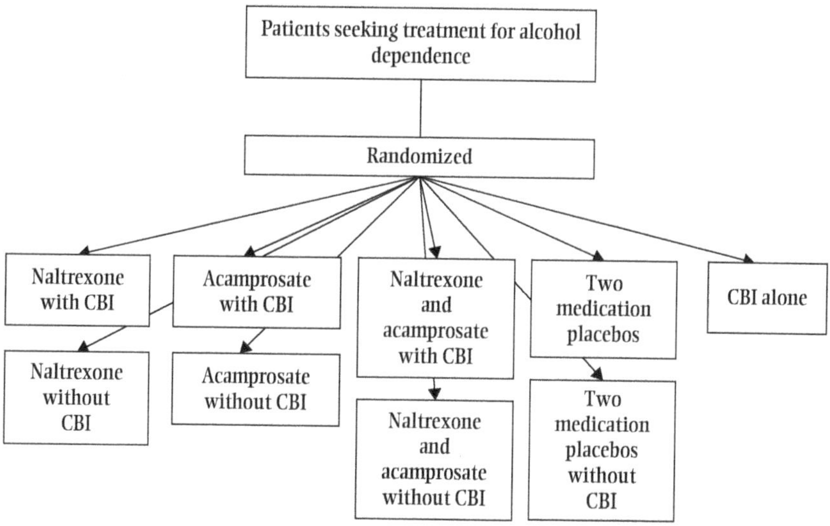

Figure 49.1 Summary of Study Design
NOTE: CBI = combined behavioral intervention.

Study Intervention: Participants randomized to the medication groups were given numbered pill packs with either the active medication and/or matching placebos. All participants took the same number of pills daily to avoid unblinding. Those randomized to naltrexone started at 25 mg daily and were titrated up to 100 mg daily over 8 days. Those randomized to acamprosate started at two pills of 500 mg three times per day and maintained this dose over the course of the study.

Those randomized to receive any of the medications or placebo also received medical management (MM). MM is a nine-session intervention focused on enhancing adherence and abstinence, delivered by licensed medical practitioners (medical doctors, nurses, etc.). Each session lasts 20 to 45 minutes.

Combined Behavioral Intervention (CBI) includes aspects of Cognitive Behavioral Therapy (CBT), 12-step facilitation (i.e., Alcoholics Anonymous), motivational interviewing, and support system involvement (i.e., family counseling). Participants randomized to the CBI groups received up to 20 sessions, each 50 minutes in length, led by therapists with at least a master's degree and 2 years of experience. The therapists determined how many sessions were appropriate for each patient. Participants received a median of 10 sessions during the study.

Follow-Up: 16 weeks. At the conclusion of the study, patients were subsequently reevaluated after 10 weeks, 9 months, and 1 year following completion of the study treatment.

Endpoints: Primary outcomes: percentage of days abstinent during trial and time until the patient's first "heavy drinking day" as previously described. Secondary outcomes: number of heavy drinking days per month, number of drinks per drinking day, alcohol cravings (via the Obsessive Compulsive Drinking Scale), serum levels of carbohydrate deficient transferrin, and medication side effects (via the Systematic Assessment for Treatment Emergent Effects).

RESULTS

- Alcohol consumption decreased overall in all groups during the 16-week intervention period. In the month before treatment, 25.2% of days were considered abstinent days (days with no alcohol consumption). During treatment, the mean proportion of abstinent days to all days observed increased to 73.1%. There was also a decrease in reported drinks per drinking day during treatment (12.6 drinks vs. 7.1 drinks).
- The naltrexone group had a significantly lower risk of a heavy drinking days compared to placebo (hazard ratio = 0.72, p = 0.02), but the acamprosate and CBI groups did not (see Tables 49.1 and 49.2).
- Those who received naltrexone alone or CBI plus placebo had significantly more abstinence days compared to those receiving MM plus placebo. However, combining naltrexone with CBI showed no added benefit (Tables 49.1 and 49.2).

Table 49.1 Summary of COMBINE's Key Findings (without CBI)

Outcome	Naltrexone	Acamprosate	Naltrexone and acamprosate	Placebo
% days abstinent	80.0%	75.6%	80.5%	73.8%
# of heavy drinking events	104	108	96	115

NOTES: COMBINE = Combined Pharmacotherapies and Behavioral Interventions for Alcohol Dependence. CBI = combined behavioral intervention.

Table 49.2 Summary of COMBINE's Key Findings (with CBI)

Outcome	Naltrexone	Acamprosate	Naltrexone and Acamprosate	Placebo	CBI only
Percent Days Abstinent	75.9%	78.2%	77.6%	79.8%	66.6%
# of Heavy Drinking Events	103	103	116	111	124

NOTES: COMBINE = Combined Pharmacotherapies and Behavioral Interventions for Alcohol Dependence. CBI = combined behavioral intervention.

- Acamprosate (with or without naltrexone or CBI) was not significantly different than placebo on any drinking measure.
- Of those taking naltrexone, 2% developed aspartate aminotransferase (AST) or alanine aminotransferase (ALT) levels at least five times the upper limit of normal. Other reported side effects included nausea/vomiting, diarrhea, somnolence, and decreased appetite.

Criticisms and Limitations: Because the trial excluded participants with comorbid mental illness and those who reported use of other substances, the results of the study may not be generalizable to patients with multiple psychiatric comorbidities.

Additionally, in this study, participants received an intensive course of psychosocial interventions that may not be feasible in a real-world clinical setting.

Other Relevant Studies and Information:

- These findings have been replicated in numerous other studies. There are also data to show efficacy of naltrexone with respect to alcohol treatment in those receiving treatment for concurrent schizophrenia,[2] depression,[3,4] and/or PTSD.[5]
- Another multisite study found similar results with the intramuscular, extended-release formulation of naltrexone (also known as Vivitrol). Those who received the injection showed a 25% reduction in the number of heavy drinking days compared to placebo.[6]
- Other studies reveal that naltrexone may be more efficacious in specific subgroups of patients. For example, smokers show a stronger response to naltrexone compared to nonsmokers.[7]
- There are a number of randomized trials have shown mixed results for the efficacy of acamprosate for alcohol use disorder.[8,9]
- A meta-analysis of 64 randomized, placebo-controlled trials from 1970 to 2009 found acamprosate to be slightly more efficacious in promoting abstinence and naltrexone slightly more efficacious in reducing heavy drinking and cravings.[10]
- The American Psychiatric Association (APA) practice guidelines recommend the use of naltrexone, disulfiram, or acamprosate, in addition to motivationally enhanced treatment or other therapies and self-help groups like Alcoholics Anonymous, for those with alcohol use disorders.[11]

Summary and Implications: The COMBINE study was a randomized controlled trial that compared medications with and without behavioral interventions. It found that daily naltrexone with nine sessions of MM is as effective as CBI (i.e., cognitive behavioral therapy, 12-step facilitation, motivational interviewing) alone. The addition of CBI to naltrexone was no more effective than naltrexone alone. Surprisingly, acamprosate was found to be no better than placebo.

CLINICAL CASE: TREATING ALCOHOL USE DISORDER

Case History

A 38-year-old man with a history of alcohol use disorder presents to an outpatient clinic after completing a 4-day inpatient alcohol detox program. His last drink was 10 days ago, and he is motivated for substance use treatment. He denies use of other substances, which has been confirmed by a recent urine toxicology screen. He does not meet DSM criteria for other psychiatric conditions requiring medication. Routine laboratory testing shows normal AST and ALT levels.

Based on the results of the COMBINE study, how should this patient be treated?

Suggested Answer

The COMBINE study found that those naltrexone or psychosocial interventions (but not necessarily acamprosate) can be useful on their own in the treatment of alcohol use disorders. Clinical practice guidelines from the APA support the use of naltrexone, acamprosate, and disulfiram in this group in addition to psychosocial interventions.

The patient in this vignette is similar to participants included in the COMBINE study. Based on the patient's preferences and particular social situation, it would be useful to consider starting naltrexone and/or referral to psychotherapy or another type of social intervention. As with any medication, this decision should be made after a careful discussion with the patient.

References

1. Anton, R. F., O'Malley, S. S., Ciraulo, D. A., Cisler, R. A., Couper, D., Donovan, D. M., . . . Zweben, A. (2006). Combined pharmacotherapies and behavioral interventions for alcohol dependence: the COMBINE study: A randomized controlled trial. *JAMA, 295*(17), 2003–2017.
2. Petrakis, I., O'Malley, S., Rounsaville, B., Poling, J., McHugh-Strong, C., & Krystal, J. H. (2004). Naltrexone augmentation of neuroleptic treatment in alcohol abusing patients with schizophrenia. *Psychopharmaology (Berl), 172*(3):291–297.
3. Petrakis, I., Ralevski, E., Nich, C., Levinson, C., Carroll, K., Poling, J., & Rounsaville, B. (2007). Naltrexone and disulfram in patients with alcohol dependence and current depression. *Journal of Clinical Psychopharmacology, 27*(2), 160–165.
4. Pettinati, H. M., Oslin, D. W., Kampman, K. M., Dundon, W. D., Xie, H., Gallis, T. L., . . . O'Brien, C. P. (2010). A double-blind, placebo-controlled trial combining sertraline and naltrexone for treating co-occurring depression and alcohol dependence. *American Journal of Psychiatry, 167*(6), 668–675.
5. Petrakis, I., Poling, J., Levinson, C., Nich, C., Carroll, K., Ralevski, E., & Rounsaville, B. (2006). Naltrexone and disulfram in patients with alcohol dependence and comorbid posttraumatic stress disorder. *Biological Psychiatry, 60*(7), 777–783.
6. Garbutt, J. C., Kranzler, H. R., O'Malley, S. S., Gastfriend, D. R., Pettinati, H. M., Silverman, B. L., . . . Ehrich, E. W. (2005). Efficacy and tolerability of long-acting injectable naltrexone for alcohol dependence. *JAMA, 293*(13), 1617.
7. Schacht, J. P., Randall, P. K., Latham, P. K., Voronin, K. E., Book, S. W., Myrick, H., & Anton, R. F. (2017). Predictors of naltrexone response in a randomized

trial: Reward-related brain activation, OPRM1 genotype, and smoking status. *Neuropsychopharmacology, 42*(13), 2640–2653.

8. Mann, K., Lehert, P., & Morgan, M. Y. (2004). The efficacy of acamprosate in the maintenance of abstinence in alcohol-dependent individuals: Results of a meta-analysis. *Alcoholism: Clinical and Experimental Research, 28*(1), 51–63.
9. Mason, B. J. (2003). Acamprosate and naltrexone treatment alcohol dependence. *European Neuropsychopharmacology, 13*(6), 469–475.
10. Maisel, N. C., Blodgett, J. C., Wilbourne, P. L., Humphreys, K., & Finney, J. W.(2013). Meta-analysis of naltrexone and acamprosate for treating alcohol use disorders: When are these medications most helpful? *Addiction, 108*(2), 275–293.
11. Kleber, H. D., Weiss, R. D., Anton, R. F., Jr., George, T. P., Greenfield, S. F., Kosten, T.R., . . . Connery, H. S. (2010). *Practice guideline for the treatment of patients with substance use disorders–second edition.* Washington, DC: American Psychiatric Association.

50

Levomethadyl Acetate versus Buprenorphine versus Methadone for Opioid Dependence

ROBERT ROSS AND BRIAN FUEHRLEIN

> Levomethadyl acetate, buprenorphine, and high dose methadone were more effective than low dose methadone in reducing the use of illicit opioids.
>
> —JOHNSON ET AL.[1]

Research Question: Which of the following is most effective for treatment of opioid dependence: levomethadyl acetate, buprenorphine, high-dose methadone, or low-dose methadone?

Funding: The National Institute of Drug Abuse

Year Study Began: 1996

Year Study Published: 2000

Study Location: Johns Hopkins University Medical Center

Who Was Studied: Adults aged 18 to 55 years with a DSM-IV diagnosis of opioid dependence with laboratory confirmed recent opioid use

Who Was Excluded: Patients with severe medical or psychiatric comorbidities, pregnancy

How Many Participants: 220

Study Overview: See Figure 50.1 for a summary of the study design.

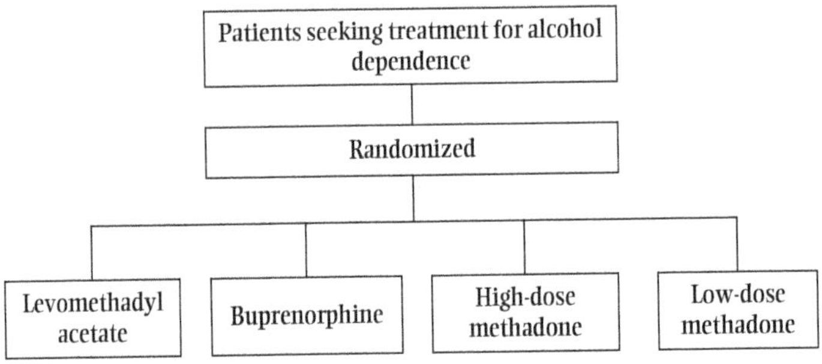

Figure 50.1 Summary of Study Design

Study Intervention: In this double-blinded study, patients in the levomethadyl acetate group were given a dose between 75 and 115 mg on Monday and Wednesday and a 40% higher dose on Friday.

Patients in the buprenorphine group underwent induction with daily dosing increasing from a starting dose of 4 mg. The dose could be titrated to maximum of 24 mg Monday and Wednesday and 32 mg Friday.

Patients in the low dose methadone group received a daily dose of 20 mg, while patients in the high dose methadone group started at 20 mg daily and were titrated to a range of 60 mg to 100 mg.

Dose increases occurred if patients had greater than 83% attendance and if greater than 33% urines were positive for opioids in a prespecified increase week. Dose increases were blinded.

Follow-Up: 17 weeks

Endpoints: Primary outcomes: retention, illicit opioid use based on urine toxicology results, and self-report of frequency and severity of opioid use. Secondary outcomes: fraction of positive cocaine tests, length of continuous abstinence from cocaine, treatment side effects, breathalyzer readings, sex-associated differences

RESULTS

- Overall study retention was 60% for levomethadyl acetate, 64% for buprenorphine, 84% for high dose methadone, and 58% for low dose methadone.
- Patient mean length of retention was significantly higher ($p < 0.001$) for those receiving levomethadyl acetate (89 days), buprenorphine (96 days), and high-dose methadone (105 days) relative to low dose methadone (70 days).
- Mean percentage of opioid positive urine screens was 52 for levomethadyl acetate, 62 for buprenorphine, 62 for high dose methadone, and 79 for low dose methadone. The difference for each group was statistically significant relative to low dose methadone ($p = 0.005$).
- Patients reported the degree of their addiction on a scale from 0 to 100 with those in the methadone group giving the highest mean rating (53) and those in the buprenorphine group giving the lowest (34) (Table 50.1).

Table 50.1 SUMMARY OF KEY FINDINGS

Outcome	Levomethadyl acetate	Buprenorphine	High dose methadone	Low dose methadone	P value[a]
Mean days of study retention (95% CI)	89 [78, 100]	96 [88, 105]	105 [98, 112]	70 [62, 79]	<0.001
Opioid positive urine screen (%/wk)	52 [44, 60]	62 [55, 70]	62 [54, 69]	79 [70, 88]	0.005
Patient rating of drug problem severity	35 [28, 43]	34 [27, 42]	38 [30, 45]	53 [45, 60]	0.002

[a] Compared to low dose methadone group.

Criticisms and Limitations: The trial did not include older patients (aged >55) or patients with comorbid serious psychiatric or medical illness requiring medications, which is common in patients who use opioids. The study results may not generalize to these groups, who make up more than half of patients who meet criteria for opioid use disorder.

Other Relevant Studies and Information:

- National Institute of Health and Care Excellence guidelines recommend either buprenorphine or methadone for treatment of opioid use disorder. The decision about which drug should be made clinically on a case-by-case basis.[2]
- World Health Organization guidelines recommend both methadone and buprenorphine but recommend methadone as the preferred agent overall.[3]
- A number of other randomized trials have concluded that methadone and buprenorphine are equally effective at reducing illicit opioid use. Some show increased retention in the methadone group, similar to the trend observed in this study.[4, 5, 6]
- Levomethadyl acetate has been shown to be associated with increased QTc interval and torsades de points. Hence, it was barred from the European market,[7] and voluntarily withdrawn from the US market (brand name Orlamm).[8]

Summary and Implications: This study found that in otherwise healthy adults with opioid use disorder, levomethadyl acetate, buprenorphine, and high-dose methadone were all more effective than low-dose methadone with respect to retention in treatment as well as rates of opioid use. Because levomethadyl has been removed from US and European markets due to safety concerns, major guidelines recommend treatment of opioid disorders with either buprenorphine or methadone.

CLINICAL CASE: LEVOMETHADYL ACETATE VERSUS BUPRENORPHINE VERSUS METHADONE FOR OPIOID DEPENDENCE

Case History

A 43-year-old man presents to an outpatient clinic for an intake appointment for treatment of opioid use disorder. He has been using 30 mg of oxycodone per day, up from 5 mg per day when he first started. He initially had a prescription after knee surgery but has been buying pills from a friend for nearly a year. The patient is tearful when describing how much money he stole from his mother, how he got fired from his job as a bank teller because he was using, and constantly craves opiates. He tried injecting heroine for the first time last week. His psychiatric review of systems is otherwise negative. He has no major medical conditions. He works as an attorney and is reluctant to try methadone because of the stigma and daily commitment.

Based on the results of this study, what is the appropriate treatment?

Suggested Answer

This study showed that levomethadyl acetate, buprenorphine, and methadone are all effective for managing opioid use disorder. The medications appear equally effective overall with some subtle differences. Levomethadyl acetate, however, is more likely to cause ventricular arrhythmias and is no longer readily available in the US and European markets.

The patient in this vignette is typical of patients included in the study, as he reaches diagnostic criteria for opiate use disorder and is seeking treatment. Thus, he should be treated initially with buprenorphine or high-dose methadone. Given the office-based nature coupled with the preferred side-effect profile, buprenorphine is often the first-line medication-assisted treatment. However, the decision to choose buprenorphine or methadone is patient specific. This study demonstrated that buprenorphine could be dosed 3 days per week, though patients often prefer daily dosing.

References

1. Johnson, R. E., Chutuape, M. A., Strain, E. C., Walsh, S. L., Stitzer, M. L., & Bigelow, G. E. (2000). A comparison of levomethadyl acetate, buprenorphine, and methadone for opioid dependence. *New England Journal of Medicine, 343*, 1290–1297.
2. National Institute for Health and Care Excellence. (2007). *National treatment Association guidance: Methadone and buprenorphine for the management of opioid dependence.* London: Author.
3. World Health Organization. (2009). *Guidelines for the psychosocially assisted pharmacological treatment of opioid dependence.* Geneva: Author.
4. Ling, W., Charuvastra, C., Collins, J. F., Batki, S., Brown, L. S., Jr., Kintaudi, P., . . . Segal, D. (1998). Buprenorphine maintenance treatment of opiate dependence: a multicenter, randomized clinical trial. *Addiction, 93*(4), 475–486.
5. Magura, S., Lee, J. D., Hershberger, J., Joseph, H., Marsch, L., & Shropshire, C., Rosenblum, A. (2009). Buprenorphine and methadone maintenance in jail and post-release: A randomized clinical trial. *Drug and Alcohol Dependence, 99*(1–3), 222–230.
6. Mattick, R. P., Ali, R., White, J. M., O'Brien, S., Wolk, S., & Danz, C. (2003). Buprenorphine versus methadone maintenance therapy: A randomized double-blind trial with 405 opioid-dependent patients. *Addiction, 98*(4), 441–452.

7. Wieneke, H., Conrads, H., Wolstein, J., Breuckmann, F., Gastpar, M., Erbel, R., & Scherbaum, N. (2009). Levo-alpha-acetylmethadol (LAAM) induced QTc-prolongation: Results from a controlled clinical trial. *European Journal of Medical Research, 14*(1), 7–12.
8. Food and Drug Administration. (2013). *US FDA safety alerts: Orlaam (levomethadyl acetate hydrochloride)*. Washington, DC: Author.

Index

Tables, figures, and boxes are indicated by an italic *t*, *f*, and *b* following the page number.

acamprosate, for alcohol dependence, 318
  with Combined Behavioral Intervention, 314–319 (*see also* alcohol dependence, pharmacotherapies with Combined Behavioral Intervention)
AIDS patients, hospitalized, delirium treatment, 106–110. *see also* delirium treatment, in AIDS patients, hospitalized
alcohol dependence
  acamprosate for, 318
  American Psychiatric Association guidelines, 318
  depression treatment with, 143–147 (*see also* depression treatment, with alcohol or drug dependence)
  naltrexone for, 318
  pharmacotherapies with Combined Behavioral Intervention, 314–319
    clinical case, 318*b*–319*b*
    criticisms and limitations, 317
    follow-up and endpoints, 316
    intervention, 315–316
    participants, 315
    relevant studies and information, 318
    research question, 314
    results, 316, 317*t*
    study design, 315*f*
    summary and implications, 318
Alzheimer's disease
  atypical antipsychotic effectiveness, 93–98
    clinical case, 98*b*
    criticisms and limitations, 96–97
    follow-up and endpoints, 95
    intervention, 94–95
    participants, 93–94
    relevant studies and information, 97
    research question, 93
    results, 95, 96*t*
    study design, 94*f*
    summary and implications, 97–98
  DOMINO-AD, 115
  memantine for, in patients on donepezil, 112–116 (*see also* memantine, for Alzheimer's disease in patients on donepezil)
antidepressants. *see also* tricyclic antidepressants; *specific types*
  benefits and initial severity, 167–171
    clinical case, 171*b*
    criticisms and limitations, 169–170
    follow-up and endpoints, 168–169
    participants, 167–168
    relevant studies and information, 170
    research question, 167
    results, 168*f*, 169

antidepressants. (*cont.*)
study design, 168*f*
summary and implications, 170
for bipolar disorder, adjunctive *vs.* mood stabilizer monotherapy, 24–29 (*see also* bipolar disorder, mood stabilizer monotherapy *vs.* adjunctive antidepressant)
QTc-interval abnormalities with, 241–246 (*see also* psychotropic drugs, QTc-interval abnormalities with)
for social phobia, 9–14 (*see also* social phobia, fluoxetine, comprehensive cognitive behavioral therapy, and placebo on)
STAR*D, 173–178 (*see also* depression treatment, STAR*D)
with substance use disorder, 143–147 (*see also* depression treatment, with alcohol or drug dependence)
suicidality with, pediatric, 149–153 (*see also* selective serotonin reuptake inhibitors (SSRIs), pediatric suicidality with; selective serotonin reuptake inhibitors (SSRIs), suicidality with, pediatric)
Antipsychotic Risk of Sudden Cardiac Death study, 274–278. *see also* antipsychotics, atypical, sudden cardiac death risks
antipsychotics
cardiac death risks, American Psychiatric Association on, 277
for dementia, morbidity and mortality, 97
EKG before, baseline, 244
metabolic risk, switching to aripiprazole for, 279–283
clinical case, 283*b*
criticisms and limitations, 282
follow-up and endpoints, 281
intervention, 280–281
participants, 280
relevant studies and information, 282–283
research question, 279
results, 281, 282*t*
study design, 280*f*
summary and implications, 283
QTc-interval abnormalities with, 241–246 (*see also* psychotropic drugs, QTc-interval abnormalities with)
American Psychiatric Association on, 244–245
Berkshire Healthcare National Health Service on, 244
for schizophrenia, after first hospitalization, oral *vs.* depot, 300–305
clinical case, 304*b*–305*b*
criticisms and limitations, 302
follow-up and endpoints, 301
implementation, 301
participants, 301
relevant studies and information, 302–304
research question, 300
results, 302, 303*t*
study design, 301*f*
summary and implications, 304
for schizophrenia, effectiveness, 253–258
clinical case, 258*b*
criticisms and limitations, 257
follow-up and endpoints, 254–255
intervention, 254
participants, 254
relevant studies and information, 257
research question, 253
results, 255, 256*t*
study design, 254*f*
summary and implications, 257
on suicidality, 298
tardive dyskinesia with
meta-analysis, 250
Yale Tardive Dyskinesia Study, 249

tardive dyskinesia with, atypical *vs.* conventional, 247–251
clinical case, 250*b*–251*b*
criticisms and limitations, 249
follow-up and endpoints, 248
implementation, 248
participants, 247–248
relevant studies and information, 249–250
research question, 247
results, 248–249, 249*t*
study design, 248*f*
summary and implications, 250
antipsychotics, atypical. *see also* *specific drugs*
for Alzheimer's disease, effectiveness, 93–98 (*see also* Alzheimer's disease, atypical antipsychotic effectiveness)
cardiac death risks, American Psychiatric Association on, 277
cost utility, 285–289 (*see also* antipsychotics, first- *vs.* second-generation, for schizophrenia)
for dementia, risk of death, 100–104
clinical case, 103*b*–104*b*
criticisms and limitations, 102
follow-up and endpoints, 101
intervention, 101
relevant studies and information, 102–103
research question, 100
results, 102, 102*t*
studies and patients, 100–101
study design, 101*f*
summary and implications, 103
FDA advisory, 102
for schizophrenia, *vs.* clozapine, 266–272, 298 (*see also* schizophrenia, clozapine for, *vs.* other atypical antipsychotics)
sudden cardiac death risks, 274–278
clinical case, 277*b*–278*b*
criticisms and limitations, 277
follow-up and endpoints, 276
implementation, 275
participants, 275
relevant studies and information, 277
research question, 274
results, 276, 276*t*
study design, 275*f*
summary and implications, 277
tardive dyskinesia with, 247–251 (*see also* antipsychotics, tardive dyskinesia with, atypical *vs.* conventional)
antipsychotics, first- *vs.* second-generation
clinical case, for schizophrenia
after first hospitalization, oral *vs.* depot, 304*b*–305*b*
clozapine *vs.* other atypical antipsychotics, 271*b*–272*b*
cost utility, first- *vs.* second-generation, 288*b*–289*b*
early-onset, first- *vs.* second-generation, 59*b*
effectiveness, 258*b*
for schizophrenia, cost utility, 285–289
clinical case, 288*b*–289*b*
criticisms and limitations, 287–288
follow-up and endpoints, 287
intervention, 286–287
participants, 286
relevant studies and information, 288
research question, 285
results, 287, 287*t*
study design, 286*f*
summary and implications, 288
for schizophrenia, early-onset, 55–59
American Academy of Child and Adolescent Psychiatry recommendations, 58
clinical case, 59*b*
criticisms and limitations, 58
follow-up and endpoints, 56–57
intervention, 56
participants, 56
relevant studies and information, 58
research question, 55
results, 57, 57*t*–58*t*
study design, 56*f*
summary and implications, 58–59

anxiety disorders. *see also specific disorders*
childhood, sertraline, cognitive behavioral therapy, or combination for
criticisms and limitations, 64
follow-up and endpoints, 62–63
intervention, 62
participants, 62
relevant studies and information, 64
research question, 61
results, 63, 63*t*–64*t*
study design, 62*f*
summary and implications, 64
comorbidities, psychiatric, 127–131 (*see also* comorbidities, psychiatric)
panic disorder, 3–7 (*see also* panic disorder, comprehensive cognitive behavioral therapy, imipramine, and combination)
social phobia, generalized, 9–14 (*see also* social phobia, fluoxetine, comprehensive cognitive behavioral therapy, and placebo on)
aripiprazole
for dementia, risk of death, 100–104 (*see also* antipsychotics, atypical, for dementia, risk of death)
on metabolic risk, switching to, 279–283 (*see also* antipsychotics, metabolic risk, switching to aripiprazole for)
attention deficit/hyperactivity disorder (ADHD)
American Academy of Pediatrics guidelines, 47
multimodal treatment, 43–48
clinical case, 48*b*
criticisms and limitations, 47
follow-up and endpoints, 45
intervention, 44–45
participants, 44
relevant studies and information, 47
research question, 43
results, 46, 46*t*–47*t*
study design, 44*f*
summary and implications, 48
avoidant personality disorder, 10-year course, *vs.* borderline personality disorder, 213–217. *see also* borderline personality disorder (BPD), 10-year course

BALANCE study, 19–23, 38. *see also* bipolar disorder, lithium + valproate *vs.* monotherapy for relapse prevention
benzodiazepines. *see also specific types*
with/without cognitive behavioral therapy, for insomnia in elderly, 135–140 (*see also* insomnia in elderly, behavioral and/or pharmacotherapy for)
benztropine + chlorpromazine, for treatment-resistant schizophrenia, 260–264. *see also* schizophrenia treatment, clozapine, treatment-resistant
bipolar disorder
mood stabilizer monotherapy *vs.* adjunctive antidepressant, 24–29
clinical case, 28*b*–29*b*
criticisms and limitations, 27
follow-up and endpoints, 26
intervention, 25–26
participants, 25
relevant studies and information, 27–28
research question, 24
results, 26–27, 26*t*
study design, 25*f*
summary and implications, 28
suicide risk, lithium, divalproex, and carbamazepine on, 30–34
clinical case, 33*b*–34*b*
criticisms and limitations, 32
follow-up and endpoints, 31
intervention, 31
participants, 30–31

relevant studies and information, 33
research question, 30
results, 31–32, 32*t*
study design, 31*f*
summary and implications, 33
bipolar I disorder
child or adolescent, American Academy of Child and Adolescent Psychiatry recommendations, 82
child or adolescent, initial treatment, 79–83
clinical case, 82*b*–83*b*
criticisms and limitations, 82
follow-up and endpoints, 81
intervention, 80–81
participants, 80
relevant studies and information, 82
research question, 79
results, 81, 81*t*
study design, 80*f*
summary and implications, 82
natural history, long-term, 35–39
clinical case, 38*b*–39*b*
criticisms and limitations, 38
follow-up and endpoints, 37
intervention, 36–37
participants, 36
relevant studies and information, 38
research question, 35
results, 37, 37*t*–38*t*
study design, 36*f*
summary and implications, 38
relapse prevention, lithium + valproate *vs.* monotherapy for, 19–23, 38
clinical case, 22*b*–23*b*
criticisms and limitations, 21–22
follow-up and endpoints, 20–21
intervention, 20
participants, 20
relevant studies and information, 22
research question, 19
results, 21, 21*t*
study design, 20*f*
summary and implications, 22
borderline personality disorder (BPD)
10-year course, 213–217, 216
clinical case, 217*b*
criticisms and limitations, 216
follow-up and endpoints, 214–215
participants, 214
relevant studies and information, 216
research question, 213
results, 215, 215*t*
study design, 214*f*
summary and implications, 216
American Psychiatric Association guidelines, 204
biological basis and heritability, 216
dialectical behavior therapy for, American Psychiatric Association on, 210
psychotherapy for, 201–205
clinical case, 205*b*
criticisms and limitations, 204
follow-up and endpoints, 202–203
intervention, 202
mentalization-based treatment, 204
participants, 201–202
relevant studies and information, 204
research question, 201
results, 203, 203*t*
study design, 202*f*
summary and implications, 204–205
suicidal behavior, dialectical behavior therapy *vs.* community treatment for, 205–211
clinical case, 210*b*–211*b*
criticisms and limitations, 209
follow-up and endpoints, 208–209
intervention, 208
participants, 208
relevant studies and information, 210
research question, 207
results, 209, 209*t*
study design, 208*f*
summary and implications, 210
transference-focused psychotherapy for, American Psychiatric Association on, 210

buprenorphine *vs.* methadone, in pregnancy, 233–237. *see also* pregnancy, buprenorphine *vs.* methadone in
bupropion, for bipolar disorder, 24–29. *see also* bipolar disorder, mood stabilizer monotherapy *vs.* adjunctive antidepressant

CAMP trial, 279–283. *see also* antipsychotics, metabolic risk, switching to aripiprazole for
CAMS (Child/Adolescent Anxiety Multimodal Study), 61–65. *see also* anxiety disorders, childhood, sertraline, cognitive behavioral therapy, or combination for
Canadian Cardiac Randomized Evaluation of Antidepressant and Psychotherapy Efficacy (CREATE) trial, 226–230
  clinical case, 229*b*–230*b*
  criticisms and limitations, 228
  follow-up and endpoints, 228
  intervention, 227–228
  participants, 227
  relevant studies and information, 229
  research question, 226
  results, 228, 228*t*
  study design, 227*f*
  summary and implications, 229
carbamazepine, for bipolar disorder, 24–29. *see also* bipolar disorder, mood stabilizer monotherapy *vs.* adjunctive antidepressant
  on suicide risk, 30–34 (*see also* bipolar disorder, suicide risk, lithium, divalproex, and carbamazepine on)
CATIE (Clinical Antipsychotics Trials of Intervention Effectiveness), 266–272, 298. *see also* schizophrenia, clozapine for, *vs.* other atypical antipsychotics
  AD (Alzheimer's Disease), 93–98 (*see also* Alzheimer's disease, atypical antipsychotic effectiveness)
  Phase 1, 253–258, 288 (*see also* antipsychotics, for schizophrenia, effectiveness)
Child/Adolescent Anxiety Multimodal Study (CAMS), 61–65. *see also* anxiety disorders, childhood, sertraline, cognitive behavioral therapy, or combination for
chlorpromazine
  + benztropine, for treatment-resistant schizophrenia, 260–264 (*see also* schizophrenia, clozapine for, treatment-resistant)
  for delirium, in hospitalized AIDS patients, 106–110 (*see also* delirium treatment, in AIDS patients, hospitalized)
  equivalents per day, 243
citalopram
  for Alzheimer's disease
    agitation in, 97
    effectiveness, 94–98
  for depression
    with coronary artery disease, 226–230 (*see also* Canadian Cardiac Randomized Evaluation of Antidepressant and Psychotherapy Efficacy (CREATE) trial)
    STAR*D, 173–178 (*see also* depression treatment, STAR*D)
  suicidality with, pediatric, 149–153 (*see also* selective serotonin reuptake inhibitors (SSRIs), pediatric suicidality with; selective serotonin reuptake inhibitors (SSRIs), suicidality with, pediatric)
Clinical Antipsychotics Trials of Intervention Effectiveness. *see* CATIE (Clinical Antipsychotics Trials of Intervention Effectiveness)

clinical cases
  alcohol dependence
    depression treatment with, 147*b*
    pharmacotherapies with Combined Behavioral Intervention, 318*b*–319*b*
  Alzheimer's disease
    atypical antipsychotic effectiveness, 98*b*
    memantine, for Alzheimer's disease in patients on donepezil, 115*b*–116*b*
  antidepressants
    benefits and initial severity, 171*b*
    for bipolar disorder, adjunctive, *vs.* mood stabilizer monotherapy, 28*b*–29*b*
    for depression, with substance use disorders, 147*b*
    QTc-interval abnormalities with, 245*b*–246*b*
    for social phobia, 13*b*–14*b*
    STAR*D, 177*b*–178*b*
    suicidality with, pediatric, 153*b*
  antipsychotics
    for dementia, risk of death, 103*b*–104*b*
    metabolic risk, switching to aripiprazole for, 283*b*
    QTc-interval abnormalities with, 245*b*–246*b*
  antipsychotics, atypical
    for Alzheimer's disease, effectiveness, 98*b*
    cost utility, first- *vs.* second-generation, 288*b*–289*b*
    sudden cardiac death risks, 277*b*–278*b*
    tardive dyskinesia with, 250*b*–251*b*
  anxiety disorders
    childhood, sertraline, cognitive behavioral therapy, *vs.* combination for, 64*b*–65*b*
    comorbidities, psychiatric, 130*b*–131*b*
    panic disorder, cognitive behavioral therapy with imipramine, 7*b*
    social phobia, fluoxetine, comprehensive cognitive behavior therapy, and placebo for, 13*b*–14*b*
  attention deficit/hyperactivity disorder, multimodal treatment, 48*b*
  bipolar disorder
    mood stabilizer monotherapy *vs.* adjunctive antidepressant, 28*b*–29*b*
    suicide risk, lithium, divalproex, and carbamazepine on, 33*b*–34*b*
  bipolar I disorder
    child or adolescent, initial treatment, 82*b*–83*b*
    natural history, long-term, 38*b*–39*b*
    relapse prevention, lithium + valproate *vs.* monotherapy for, 22*b*–23*b*
  borderline personality disorder
    10-year course, 217*b*
    psychotherapy for, 205*b*
    suicidal behavior, dialectical behavior therapy *vs.* community treatment for, 210*b*–211*b*
  comorbidities, psychiatric, 130*b*–131*b*
  CREATE trial, 229*b*–230*b*
  delirium, in AIDS patients, hospitalized, 110*b*
  dementia, atypical antipsychotics on risk of death, 103*b*–104*b*
  depression
    with alcohol or drug dependence, 147*b*
    antidepressants, benefits and initial severity, 171*b*
    antidepressants, with substance use disorders, 147*b*
    cardiac function and, on health-related quality of life, 224*b*–225*b*
    cognitive therapy *vs.* paroxetine for, 182*b*–183*b*
    electroconvulsive therapy, efficacy and safety, 164*b*–165*b*

clinical cases (*cont.*)
imipramine *vs.* cognitive behavioral therapy *vs.* supportive therapy for, 159*b*
NIMH collaborative research program, 159*b*
STAR*D, 177*b*–178*b*
depression, adolescent
with SSRI resistance, 53*b*–54*b*
TADS, 88*b*
insomnia in elderly, behavioral and/or pharmacotherapy for, 139*b*–140*b*
mental and substance use disorders, global burden, 125*b*–126*b*
obsessive-compulsive disorder
child and adolescent, cognitive behavioral therapy, sertraline *vs.* combination for, 77*b*
exposure and ritual prevention, clomipramine, *vs.* combination for, 190*b*–191*b*
SSRI dose-response relationships, adult, 195*b*–196*b*
opioid disorders
levomethadyl acetate *vs.* buprenorphine *vs.* methadone for, 324*b*–325*b*
methadone maintenance *vs.* detoxification and psychosocial treatment, 312*b*–313*b*
in pregnancy, buprenorphine *vs.* methadone for, 324*b*–325*b*
panic disorder, comprehensive CBT, imipramine, and combination for, 7*b*
schizophrenia
early-onset, 59*b*
psychosis conversion to, factors, 293*b*–294*b*
schizophrenia, antipsychotics for
after first hospitalization, oral *vs.* depot, 304*b*–305*b*
cost utility, first- *vs.* second-generation, 288*b*–289*b*
effectiveness, 258*b*
first- *vs.* second-generation, early-onset, 59*b*
schizophrenia, clozapine for
vs. other atypical antipsychotics, 271*b*–272*b*
suicidality with, 298*b*–299*b*
treatment-resistant, 263*b*–264*b*
selective serotonin reuptake inhibitors
for depression with coronary artery disease, 229*b*–230*b*
for SSRI-resistant adolescents, 53*b*–54*b*
substance use disorder with, 147*b*
suicidality with, adolescent, predictors, 71*b*–72*b*
suicidality with, pediatric, 153*b*
social phobia, fluoxetine, comprehensive CBT, and placebo on, 13*b*–14*b*
substance use disorders
depression with, antidepressants for, 147*b*
global burden, 125*b*–126*b*
substance use disorders, opioid
methadone *vs.* detoxification and psychosocial treatment, 309–313
pregnancy with, buprenorphine *vs.* methadone for, 236*b*–237*b*
suicidality
adolescent, predictors, 71*b*–72*b*
in bipolar disorders, lithium, divalproex, and carbamazepine on, 33*b*–34*b*
in borderline personality disorder, dialectical behavior therapy *vs.* community treatment for, 210*b*–211*b*
in schizophrenia, with clozapine, 298*b*–299*b*
tardive dyskinesia with antipsychotics, atypical *vs.* conventional, 250*b*–251*b*
clomipramine, *vs.* exposure and ritual prevention or combination, for obsessive-compulsive disorder, 187–191. *see also*

obsessive-compulsive disorder (OCD), exposure and ritual prevention...
clozapine
  mortality with, *vs.* other antipsychotics, 298
  for schizophrenia, 263
    after first hospitalization, 300–305 (*see also* antipsychotics, for schizophrenia, after first hospitalization)
    American Psychiatric Association guidelines, 271
    mortality rate, 271
    vs. other atypical antipsychotics, 266–272, 298 (*see also* schizophrenia, clozapine for, *vs.* other atypical antipsychotics)
    on suicidality, 295–299 (*see also* International Suicide Prevention Trial (InterSePT))
    treatment-resistant, 260–264 (*see also* schizophrenia treatment, clozapine, treatment-resistant)
  tardive dyskinesia with, 249, 250
cognitive behavioral therapy (CBT)
  for alcohol dependence, 314–319 (*see also* alcohol dependence, pharmacotherapies with Combined Behavioral Intervention)
  for anxiety
    childhood, *vs.* sertraline or combination, 61–65 (*see also* anxiety disorders, childhood, sertraline, cognitive behavioral therapy, or combination for)
    generalized social phobia, 9–14 (*see also* social phobia, fluoxetine, comprehensive cognitive behavioral therapy, and placebo for)
    panic disorder, with or without imipramine, 3–7 (*see also* panic disorder, comprehensive cognitive behavioral therapy, imipramine, and combination)
  comprehensive, for generalize social phobia, 9–14 (*see also* social phobia, fluoxetine, comprehensive cognitive behavioral therapy, and placebo for)
  for depression, adolescent, 84–88 (*see also* depression treatment, adolescent, TADS)
    SSRI resistant, 50–54 (*see also* depression treatment, adolescent, SSRI resistant)
  for depression, *vs.* interpersonal therapy, 227
  for insomnia
    American College of Physicians recommendation, 138
    in elderly, with/without temazepam, 135–140 (*see also* insomnia in elderly, behavioral and/or pharmacotherapy for)
  for obsessive-compulsive disorder
    exposure and ritual prevention *vs.* clomipramine and combination, 187–191 (*see also* obsessive-compulsive disorder (OCD), exposure and ritual prevention...)
    vs. sertraline or combination, 73–77 (*see also* obsessive-compulsive disorder (OCD), child and adolescent, cognitive behavioral therapy, sertraline *vs.* combination for)
  for suicidality, predictors of suicidal events with, 67–72 (*see also* suicidality, adolescent, predictors)
cognitive therapy. *see also specific types*
  for depression, *vs.* paroxetine, 179–183 (*see also* major depressive disorder, cognitive therapy *vs.* paroxetine for)
Collaborative Longitudinal Personality Disorders Study, 213–217. *see also* borderline personality disorder (BPD), 10-year course

Combined Behavioral Intervention (CBI), 316
  for alcohol dependence, 314–319 (*see also* alcohol dependence, pharmacotherapies with Combined Behavioral Intervention)
COMBINE study, 314–319. *see also* alcohol dependence, pharmacotherapies with Combined Behavioral Intervention
community treatment
  for attention deficit/hyperactivity disorder, 43–48 (*see also* attention deficit/hyperactivity disorder (ADHD), multimodal treatment)
  for borderline personality disorder, suicidal behavior in, 205–211 (*see also* borderline personality disorder (BPD), suicidal behavior...)
comorbidities, psychiatric, prevalence and severity, 127–131
  clinical case, 130*b*–131*b*
  criticisms and limitations, 129
  endpoints, 128
  participants, 127–128
  relevant studies and information, 130
  research question, 127
  results, 129, 129*t*
  study design, 128*f*
  summary and implications, 130
Comparison of Antipsychotics for Metabolic Problems in Schizophrenia or Schizoaffective Disorder (CAMP), 279–283. *see also* antipsychotics, metabolic risk, switching to aripiprazole for
comprehensive cognitive behavioral therapy, for generalized social phobia, 9–14. *see also* social phobia, fluoxetine, comprehensive cognitive behavioral therapy, and placebo for
coronary artery disease, depression with
  on health-related quality of life, 221–225 (*see also* depression, cardiac function and, on health-related quality of life)
  interpersonal therapy and/or citalopram for, 226–230 (*see also* Canadian Cardiac Randomized Evaluation of Antidepressant and Psychotherapy Efficacy (CREATE) trial)
  screening recommendations, 224, 229
Cost Utility of the Latest Antipsychotic Drugs in Schizophrenia Study (CUtLASS)
  CUtLASS 1, 257, 285–289 (*see also* antipsychotics, first- *vs.* second-generation, for schizophrenia)
  CUtLASS 2, 288
CREATE trial, 226–230. *see also* Canadian Cardiac Randomized Evaluation of Antidepressant and Psychotherapy Efficacy (CREATE) trial

delirium treatment, American Psychiatric Association guidelines, 109–110
delirium treatment, in AIDS patients, hospitalized, 106–110
  clinical case, 110*b*
  criticisms and limitations, 109
  follow-up and endpoints, 108
  intervention, 107–108
  participants, 107
  relevant studies and information, 109–110
  research question, 106
  results, 108, 108*t*–109*t*
  study design, 107*f*
  summary and implications, 110
depression
  cardiac function and, on health-related quality of life, 221–225
    American Heart Association screening, 224, 229
    clinical case, 224*b*–225*b*

criticisms and limitations, 224
follow-up and endpoints, 223
participants, 222
relevant studies and information, 224
research question, 221
results, 223, 223*t*
study design, 222–223, 222*f*
summary and implications, 224
major depressive disorder,10-year course, *vs.* borderline personality disorder, 213–217 (*see also* borderline personality disorder (BPD), 10-year course)
depression treatment
with alcohol or drug dependence, 143–147
clinical case, 147*b*
criticisms and limitations, 146
follow-up and endpoints, 144
intervention, 144
participants, 144
relevant studies and information, 146
research question, 143
results, 145, 145*t*
study design, 144*f*
summary and implications, 146
American Psychiatric Association guidelines, 146, 182
antidepressant, benefits and initial severity, 167–171 (*see also* antidepressants, benefits and initial severity)
cognitive therapy *vs.* paroxetine, major depressive disorder, 179–183 (*see also* major depressive disorder, cognitive therapy *vs.* paroxetine for)
electroconvulsive therapy, efficacy and safety, 161–165
clinical case, 164*b*–165*b*
criticisms and limitations, 163–164
follow-up and endpoints, 162
participants, 161–162
relevant studies and information, 164
research question, 161
results, 162, 163*t*
study design, 162
summary and implications, 164
NICE criteria, 168–170
NIMH collaborative research program, 155–159, 182
clinical case, 159*b*
criticisms and limitations, 158
follow-up and endpoints, 157
intervention, 156–157
participants, 156
relevant studies and information, 158
research question, 155
results, 157, 157*t*
study design, 156*f*
summary and implications, 158
SSRIs, with coronary artery disease, 226–230 (*see also* Canadian Cardiac Randomized Evaluation of Antidepressant and Psychotherapy Efficacy (CREATE) trial)
STAR*D, 173–178
clinical case, 177*b*–178*b*
criticisms and limitations, 177
follow-up and endpoints, 176
intervention, 175–176
participants, 174
relevant studies and information, 177
research question, 173
results, 176, 176*t*
study design, 173, 174*f*
summary and implications, 177
unresponsive depression, American Psychiatric Association guidelines, 177
depression treatment, adolescent
American Academy of Child and Adolescent Psychiatry recommendations, 87
SSRI resistant, 50–54
clinical case, 53*b*–54*b*
criticisms and limitations, 53

depression treatment, adolescent (*cont.*)
- follow-up and endpoints, 52
- intervention, 51–52
- participants, 51
- relevant studies and information, 53
- research question, 50
- results, 52, 52*t*–53*t*
- study design, 51*f*
- summary and implications, 53
- TADS (Treatment for Adolescents with Depression Study), 84–88
  - clinical case, 88*b*
  - criticisms and limitations, 87
  - follow-up and endpoints, 86
  - intervention, 85–86
  - participants, 84–85
  - relevant studies and information, 87
  - research question, 84
  - results, 86–87, 86*t*
  - study design, 85*f*
  - summary and implications, 87

detoxification and psychosocial treatment, *vs.* methadone maintenance, for opioid disorders, 309–313. *see also* opioid disorders, methadone maintenance...

dextroamphetamine, with/without behavioral treatment for attention deficit/hyperactivity disorder, 43–48. *see also* attention deficit/ hyperactivity disorder (ADHD), multimodal treatment

dialectical behavior therapy (DBT), for borderline personality disorder, 201–205. *see also* borderline personality disorder (BPD), psychotherapy for
- American Psychiatric Association on, 210
- suicidal behavior in, 205–211 (*see also* borderline personality disorder (BPD), suicidal behavior...)

disability-adjusted life years (DALY), mental and substance use disorders, 122*f*, 123–124, 124*t*

divalproex, for bipolar disorder
- child or adolescent, initial treatment, 79–83 (*see also* bipolar I disorder, child or adolescent, initial treatment)
- on suicide risk, 30–34 (*see also* bipolar disorder, suicide risk, lithium, divalproex, and carbamazepine on)

DOMINO-AD (Donepezil and Memantine in Moderate to Severe Alzheimer's Disease), 115

donepezil, plus memantine for Alzheimer's disease, 112–116. *see also* memantine, for Alzheimer's disease in patients on donepezil
- DOMINO-AD, 115

droperidol, QTc-interval abnormalities with, 241–246. *see also* psychotropic drugs, QTc-interval abnormalities with

drug dependence. *see* substance use disorders; *specific types*

electroconvulsive therapy, on depression, 161–165. *see also* depression treatment, electroconvulsive therapy, efficacy and safety

Enhancing Recovery in Coronary Heart Disease Patients (ENRICHD), 229

European Prediction of Psychosis Study, 292

exposure and ritual prevention, for obsessive-compulsive disorder, *vs.* clomipramine and combination, 187–191. *see also* obsessive-compulsive disorder (OCD), exposure and ritual prevention...

FIN11 study, 298

fluoxetine
- for depression
  - adolescent, 84–88 (*see also* depression treatment, adolescent, TADS)

benefits and initial severity, 167–171 (*see also* antidepressants, benefits and initial severity)
for social phobia, generalized, 9–14 (*see also* social phobia, fluoxetine, comprehensive cognitive behavioral therapy, and placebo on for)
suicidality with, pediatric, 149–153 (*see also* selective serotonin reuptake inhibitors (SSRIs), pediatric suicidality with; selective serotonin reuptake inhibitors (SSRIs), suicidality with, pediatric)
fluvoxamine, pediatric suicidality with, 149–153. *see also* selective serotonin reuptake inhibitors (SSRIs), suicidality with, pediatric

global burden, mental and substance use disorders, 121–126. *see also* mental and substance use disorders, global burden

haloperidol
for behavioral disorders in elderly, risk of death with, 102
for delirium, in hospitalized AIDS patients, 106–110 (*see also* delirium treatment, in AIDS patients, hospitalized)
for schizophrenia, after first hospitalization, 300–305 (*see also* antipsychotics, for schizophrenia, after first hospitalization)
health-related quality of life, depression symptoms and, 221–225. *see also* depression, cardiac function and, on health-related quality of life
Heart and Soul Study, 221–225. *see also* depression, cardiac function and, on health-related quality of life

imipramine
for depression, with clinical management, 155–159, 182 (*see also* depression treatment, NIMH collaborative research program)
for panic disorder, *vs.* cognitive behavioral therapy or combination, 3–7 (*see also* panic disorder, comprehensive cognitive behavioral therapy, imipramine, and combination)
impulse control disorders, psychiatric comorbidities. *see also* comorbidities, psychiatric
impulse control disorders, psychiatric comorbidities, prevalence and severity, 127–131
insomnia in elderly, behavioral and/or pharmacotherapy for, 135–140
clinical case, 139*b*–140*b*
criticisms and limitations, 138
follow-up and endpoints, 137
intervention, 136
participants, 135–136
relevant studies and information, 138–139
research question, 135
results, 137–138, 138*t*
study design, 136*f*
summary and implications, 139
International Suicide Prevention Trial (InterSePT), 271, 295–299
suicidality in, clozapine for, 295–299
clinical case, 298*b*–299*b*
criticisms and limitations, 297–298
follow-up and endpoints, 296
intervention, 296
participants, 296
relevant studies and information, 298
research question, 295
results, 297, 297*t*
study design, 296*f*
summary and implications, 298

interpersonal therapy (IPT), for depression, 155–159, 182. *see also* depression treatment, NIMH collaborative research program
vs. cognitive behavioral therapy, 227
with coronary artery disease, 226–230 (*see also* Canadian Cardiac Randomized Evaluation of Antidepressant and Psychotherapy Efficacy (CREATE) trial)

levomethadyl acetate *vs.* buprenorphine *vs.* methadone, for opioid dependence, 321–325. *see also* opioid disorders, levomethadyl acetate *vs.* buprenorphine *vs.* methadone for
lithium, for bipolar disorder, 24–29
child or adolescent, initial treatment, 79–83 (*see also* bipolar I disorder, child or adolescent, initial treatment)
on suicide risk, 30–34 (*see also* bipolar disorder, suicide risk, lithium, divalproex, and carbamazepine on)
+ valproate, relapse prevention, 19–23, 38 (*see also* bipolar disorder, relapse prevention, lithium + valproate *vs.* monotherapy for)
+ valproic acid, 24–29 (*see also* bipolar disorder, mood stabilizer monotherapy *vs.* adjunctive antidepressant)
Longitudinal Interval Follow-up Evaluation (LIFE), 36–37
lorazepam, for delirium, in hospitalized AIDS patients, 106–110. *see also* delirium treatment, in AIDS patients, hospitalized

M180 study, 309–313. *see also* opioid disorders, methadone maintenance *vs.* detoxification and psychosocial treatment
major depressive disorder (MDD). *see also* depression
10-year course, *vs.* borderline personality disorder, 213–217 (*see also* borderline personality disorder (BPD), 10-year course)
cognitive therapy *vs.* paroxetine for, 179–183
clinical case, 182*b*–183*b*
criticisms and limitations, 181–182
follow-up and endpoints, 180–181
intervention, 180
participants, 179–180
relevant studies and information, 182
research question, 179
results, 181, 181*t*
study design, 180*f*
summary and implications, 182
mania, child or adolescent, American Academy of Child and Adolescent Psychiatry treatment recommendations, 82
McLean Study of Adult Development (MSAD), 216
memantine, for Alzheimer's disease in patients on donepezil, 112–116
clinical case, 115*b*–116*b*
criticisms and limitations, 115
DOMINO-AD, 115
follow-up and endpoints, 114
intervention, 113
participants, 113
relevant studies and information, 115
research question, 112
results, 114, 114*t*
study design, 113*f*
summary and implications, 115
mental and substance use disorders, global burden, 121–126
clinical case, 125*b*–126*b*
criticisms and limitations, 124–125
endpoints, 123
intervention, 123
participants, 122
relevant studies and information, 125

- research question, 121
- results, 123–124, 124*t*
- study design, 122*f*
- summary and implications, 125

mental health disorders. *see also* *specific types*
- comorbidities, psychiatric, 127–131 (*see also* comorbidities, psychiatric)

mentalization-based treatment (MBT), for borderline personality disorder, 204

methadone, for opioid disorders
- *vs.* buprenorphine
  - effectiveness, 312
  - in pregnancy, 233–237 (*see also* pregnancy, buprenorphine *vs.* methadone in)
- *vs.* detoxification and psychosocial treatment, 309–313 (*see also* opioid disorders, methadone maintenance...)
- Substance Abuse and Mental Health Services Administration guidelines, 312

methylphenidate, with/without behavioral treatment for attention deficit/hyperactivity disorder, 43–48. *see also* attention deficit/hyperactivity disorder (ADHD), multimodal treatment

mirtazapine, suicidality with, pediatric, 149–153. *see also* selective serotonin reuptake inhibitors (SSRIs), pediatric suicidality with; selective serotonin reuptake inhibitors (SSRIs), suicidality with, pediatric

molindone, for schizophrenia, early-onset, 55–59. *see also* schizophrenia, early-onset

mood disorders. *see also* *specific types*
- American Psychiatric Association guidelines, 146
- comorbidities, psychiatric, 127–131 (*see also* comorbidities, psychiatric)

mood stabilizer, for bipolar disorder. *see also specific types*
- *vs.* adjunctive antidepressant, 24–29 (*see also* bipolar disorder, mood stabilizer monotherapy *vs.* adjunctive antidepressant)
- suicide risk with lithium, divalproex, and carbamazepine, 30–34 (*see also* bipolar disorder, suicide risk, lithium, divalproex, and carbamazepine on)

MOTHER trial, 233–237. *see also* pregnancy, buprenorphine *vs.* methadone in

MTA Cooperative Group trial, multimodal treatment for attention deficit/hyperactivity disorder, 43–48. *see also* attention deficit/hyperactivity disorder (ADHD), multimodal treatment

naltrexone
- for alcohol dependence, 318
- for alcohol dependence, with Combined Behavioral Intervention, 314–319 (*see also* alcohol dependence, pharmacotherapies with Combined Behavioral Intervention)

National Comorbidity Study (NCS), 130

National Comorbidity Study Adolescents (NCS-A), 130

National Comorbidity Survey Replication (NCS-R), 127–131. *see also* comorbidities, psychiatric

National Institute of Mental Health (NIMH) Treatment of Depression Collaborative Research Program, 155–159, 182. *see also* depression treatment, NIMH collaborative research program

nefazodone, for depression, 167–171. *see also* antidepressants, benefits and initial severity
neonatal abstinence syndrome, prenatal buprenorphine *vs.* methadone on, 233–237. *see also* pregnancy, buprenorphine *vs.* methadone in
neuroleptics. *see also specific types*
  for delirium, in hospitalized AIDS patients, 106–110 (*see also* delirium treatment, in AIDS patients, hospitalized)
NICE criteria, depression, 168–170
North American Prodrome Longitudinal study, 290–294. *see also* schizophrenia, psychosis conversion to, factors

obsessive-compulsive disorder (OCD)
  10-year course, *vs.* borderline personality disorder, 213–217 (*see also* borderline personality disorder (BPD), 10-year course)
  American Psychiatry Association guidelines, 190
  exposure and ritual prevention, clomipramine, *vs.* combination for, 187–191
    clinical case, 190*b*–191*b*
    criticisms and limitations, 190
    follow-up and endpoints, 189
    intervention, 188–189
    participants, 188
    relevant studies and information, 190
    research question, 187
    results, 189, 189*t*
    study design, 188*f*
    summary and implications, 190
  sertraline on, 195
  SSRI dose-response relationship, adult, 192–196
    clinical case, 195*b*–196*b*
    criticisms and limitations, 195
    follow-up and endpoints, 193–194
    intervention, 193
    participants, 193
    relevant studies and information, 195
    research question, 192
    results, 194, 194*t*
    study design, 193*f*
    summary and implications, 195
obsessive-compulsive disorder (OCD), child and adolescent
  American Academy of Child and Adolescent Psychiatry treatment recommendations, 76
  cognitive behavioral therapy, sertraline, *vs.* combination for, 73–77
    clinical case, 77*b*
    criticisms and limitations, 76
    follow-up and endpoints, 75
    intervention, 74–75
    participants, 74
    relevant studies and information, 76
    research question, 73
    results, 75, 75*t*
    study design, 74*f*
    summary and implications, 76
  psychiatric co-morbidities, 76
olanzapine
  for Alzheimer's disease, effectiveness, 93–98 (*see also* Alzheimer's disease, atypical antipsychotic effectiveness)
  for dementia, risk of death, 100–104 (*see also* antipsychotics, atypical, for dementia, risk of death)
  on metabolic risk, *vs.* aripiprazole, 279–283 (*see also* antipsychotics, metabolic risk, switching to aripiprazole for)
  for schizophrenia
    after first hospitalization, 300–305 (*see also* antipsychotics, for schizophrenia, after first hospitalization)
    vs. clozapine, 266–272, 298 (*see also* schizophrenia, clozapine for, *vs.* other atypical antipsychotics)

early-onset, 55–59 (*see also* schizophrenia, early-onset)
effectiveness, 253–258 (*see also* antipsychotics, for schizophrenia, effectiveness)
on suicidality, *vs.* clozapine, 295–299 (*see also* International Suicide Prevention Trial (InterSePT))
weight gain from, 257, 282
opioid disorder treatment
levomethadyl acetate *vs.* buprenorphine *vs.* methadone, 321–325
clinical case, 324*b*–325*b*
criticisms and limitations, 323
follow-up and endpoints, 322
intervention, 322
participants, 321–322
relevant studies and information, 324
research question, 321
results, 323, 323*t*
study design, 322*f*
summary and implications, 324
methadone maintenance, SAMHSA guidelines, 312
methadone maintenance *vs.* buprenorphine
effectiveness, 312
in pregnancy, 233–237 (*see also* pregnancy, buprenorphine *vs.* methadone in)
methadone maintenance *vs.* detoxification and psychosocial treatment, 309–313
clinical case, 312*b*–313*b*
criticisms and limitations, 312
follow-up and endpoints, 310–311
intervention, 310
participants, 310
relevant studies and information, 312
research question, 309
results, 311, 311*t*
study design, 310*f*
summary and implications, 312
in pregnancy
American College of Obstetrics and Gynecology on, 236
prenatal buprenorphine *vs.* methadone, 233–237 (*see also* pregnancy, buprenorphine *vs.* methadone in)

panic disorder, comprehensive cognitive behavioral therapy, imipramine, and combination for, 3–7
clinical case, 7*b*
criticisms and limitations, 6
follow-up and endpoints, 5
intervention, 4
participants, 3–4
relevant studies and information, 6
research question, 3
results, 5–6, 5*t*
study design, 4*f*
summary and implications, 6–7
paroxetine
for bipolar disorder, 24–29 (*see also* bipolar disorder, mood stabilizer monotherapy *vs.* adjunctive antidepressant)
for depression
benefits and initial severity, 167–171 (*see also* antidepressants, benefits and initial severity)
vs. cognitive therapy, 179–183 (*see also* major depressive disorder, cognitive therapy *vs.* paroxetine for)
suicidality with, pediatric, 149–153 (*see also* selective serotonin reuptake inhibitors (SSRIs), pediatric suicidality with; selective serotonin reuptake inhibitors (SSRIs), suicidality with, pediatric)
Pediatric OCD Treatment Study, 73–77, 190. *see also* obsessive-compulsive disorder (OCD), child and adolescent, cognitive behavioral therapy, sertraline *vs.* combination for

perphenazine, for schizophrenia
after first hospitalization, 300–305 (*see also* antipsychotics, for schizophrenia, after first hospitalization)
effectiveness, 253–258 (*see also* antipsychotics, for schizophrenia, effectiveness)
POTS (Pediatric OCD Treatment Study), 73–77, 190. *see also* obsessive-compulsive disorder (OCD), child and adolescent, cognitive behavioral therapy, sertraline *vs.* combination for
pregnancy, buprenorphine *vs.* methadone in, 233–237
clinical case, 236*b*–237*b*
criticisms and limitations, 236
follow-up and endpoints, 234–235
intervention, 234
participants, 234
relevant studies and information, 236
research question, 233
results, 235, 235*t*
study design, 234*f*
summary and implications, 236
psychiatric comorbidities, prevalence and severity, 127–131. *see also* comorbidities, psychiatric, prevalence and severity
psychosis
conversion to schizophrenia from, factors, 290–294 (*see also* schizophrenia, psychosis conversion to, factors)
European Prediction of Psychosis Study, 292
first episode, treatment, 257
prevention or delay, pharmacologic trials, 293
psychotropic drugs. *see also* *specific types*
QTc-interval abnormalities with, 241–246
American Psychiatric Association on, 244–245
Berkshire Healthcare National Health Service on, 244
clinical case, 245*b*–246*b*
criticisms and limitations, 244
follow-up and endpoints, 243
implementation, 242–243
participants, 242
relevant studies and information, 244–245
research question, 241
results, 243, 243*t*–244*t*
study design, 242*f*
summary and implications, 245

QTc-interval abnormalities, with psychotropic medications, 241–246. *see also* psychotropic drugs, QTc-interval abnormalities with
quetiapine
for Alzheimer's disease, effectiveness, 93–98 (*see also* Alzheimer's disease, atypical antipsychotic effectiveness)
for dementia, risk of death, 100–104 (*see also* antipsychotics, atypical, for dementia, risk of death)
on metabolic risk, *vs.* aripiprazole, 279–283 (*see also* antipsychotics, metabolic risk, switching to aripiprazole for)
for schizophrenia
after first hospitalization, 300–305 (*see also* antipsychotics, for schizophrenia, after first hospitalization)
vs. clozapine, 266–272, 298 (*see also* schizophrenia, clozapine for, *vs.* other atypical antipsychotics)
effectiveness, 253–258 (*see also* antipsychotics, for schizophrenia, effectiveness)

risperidone
for Alzheimer's disease, effectiveness, 93–98 (*see also* Alzheimer's

disease, atypical antipsychotic effectiveness)
for bipolar I disorder, child or adolescent, initial treatment, 79–83 (*see also* bipolar I disorder, child or adolescent, initial treatment)
for dementia, risk of death, 100–104 (*see also* antipsychotics, atypical, for dementia, risk of death)
on metabolic risk
vs. aripiprazole, 279–283 (*see also* antipsychotics, metabolic risk, switching to aripiprazole for)
vs. ziprasidone, 282
for schizophrenia
after first hospitalization, 300–305 (*see also* antipsychotics, for schizophrenia, after first hospitalization)
vs. clozapine, 266–272, 298 (*see also* schizophrenia, clozapine for, *vs.* other atypical antipsychotics)
early-onset, 55–59 (*see also* schizophrenia, early-onset)
effectiveness, 253–258 (*see also* antipsychotics, for schizophrenia, effectiveness)
rosuvastatin, on dyslipidemia with schizophrenia, 282–283

schema-focused therapy, for borderline personality disorder, 204
schizophrenia
dyslipidemia with, rosuvastatin on, 282–283
psychosis conversion to, factors, 290–294
clinical case, 293*b*–294*b*
criticisms and limitations, 293
follow-up and endpoints, 291
intervention, 291
participants, 290–291
relevant studies and information, 293
research question, 290
results, 292, 292*t*
study design, 291*f*
summary and implications, 293
Schizophrenia Patients Outcome Research Team, 257
schizophrenia treatment
American Psychiatric Association guidelines, 283, 288
CUtLASS 1, 257, 285–289 (*see also* antipsychotics, first- *vs.* second-generation, for schizophrenia)
CUtLASS 2, 288
European First Episode Schizophrenia Trial (EUFEST), 302
psychosis treatment, first episode, 257
schizophrenia treatment, antipsychotics
effectiveness, 253–258 (*see also* antipsychotics, for schizophrenia, effectiveness)
first- *vs.* second-generation, with early-onset schizophrenia, 55–59
American Academy of Child and Adolescent Psychiatry recommendations, 58
clinical case, 59*b*
criticisms and limitations, 58
follow-up and endpoints, 56–57
intervention, 56
participants, 56
relevant studies and information, 58
research question, 55
results, 57, 57*t*–58*t*
study design, 56*f*
summary and implications, 58–59
oral *vs.* depot, after first hospitalization, 300–305 (*see also* antipsychotics, for schizophrenia, after first hospitalization)
schizophrenia treatment, clozapine, 263
American Psychiatric Association guidelines, 271
mortality rate, 271
vs. other atypical antipsychotics, 266–272, 298
clinical case, 271*b*–272*b*
criticisms and limitations, 269

schizophrenia treatment, clozapine (*cont.*)
follow-up and endpoints, 267
intervention, 267
participants, 267
relevant studies and information, 269–271
research question, 266
results, 269, 270*t*
study design, 268*f*
summary and implications, 271
suicidality, 295–299
clinical case, 298*b*–299*b*
criticisms and limitations, 297–298
follow-up and endpoints, 296
intervention, 296
participants, 296
relevant studies and information, 298
research question, 295
results, 297, 297*t*
study design, 296*f*
summary and implications, 298
treatment-resistant schizophrenia, 260–264
clinical case, 263*b*–264*b*
criticisms and limitations, 262–263
follow-up and endpoints, 261–262
intervention, 261
participants, 260–261
relevant studies and information, 263
research question, 260
results, 262, 262*t*
study design, 261*f*
summary and implications, 263
selective serotonin reuptake inhibitors (SSRIs). *see also* Canadian Cardiac Randomized Evaluation of Antidepressant and Psychotherapy Efficacy (CREATE) trial
for depression
with coronary artery disease, 226–230
SSRI-resistant adolescent, new SSRI, 50–54 (*see also* depression treatment, adolescent, SSRI resistant)
with substance use disorder, 143–147 (*see also* depression treatment, with alcohol or drug dependence)
for obsessive-compulsive disorder, adult dose–response relationship, 192–196
suicidality with, pediatric, 149–153
adolescent predictors, 67–72 (*see also* suicidality, adolescent, predictors)
clinical case, 153*b*
criticisms and limitations, 152
follow-up and endpoints, 150–151
participants, 150
relevant studies and information, 152
research question, 149
results, 151, 151*t*
study design, 150*f*
summary and implications, 152–153
suicidality with, spontaneously reported, 151
Texas Medication Algorithm, 69
Sequenced Treatment Alternatives to Relive Depression (STAR*D), 173–178. *see also* depression treatment, STAR*D
sertraline
for anxiety in childhood, *vs.* cognitive behavior therapy or combination, 61–65 (*see also* anxiety disorders, childhood, sertraline, cognitive behavioral therapy, *vs.* combination for)
for depression, with coronary artery disease, 226–230 (*see also* Canadian Cardiac Randomized Evaluation of Antidepressant and Psychotherapy Efficacy (CREATE) trial)
for obsessive-compulsive disorder, 195
vs. cognitive behavioral therapy or combination, 73–77 (*see also*

obsessive-compulsive disorder (OCD), child and adolescent, cognitive behavioral therapy, sertraline *vs.* combination for)
suicidality with, pediatric, 149–153 (*see also* selective serotonin reuptake inhibitors (SSRIs), pediatric suicidality with; selective serotonin reuptake inhibitors (SSRIs), suicidality with, pediatric)
Sertraline Antidepressant Heart-Attack Randomized Trial (SADHART), 229
social phobia, fluoxetine, comprehensive cognitive behavioral therapy, and placebo on, 9–14
clinical case, 13*b*–14*b*
criticisms and limitations, 12
follow-up and endpoints, 11
intervention, 10–11
participants, 10
relevant studies and information, 12–13
research question, 9
results, 11–12, 11*t*
study design, 10*f*
summary and implications, 13
STAR*D, 173–178. *see also* depression treatment, STAR*D
STEP-BD (Systemic Treatment Enhancement Program-Bipolar Disorder), 24–29, 38. *see also* bipolar disorder, mood stabilizer monotherapy *vs.* adjunctive antidepressant
Structured Interview for Prodromal Syndromes (SIPS) criteria, 291, 292
substance use disorders. *see also* opioid disorders
comorbidities, psychiatric, 127–131 (*see also* comorbidities, psychiatric)
depression with
American Psychiatric Association guidelines, 146
antidepressants on, 143–147 (*see also* depression treatment, with alcohol or drug dependence)
global burden, 121–126 (*see also* mental and substance use disorders, global burden)
sudden cardiac death, with typical antipsychotics, 274–278, 277. *see also* antipsychotics, atypical, sudden cardiac death risks
suicidality
adolescent, predictors, 67–72
clinical case, 71*b*–72*b*
criticisms and limitations, 70
follow-up and endpoints, 69
intervention, 68–69
participants, 68
relevant studies and information, 70–71
research question, 67
results, 69–70
study design, 68*f*
summary and implications, 71
with antidepressants, in pediatric patients, 149–153 (*see also* selective serotonin reuptake inhibitors (SSRIs), pediatric suicidality with; selective serotonin reuptake inhibitors (SSRIs), suicidality with, pediatric)
antipsychotics on, 298
in bipolar disorder, lithium, divalproex, and carbamazepine on, 30–34 (*see also* bipolar disorder, suicide risk, lithium, divalproex, and carbamazepine on)
in borderline personality disorder, dialectical behavior therapy *vs.* community treatment for, 205–211 (*see also* borderline personality disorder (BPD), dialectical behavior therapy *vs.* community treatment)

suicidality (*cont.*)
International Suicide Prevention Trial (InterSePT), 271
in schizophrenia, clozapine for, 295–299 (*see also* schizophrenia, suicidality in, clozapine for)
supportive therapy
for borderline personality disorder, 201–205 (*see also* borderline personality disorder (BPD), psychotherapy for)
for depression, *vs.* imipramine and cognitive behavioral therapy vs, 159*b*
Systemic Treatment Enhancement Program-Bipolar Disorder, 24–29, 38. *see also* bipolar disorder, mood stabilizer monotherapy *vs.* adjunctive antidepressant
Systems Training for Emotional Predictability and problem Solving (STEPS), for borderline personality disorder, 204

TADS (Treatment for Adolescents with Depression Study), 84–88, 151. *see also* depression treatment, adolescent, TADS
tardive dyskinesia, with atypical *vs.* conventional antipsychotics, 247–251. *see also* antipsychotics, tardive dyskinesia with, atypical *vs.* conventional
TASA (Treatment of Adolescent Suicide Attempters) study, 67–71. *see also* suicidality, adolescent, predictors
TD Incidence Study, 247–251. *see also* antipsychotics, tardive dyskinesia with, atypical *vs.* conventional
TEAM (Treatment of Early Age Mania) study, 79–83. *see also* bipolar I disorder, child or adolescent, initial treatment
temazepam, with/without cognitive behavioral therapy, for insomnia in elderly, 135–140. *see also* insomnia in elderly, behavioral and/or pharmacotherapy for
TEOSS (Treatment of Early-Onset Schizophrenia Spectrum Disorders) trial, 55–59. *see also* schizophrenia, early-onset
Texas Medication Algorithm, 69
thioridazine, QTc-interval abnormalities with, 241–246. *see also* psychotropic drugs, QTc-interval abnormalities with
TORDIA (Treatment of Resistant Depression in Adolescents) trial, 50–54. *see also* depression treatment, adolescent, SSRI resistant
transference-focused psychotherapy (TFP), for borderline personality disorder, 201–205. *see also* borderline personality disorder (BPD), psychotherapy for
American Psychiatric Association on, 210
Treatment for Adolescents with Depression Study, 84–88, 151. *see also* depression treatment, adolescent, TADS
Treatment of Adolescent Suicide Attempters study, 67–71. *see also* suicidality, adolescent, predictors
Treatment of Early Age Mania study, 79–83. *see also* bipolar I disorder, child or adolescent, initial treatment
Treatment of Early-Onset Schizophrenia Spectrum Disorders trial, 55–59. *see also* schizophrenia, early-onset
Treatment of Resistant Depression in Adolescents trial, 50–54. *see also* depression treatment, adolescent, SSRI resistant
tricyclic antidepressants
for depression with substance use disorder, 143–147 (*see also* depression treatment, with alcohol or drug dependence)

QTc-interval abnormalities with, 241–246 (*see also* psychotropic drugs, QTc-interval abnormalities with)

valproate + lithium, for bipolar I disorder, relapse prevention, 19–23, 38. *see also* bipolar disorder, relapse prevention, lithium + valproate *vs.* monotherapy for
valproic acid, for bipolar disorder, 24–29. *see also* bipolar disorder, mood stabilizer monotherapy *vs.* adjunctive antidepressant
venlafaxine
for depression
adolescent, SSRI resistant, 50–54 (*see also* depression treatment, adolescent, SSRI resistant)
benefits and initial severity, 167–171 (*see also* antidepressants, benefits and initial severity)
suicidality with, pediatric, 149–153 (*see also* selective serotonin reuptake inhibitors (SSRIs), pediatric suicidality with; selective serotonin reuptake inhibitors (SSRIs), suicidality with, pediatric)

years lived with disability (YLD), mental and substance use disorders, 122*f*, 123–124, 124*t*
years of life lost to premature mortality (YLL), mental and substance use disorders, 122*f*, 123–124, 124*t*

ziprasidone
on metabolic risk, *vs.* risperidone or olanzapine, 282
for schizophrenia
vs. clozapine, 266–272, 298 (*see also* schizophrenia, clozapine for, *vs.* other atypical antipsychotics)
effectiveness, 253–258 (*see also* antipsychotics, for schizophrenia, effectiveness)
zuclopenthixol, for schizophrenia
after first hospitalization, 300–305 (*see also* antipsychotics, for schizophrenia, after first hospitalization)
cost utility, 286
oral *vs.* depot, 301